A Practical Guide to Skin Cancer

Allison Hanlon

Editor

A Practical Guide to Skin Cancer

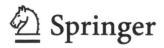 Springer

Editor
Allison Hanlon, MD, PhD
Department of Medicine
Division of Dermatology
Vanderbilt University Medical Center
Nashville, TN, USA

ISBN 978-3-319-74901-3   ISBN 978-3-319-74903-7   (eBook)
https://doi.org/10.1007/978-3-319-74903-7

Library of Congress Control Number: 2018935275

Printed on acid-free paper

This Springer imprint is published by the registered company is Springer International Publishing AG part of Springer Nature.
The registered company address is: Gewerbestrasse 11, 6330 Cham, Switzerland

To Gar Bo, Alannah and Mary, thank you for your encouragement, patience and love.

Contents

Contributors

Saud Aleissa, MD Department of Dermatology, Tufts Medical Center, Boston, MA, USA

Eileen Larkin Axibal, MD Department of Dermatology, University of Colorado Denver, Aurora, CO, USA

Trisha Bhat, BA Washington University in St. Louis, School of Medicine, St. Louis, MO, USA

Jeremy S. Bordeaux, MD, MPH University Hospitals Cleveland Medical Center and Case Western Reserve University School of Medicine, Cleveland, OH, USA

Mariah Ruth Brown, MD Department of Dermatology, University of Colorado Denver, Aurora, CO, USA

Jose A. Cervantes, MD Tucson Hospital Medical Education Program, Tucson Medical Center, Tucson, AZ, USA

Maggie Chow, MD, PhD Department of Dermatology, University of Southern California, Los Angeles, CA, USA

Anna S. Clayton, MD Dermatology, Vanderbilt University of Medicine, Nashville, TN, USA

Charles Thomas Darragh, MD Dermatology, Vanderbilt University of Medicine, Nashville, TN, USA

Jennifer Divine, MD Divine Dermatology and Surgical Institute, Fort Collins, CO, USA

Matthew C. Fox, MD Division of Dermatology, Dell Medical School, University of Texas at Austin, Austin, TX, USA

Allison Hanlon, MD, PhD Department of Medicine, Division of Dermatology, Vanderbilt University Medical Center, Nashville, TN, USA

Shauna Higgins, MD Department of Dermatology, University of Southern California, Los Angeles, CA, USA

Kavita Mariwalla, MD Mariwalla Dermatology, West Islip, NY, USA

Paul R. Massey, MD Division of Dermatology, Dell Medical School, University of Texas at Austin, Austin, TX, USA

Vineet Mishra, MD Department of Medicine, University of Texas Health Science Center – San Antonio, San Antonio, TX, USA

Amy Musiek, MD Dermatology, Washington University in St. Louis, School of Medicine, St. Louis, MO, USA

Bichchau Michelle Nguyen, MD, MPH Department of Dermatology, Tufts Medical Center, Boston, MA, USA

Claire Noell, MD Department of Dermatology, Tufts Medical Center, Boston, MA, USA

Allison Pye, MD Dermatology, McGovern Medical School, UT Houston, Houston, TX, USA

Anthony C. Soldano, MD Division of Dermatology, Dell Medical School, University of Texas at Austin, Austin, TX, USA

Mary L. Stevenson, MD The Ronald O. Perelman Department of Dermatology, NYU Langone Medical Center, New York, NY, USA

Sheena Tsai, MPH University Hospitals Cleveland Medical Center and Case Western Reserve University School of Medicine, Cleveland, OH, USA

Daniel Wallis, MD Dermatology, Texas Tech University Health Sciences Center, Lubbock, TX, USA

Ashley Wysong, MD Department of Dermatology, University of Southern California, Los Angeles, CA, USA

Sarah Yagerman, MD The Ronald O. Perelman Department of Dermatology, NYU Langone Medical Center, New York, NY, USA

Nathalie C. Zeitouni, MDCM, FRCPC Dermatology, St. Joseph's Hospital and Medical Center, Dignity Health, Phoenix, AZ, USA

Jeffrey P. Zwerner, MD/PhD Department of Medicine, Division of Dermatology, Vanderbilt University, Nashville, TN, USA

Chapter 1
Skin Cancer: At-Risk Populations and Prevention

Claire Noell, Saud Aleissa, and Bichchau Michelle Nguyen

Abstract Skin cancer is the most common malignancy worldwide. Genetic and environmental factors increase the risk of developing skin cancer. Identifying at-risk individuals is important in skin cancer diagnosis and management. This chapter discusses in detail the risk factors, at-risk populations, and prevention of skin cancer.

Keywords Basal cell carcinoma · Squamous cell carcinoma · Melanoma · Skin cancer · Prevention · At-risk populations · Risk factors

Abbreviations

AIDS	Acquired immunodeficiency syndrome
ART	Antiretroviral therapy
BAP	BRCA1 associated protein-1
BCC	Basal cell carcinoma
BCNS	Basal cell nevus syndrome
BRAF	B-Raf proto-oncogene
BRCA	Breast cancer susceptibility gene
CDK	Cyclin-dependent kinase
CDKN	Cyclin-dependent kinase inhibitor
CLL	Chronic lymphocytic leukemia
DNA	Deoxyribonucleic acid
EVER	Epidermodysplasia verruciformis gene
HAART	Highly active antiretroviral therapy
HIV	Human immunodeficiency virus
MAPK	Mitogen-activated protein kinase
MC1R	Melanocortin-1 receptor

C. Noell (✉) · S. Aleissa · B. M. Nguyen
Department of Dermatology, Tufts Medical Center, Boston, MA, USA
e-mail: cnoell@tuftsmedicalcenter.com

MITF   Microphthalmia-associated transcription factor
NMSC   Non-melanoma skin cancer
OCA   Oculocutaneous albinism
PTEN   Phosphatase and tensin homolog
PUVA   Psoralen and ultraviolet A
RR   Relative risk
SCC   Squamous cell carcinoma
SHH   Sonic hedgehog
TNF   Tumor necrosis factor
UV   Ultraviolet

Non-melanoma Skin Cancer: Risk Factors, At-Risk Populations, and Prevention

Basal cell carcinomas and cutaneous squamous cell carcinomas are the most common cancers in the United States [1]. The precise incidence of these cancers is unknown, as they are typically not reported to cancer registries. Recent data from the American Cancer Society estimates that 3.3 million people were diagnosed with non-melanoma skin cancers in 2012, with basal cell carcinomas comprising 80% [2].

Risk Factors

Ultraviolet Radiation

Ultraviolet (UV) radiation is a well-known risk factor in the development of non-melanoma skin cancers (Table 1.1). Ultraviolet radiation is comprised of wavelengths 100–400 nm and is subdivided into UVA, UVB, and UVC. Ultraviolet exposure consists of 95% UVA and 5% UVB as UVC is filtered out completely by the ozone layer [3]. A study evaluating the relationship between non-melanoma skin cancers and ultraviolet B exposure in Maryland shore watermen found that squamous cell carcinomas are significantly associated with cumulative ultraviolet B radiation, which is further increased with high levels of exposure; the association with basal cell carcinoma was unclear [4].

Indoor tanning, largely composed of ultraviolet A, is a modifiable risk factor shown to significantly increase the risk of skin cancer. A meta-analysis of indoor tanning and non-melanoma skin cancer evaluated studies comparing populations ever using versus never using indoor tanning. It demonstrated that the relative risks of developing squamous cell carcinoma and basal cell carcinoma were 1.67 and 1.29, respectively, in patients who had ever used tanning beds; the relative risks were further increased to 2.02 and 1.40 in patients reporting use before 25 years of age [5].

Table 1.1 Non-melanoma
skin cancer risk factors

Environmental
UV radiation
Indoor tanning
Ionizing radiation
Psoralen UVA (PUVA) therapy
Chemical exposures
Arsenic
Polycyclic aromatic hydrocarbons
Chronic cutaneous inflammation
Immunosuppression
Fair phenotype
Previous history of skin cancer

In contrast, the association between non-melanoma skin cancer and narrowband ultraviolet B therapy appears to be less clear. Several small studies found varying levels of association, while a large retrospective analysis reviewing the Scottish Cancer Registry records of 3867 patients who received a median of 29 narrowband UVB treatments determined that its use was not significantly associated with the development of skin cancers; a notable limitation of this study was that only a small fraction of the study population (352) had received >100 treatments [6].

Psoralen, a phototoxic drug, and ultraviolet A (PUVA) is an effective and established treatment modality most notably for psoriasis, but long-term therapy has been limited due to its cutaneous carcinogenicity. A 30-year prospective cohort study by Stern followed the development of biopsy-proven non-melanoma skin cancers in 1380 psoriasis patients treated with PUVA, with 25% developing 2973 squamous cell carcinomas. Patients exposed to 351–450 and more than 450 treatments had, respectively, 6-fold and almost 35-fold increased risks of squamous cell carcinoma compared to those who had received fewer than 50 treatments, suggesting a dose-dependent relationship. The association between basal cell carcinomas and PUVA was not found to be significant [7].

Ionizing Radiation

While ionizing radiation was historically used to treat benign conditions such as acne, it carries an increased risk of non-melanoma skin cancer. A case-control study using surveys in New Hampshire evaluated the relative risk of non-melanoma skin cancer after receiving therapeutic ionizing radiation. The risk of non-melanoma skin cancer was further increased in patients who first received treatment prior to 20 years of age compared to older populations. The risk for both basal and squamous cell carcinomas was highest in patients receiving treatment for acne, and there was a twofold increased risk of basal cell carcinoma only in patients receiving radiation for cancer treatment. The risk of developing squamous cell carcinoma was only increased in patients with lighter skin types [8].

Survivors of childhood malignancies treated with radiation therapy have an increased risk of non-melanoma skin cancer. A survey of 13,132 5-year survivors from the Childhood Cancer Survivor Study demonstrated that radiation therapy increases the risk of non-melanoma skin cancer to greater than sixfold. Two hundred thirteen participants developed 615 occurrences of non-melanoma skin cancer (97% basal cell carcinomas and 1% squamous cell carcinomas). Forty-six percent of the patients had multiple skin cancers, with a median onset age of 31 years [9].

Medications

Voriconazole, a potent antifungal typically used to treat fungal infections and for prophylaxis in immunosuppressed patients, has been linked with photosensitivity and squamous cell carcinoma. In a retrospective analysis of 3 academic centers, 8 pediatric and adult patients on long-term voriconazole developed 51 squamous cell carcinomas [10]. A recent larger, single-institution study evaluating the relationship between squamous cell carcinomas and long-term antifungal prophylaxis in lung transplant patients demonstrated a significantly increased risk of squamous cell carcinoma incidence in patients exposed to voriconazole-containing regimens independent of other risk factors; furthermore, cumulative voriconazole exposure increased the risk of recurrent squamous cell carcinoma [11].

The growth of squamous cell carcinomas and keratoacanthomas is a common development in patients with melanoma treated with (B-Raf proto-oncogene) BRAF inhibitors. Molecular analysis has demonstrated that a significant number of these malignancies contain Ras gene mutations; the proposed mechanism is the paradoxical activation of mitogen-activated protein kinase (MAPK) signaling, leading to increased growth [12].

Chemical Exposures

The association between arsenic-contaminated drinking water and incidence of several malignancies, including non-melanoma skin cancer, has been reported in developing countries, as well as in the United States. A retrospective study using the National Taiwan Cancer Registry Center evaluated the incidence of non-melanoma skin cancers in the black foot disease endemic areas of Taiwan (an established disease resulting from arsenic-containing water wells) compared to other areas between 1979 and 2007. During this interval, there were 11,191 occurrences of squamous cell carcinoma and 13,684 occurrences of basal cell carcinoma. There was a four- to sixfold increase in squamous cell carcinomas and three- to fourfold increase in basal cell carcinomas in black foot endemic areas compared to the remaining areas [13]. Arsenic ingestion through private wells in the United States can also increase the risk of skin cancer. A meta-analysis of six studies evaluating arsenic levels and skin cancer within the United States was conducted, which suggested that even arsenic concentrations below the maximum level permitted by the Environmental Protection Agency may increase the risk [14].

Exposure to arsenic and other carcinogens can occur during the production and use of pesticides, herbicides, and fungicides, leading to an increased risk of squamous cell carcinoma. Finally, contact with polycyclic aromatic hydrocarbons, a by-product of the manufacturing of coal products, steel, iron, and diesel exhaust fumes, increases the risk of squamous cell carcinoma, but not basal cell carcinoma [15].

Pre-existing Lesions and Conditions

Chronic inflammation in conditions such as non-healing wounds/ulcerations, burns, venous stasis, discoid lupus erythematosus, lichen sclerosus, and lichen planus can stimulate malignant transformation, typically squamous cell carcinoma. The term "Marjolin's ulcer" was classically used to describe the development of squamous cell carcinoma in burn scars. In 1 study following 21 Marjolin's ulcer patients, 16 developed squamous cell carcinoma, while 4 had basal cell carcinoma and 1 had basosquamous cell carcinoma. Transformation can occur over weeks to decades, with an average interval of 19 years in the study described [16]. Discoid lupus-related squamous cell carcinomas tend to occur earlier and in sun-exposed areas, with the lip being the most common location [17]. The hyperkeratotic and erosive variants of lichen planus carry malignant potential necessitating periodic surveillance, with a reported transformation incidence of 0.4–1.5% in oral lichen planus [18]. Vulvar lichen sclerosus has also been shown to hold malignant potential, with an increasing risk of vulvar squamous cell carcinoma of up to 6.7% after 20 years [19].

Porokeratosis is a disorder of keratinization encompassing several subtypes of lesions with a cornoid lamella, a distinct raised border of angled hyperkeratosis. While historically thought to be a benign condition, certain subtypes carry an increased risk of skin cancer. A literature review following 30 years of porokeratosis revealed that the linear subtype carries the highest risk of skin cancer with a 19% malignant transformation rate, while punctate porokeratosis and disseminated actinic superficial porokeratosis confer the lowest risk (3.4% and 0%, respectively) [20].

While rare, basal cell carcinoma is the most common malignancy that can develop within nevus sebaceus, a benign congenital tumor. In a retrospective microscopic analysis of 596 cases, 0.8% was found to contain basal cell carcinomas; syringocystadenoma papilliferum and trichoblastoma were the most common benign neoplasms [21].

At-Risk Populations

History of Non-melanoma Skin Cancer

Patients with a history of non-melanoma skin cancer have an increased risk of developing subsequent skin cancers. The 3-year cumulative risk of a second squamous cell carcinoma is 18%, while the risk of a second basal cell carcinoma is 44%, demonstrating the need for continued monitoring for subsequent skin cancers in these patients [22].

Skin Types

Skin types play an important role in determining the risk of non-melanoma skin cancer in certain populations. Fitzpatrick skin types I and II, as seen in Caucasians, have the highest risk of both basal cell and squamous cell carcinomas overall [23]. Basal cell carcinomas are the most common skin cancer seen in Caucasians, Hispanics, Japanese, and Chinese [24], while squamous cell carcinoma is the most common skin cancer found in African-Americans. Squamous cell carcinomas in African-Americans tend to be more aggressive, with increased mortality and overall worse prognosis [25]. Similarly, squamous cell carcinomas in Asian populations tend to occur in sun-protected areas and have an increased risk of metastasis as they are usually advanced at the time of diagnosis [24].

Immunosuppressed Populations: Organ Transplant, Immunosuppressive Medications, Cancer, and HIV

Due to the need for lifelong immunosuppression, organ transplant patients are at an increased risk for skin cancers. A cohort study of 26 transplant centers following 10,649 organ transplant patients revealed an increased overall incidence rate of 1437 per 100,000 person-years. Squamous cell carcinoma was the most common, accounting for 94% of the skin cancers. The incidence of squamous cell carcinoma in transplant patients was 1355 per 100,000 person-years, compared to the rate in the general population of 38 per 100,000. The study also highlighted predictors of posttransplant skin cancer, including a history of pretransplant skin cancer and undergoing a thoracic transplant due to requiring higher levels of immunosuppression [26]. The type of immunosuppressant can also affect a patient's risk for skin cancers. Patients on the antimetabolite drug azathioprine were more than twice as likely to develop squamous cell carcinomas, while patients taking mycophenolate were recently found to have a lower risk. Azathioprine was not significantly associated with basal cell carcinomas [27]. In contrast, sirolimus historically has been shown to have a protective effect against skin cancers in transplant patients, with the largest decrease in risk of non-melanoma skin cancer and other malignancies seen in transplant patients who converted from other immunosuppressants to sirolimus-containing regimens [28].

Immunomodulating agents and immunosuppressants used in treating autoimmune conditions such as psoriasis, inflammatory bowel disease, and rheumatoid arthritis have also shown to carry an increased risk of skin cancer. Methotrexate use for rheumatoid arthritis increases the likelihood of a second non-melanoma skin cancer in patients, and combining tumor necrosis factor-α (TNF) inhibitors with methotrexate further increases that risk. More studies are needed to conclude whether TNF inhibitors increase the risk of skin cancer when used as monotherapy [29].

Patients with hematologic malignancies, particularly chronic lymphocytic leukemia (CLL), are predisposed to develop skin cancers. The risk of skin cancer in CLL patients alone is increased eightfold [30]. Furthermore, these skin cancers tend to demonstrate more aggressive behavior, with studies demonstrating a 7-fold and 14-fold increased likelihood of recurrence of squamous cell and basal cell carcinomas previously treated with Mohs micrographic surgery, respectively [31, 32].

Finally, patients with human immunodeficiency virus/acquired immunodeficiency syndrome (HIV/AIDS) are immunocompromised and therefore at a higher risk of skin cancers. Several studies have shown that HIV/AIDS patients have an almost threefold increased incidence of non-melanoma skin cancers, with male patients over three times as likely. Fortunately starting antiretroviral therapy (ART) in these patients is protective, with treated patients carrying a decreased risk compared to ART-naïve patients [33].

Genodermatoses with Increased Risk of Basal Cell Carcinomas

There are several familial cancer syndromes that carry an increased risk of skin cancer (Table 1.2). Basal cell nevus syndrome (BCNS), or Gorlin's syndrome, is an autosomal dominant disorder caused by germline inactivating mutations in *PTCH1*, leading to unchecked sonic hedgehog (SHH) signaling and increased cell proliferation. Patients with BCNS characteristically develop multiple basal cell carcinomas, which can initially appear within the first two decades of life with a

Table 1.2 Genodermatoses associated with non-melanoma skin cancer	Basal cell carcinoma
	Basal cell nevus syndrome (Gorlin)
	Bazex-Dupré-Christol syndrome
	Squamous cell carcinoma
	Xeroderma pigmentosum
	Oculocutaneous albinism
	Epidermodysplasia verruciformis

median number of 8, though some patients can have >1000 basal cell carcinomas. They also develop several benign and malignant neoplasms, including medulloblastomas, fibrosarcomas, rhabdomyosarcomas, meningiomas, and odontogenic keratocysts, as well as cardiac and ovarian fibromas. Characteristic developmental defects include palmoplantar pits, craniofacial anomalies such as frontal bossing, bifid ribs, spina bifida occulta, corpus callosum dysgenesis, calcification of the falx cerebri, and coarse facies [34].

Bazex-Dupré-Christol syndrome (follicular atrophoderma with basal cell carcinomas) is an X-linked dominant disorder with increased development of basal cell carcinomas. The constellation of findings includes follicular atrophoderma, basal cell carcinomas, and hypotrichosis, as well as less common features such as milia, hypohidrosis, facial hyperpigmentation, and trichoepitheliomas. Patients usually develop basal cell carcinomas within the second decade of life, which can have atypical features [35].

Lastly, Rombo syndrome is another autosomal dominant syndrome with an increased risk of basal cell carcinomas. Features of Rombo syndrome usually manifest prior to 10 years of age (a later onset than seen in Bazex-Dupré-Christol syndrome) and include vermiculate atrophoderma, telangiectasias, hypotrichosis, milia, and basal cell carcinomas [36].

Genodermatoses with Increased Risk of Squamous Cell Carcinomas

Xeroderma pigmentosum is a collection of disorders with defects in deoxyribonucleic acid (DNA) repair, making affected patients exquisitely sensitive to the damaging effects of UV radiation and thereby at greater than 20,000-fold increased risk of skin cancers. Sun exposure in these patients can lead to non-melanoma skin cancer development prior to 10 years of age [37, 38].

Oculocutaneous albinism (OCA) is characterized by mutations leading to absent or reduced melanin production, leaving patients vulnerable to DNA damage and subsequent skin cancers. These patients can have absent to variable levels of pigmentation and are at an increased risk of non-melanoma skin cancers without adequate photoprotection; squamous cell carcinomas are overwhelmingly the most common [39].

Epidermodysplasia verruciformis is a rare, autosomal recessive disorder due to epidermodysplasia verruciformis 1 or 2 genes (EVER1 or EVER2), rendering them more susceptible to human papillomavirus infections. Patients present with diffuse scattered verrucous lesions on their extremities during infancy or childhood. Half of these patients develop squamous cell carcinomas, typically in a sun-exposed distribution [40].

Melanoma: Risk Factors, At-Risk Populations, and Prevention

Melanoma is a skin cancer with significant morbidity and mortality. Each year over 65,000 people are diagnosed with melanoma, and over 9000 people die from the disease each year [41]. It is the fifth leading cancer among men and the seventh among women. Malignant melanoma incidence rate is increasing in the United States, surpassing the rates of any other potentially preventable cancer. The increase in incidence may be partially due to improved detection with increased screening and better reporting systems [42].

Although melanoma only represents 5% of all new skin cancer diagnoses, it accounts for the majority of deaths related to skin cancer [43]. Death rates and mortality have been largely unchanged over the years, with the exception of white men [44].

This incidence rate differs among different ethnic groups. Among whites it is approximately 18.4 per 100,000 persons. Among Hispanics the incidence rate is 2.3. From 2008 to 2012, 6623 cases of melanoma were diagnosed among Hispanics. The incidence rate among other ethnic groups was 0.8, 1.6, and 1.0 for African-Americans, American Indians, and Asians, respectively. Lower extremity and acral lentiginous melanomas were the more common sites of presentation in these groups. The diagnosis of acral melanoma is often delayed, resulting in more advanced stages of disease at presentation [45].

Per the CDC, skin cancer costs an estimated $1.7 billion to treat and results in $3.8 billion in lost productivity [46].

Risk Factors (Table 1.3)

UV Radiation and History of Sunburn

Numerous clinical and epidemiological studies have demonstrated a correlation between increased incidence of melanoma and sun exposure. Sunburn history, defined by five or more severe sunburns in childhood, has shown to play a considerable role as a risk factor for melanoma and can carry a relative risk of 2.02 [47–49].

Table 1.3 Melanoma risk factors

Greater than five sunburns
Indoor tanning
Psoralen UVA (PUVA) phototherapy
Fair phenotype
Parkinson disease
Immunosuppression
Personal and/or family history of melanoma

The link with sun exposure in melanoma is strongly associated with intermittent sun exposure [48], in contrast to non-melanoma skin cancers (NMSC) where cumulative sun exposure plays a larger role. This explains the higher incidence of NMSC in areas maximally exposed to the sun [47]. Furthermore, there is a higher incidence of melanoma in equatorial regions, where ultraviolet B radiation (UVB, wavelengths 290–320 nm) is most intense. This suggests that UVB may play a larger role in the development of melanoma than ultraviolet A (UVA, wavelengths 320–400 nm) [50, 51].

Indoor Tanning

Indoor tanning has emerged as a popular trend, gaining in popularity over the last 50 years, especially among adults aged 18–25 years. The UVA output of some of these devices can be up to four times higher than midday sunlight [46]. Up to one third of young white females reported indoor tanning in the past year. Melanoma incidence is increasing at a faster rate among this group, suggesting that indoor tanning is a likely driver of these diverging trends [52].

PUVA

UV exposure can be iatrogenic as well. Phototherapy and especially PUVA have been used to treat a variety of dermatological conditions. The risk of melanoma appears to increase with the passage of time (RR of 2.3), approximately 15 years after first exposure to PUVA, with the highest incidence in patients receiving >250 treatments (RR of 5.5). These data emphasize the importance of long-term monitoring in these patients [53, 54].

Nevi

Some studies have demonstrated the association between melanoma and the number, size, and type of nevi, illustrating an increased risk with the presence of 25–100 nevi or 1 atypical nevus. (Olsen, 2010) Newer studies, however, have shown that this relationship is not as strong as previously thought, suggesting that physicians and patients should not rely on the total number of nevi as the sole criteria in determining a patient's risk status [55].

Moreover, the risk of melanoma in congenital nevi is strongest with large congenital nevi, defined as greater than 20 centimeters, compared to small and medium congenital nevi, with a lifetime incidence of developing melanoma of around 2% [56, 57].

Phenotypes and Lentigines

Other phenotypic traits, like the Fitzpatrick skin phototype scale describing a patient's ability to tan, hair color, freckles, and eye color, can also affect individual skin cancer risk. The risk of melanoma is 3.5 times higher in red-haired individuals and almost doubled in blond-haired individuals compared to dark-haired counterparts. Light eye color (green, hazel, blue) versus dark showed an approximately 1.5-fold relative risk. Lastly, individuals with high freckle density showed twice the risk compared to lower density individuals [58].

Parkinson Disease

Melanoma can be associated with other comorbidities. Parkinson disease has an overall decreased risk of cancer diagnoses, with the exceptions of breast cancer and melanoma [59]. These patients have a statistically significant increase in the incidence of melanoma with a relative risk almost twice as high compared to the general population [60]. Some have proposed a link between the use of levodopa in the treatment of Parkinson disease and the development of melanoma; however, that increase in prevalence often precedes both the neurologic onset of the disease and initiation of treatment [61]. Another proposed mechanism is the mutation of the melanocortin-1 receptor (MC1R) gene, as it is more likely to develop in patients with Parkinson disease than in controls [59].

At-Risk Populations

Immunosuppressed Patients: Organ Transplant, Lymphoma, and HIV

Immunosuppressed populations, including those on immunosuppressants or those with solid organ transplantation, hematologic malignancies, or HIV, carry a higher risk of melanoma. In solid organ transplant recipients on immunosuppressive therapies, the risk of melanoma is two- to fivefold higher than the general population. Such an increase can be due to the direct carcinogenic effect of these medications or partially due to increased screening of this population, as they are at a higher risk of developing non-melanoma skin cancer [62].

Malignant melanoma was first reported in patients with lymphoma in 1973. Patients with chronic lymphocytic leukemia or small lymphocytic lymphoma have a two- to threefold increased risk of developing malignant melanoma [63]. A large retrospective cohort study showed the posttransplant incidence rate of melanoma is about 125 per 100,000 person-years [26].

Since the emergence of HIV/AIDS in the 1980s, a modest increase in the incidence of melanoma was reported prior to the introduction of highly active antiretroviral therapy (HAART) in the latter part of the 1990s. In the HAART era, the incidence of melanoma in the HIV population remains as high as 50%. That risk, however, is possibly confounded by increased longevity and closer surveillance in these patients [64].

Personal History of Skin Cancer

Patients with a personal history of melanoma should be monitored closely, as the risk of developing a second melanoma can be as high as 8% [65]. The increased risk is observed for patients with both invasive and in situ melanomas [66].

Personal history of NMSC also increases the risk of melanoma, likely due to the fact that both conditions have similar risk factors. Some studies have reported that a history of NMSC can increase the risk of melanoma from 2.80 to 6.55 times compared to those without a history of NMSC [58]. Some studies have also demonstrated not only an increase in the risk but also an increase in the mortality associated with melanoma in patients with a history of basal cell or squamous cell carcinomas [67, 68].

Family History of Melanoma

Family history of melanoma is associated with a higher risk of developing the disease. Approximately 8–12% of all patients diagnosed with melanoma have a family history of the disease independent of any known mutations [69, 70]. The relative risk of developing melanoma approximately doubles with a positive family history in one first-degree relative [71] but can increase ninefold if two first-degree relatives are affected [60].

Familial Syndromes (Table 1.4)

Hereditary melanoma syndromes (familial atypical multiple mole syndromes) are a group of autosomal dominant disorders that present clinically with hundreds of dysplastic nevi and a high incidence of melanoma [70].

Over the years, numerous genes have been studied and identified as a cause of germline mutations that increase the risk of melanoma (Table 1.4). Depending on the specific mutation, that risk can be between 4- and 1000-fold [70]. Germline mutations represent about 10% of all melanomas diagnosed worldwide [72]. These mutations work by three main mechanisms: activation of oncogenes, loss of tumor suppressor genes, and chromosomal instability [73].

Table 1.4 Genetic syndromes and mutations associated with melanoma syndromes	Familial atypical multiple mole syndrome
	Xeroderma pigmentosum
	PTEN mutations (Cowden syndrome and Bannayan-Riley-Ruvalcaba syndrome)
	Oculocutaneous albinism type 2
	Genetic mutations
	Microphthalmia-associated transcription factor (MITF)
	Melanocortin-1 receptor (MCR1)
	CDKN2A
	CDK4
	BRCA1
	BRCA2
	BAP1 in uveal melanoma

Some of the most well-established gene mutations are cyclin-dependent kinase inhibitor 2A (CDKN2A) and less commonly cyclin-dependent kinase 4 (CDK4). They control the transition between the growth phase in the cell cycle (G_1) and the synthesis phase (S_1). They carry a 60–90% lifetime risk of melanoma and have been associated with pancreatic cancer [70]. Testing for this mutation is recommended for patients with a diagnosis or family history of three melanomas, two melanomas, and one pancreatic cancer or one melanoma and two pancreatic cancers [47, 74].

Patients with BRCA1 (breast cancer susceptibility gene 1) or BRCA2 mutations have a twofold increase in melanoma due to mutations affecting DNA repair and stability. These mutations are also associated with breast, ovarian, prostate, and pancreatic cancers, necessitating close monitoring [70].

BAP1 (BRCA1 associated protein-1/ubiquitin carboxy-terminal hydrolase) mutations are more commonly associated with uveal melanoma than cutaneous melanoma. They are also associated with mesothelioma and tumors of the kidney, gallbladder, and brain [75].

MITF (microphthalmia-associated transcription factor) mutations have also been associated with an increased melanoma risk and feature a high nevus count in association with renal cell carcinomas [76].

MCR1 (melanocortin-1 receptor) mutations increase the risk of melanoma through increased pheomelanin production, which is less protective against UV radiation than eumelanin. This imbalance alters skin pigmentation, leading to red hair and fair skin [77].

Xeroderma pigmentosum is a rare autosomal dominant disease that affects approximately 1 in 250,000 births. It is caused by a mutation in DNA repair genes that are responsible for nucleotide excision repair, which play a major role in UV-induced DNA damage repair by removing radiation-induced pyrimidine dimers. This leads to extreme, early onset photosensitivity and significant incidence of basal cell carcinoma, squamous cell carcinoma, and melanoma (600- to 8000-fold risk) [38].

Cowden and Bannayan-Riley-Ruvalcaba syndromes are a group of phosphatase and tensin homolog (PTEN) hamartoma tumor syndromes that are associated with melanoma [78, 79].

Oculocutaneous albinism type 2 is the most common subtype of albinism, which carries an increased risk of melanoma. It is caused by mutation in the OCA2 gene, leading to defects in melanin synthesis and a subsequent increase in melanoma [80]. A substantial challenge in this population is that they can present with the amelanotic variant of melanoma. Amelanotic melanoma typically lacks the usual clinical and dermatoscopic signs of melanoma, which often lead to delays in diagnosis and worse outcomes [81].

Prevention and Screening of Non-melanoma Skin Cancer and Melanoma

Skin cancer prevention focuses on decreasing risk factors through photoprotection, immunosuppression changes, and keratinocyte development.

Consistent and appropriate application of sunscreen has been shown to decrease the number of precancerous actinic keratoses and squamous cell carcinomas after 1–4 years of follow-up [82–84]. Unfortunately, sunscreen has not demonstrated the same beneficial effect with basal cell carcinomas [84]. The relationship between sunscreen and melanoma reduction is unclear and requires more probative studies [85]. This incongruence illustrates the need for additional photoprotection other than sunscreen, which includes photo-protective clothing, limiting sun exposure outdoors at times of highest UV radiation, and seeking shade. Vitamin D deficiency can develop in patients who follow strict sun protection making supplementation necessary.

The degree and duration of immunosuppression in solid organ transplant recipients are associated with increased incidence of skin cancer [86]. In collaboration with the transplant team, there is a reduction of immunosuppression to mimimal levels for graft tolerance. In patients with metastatic, rapidly aggressive, or increasing numbers of skin cancers, a change in immunosuppression to a mTOR inhibitor may be indicated [87, 88].

Retinoids, a vitamin A derivative, affect keratinocyte differentiation and proliferation [89]. The oral retinoid acitretin is advantageous in reducing actinic keratoses and squamous cell carcinomas. A prospective trial evaluating renal transplant patients given oral acitretin for 1 year demonstrated a significantly decreased incidence of squamous cell carcinomas, with a similar but not statistically significant reduction in basal cell carcinomas [90]. Acitretin also reduced the number of actinic keratoses by nearly 50% in renal transplant patients receiving varying doses of the drug [91]. With regard to longitudinal benefits, a retrospective study of renal transplant patients receiving acitretin for 1–16 years demonstrated a significant decrease in the number of squamous cell carcinomas within the first 3 years of taking acitretin [92].

Once discontinued, acitretin is no longer effective, and tumor development recurs. While oral retinoids are beneficial as a chemopreventive agent, topical retinoids, such as tretinoin, are not effective in reducing squamous cell carcinoma incidence [93].

Nicotinamide, vitamin B3, is a precursor of nicotinamide adenine dinucleotide and necessary cofactor in adenosine triphosphate production (ATP). UV radiation depletes cellular ATP as well as damages DNA. ATP is needed for DNA repair. Nicotinamide replenishes ATP thereby enhancing DNA repair [94]. In an Australian study, oral nicotinamide 500 mg twice a day reduced the incidence of NMSC in high-risk skin cancer patients by 23 percent relative rate reduction. Subjects with the highest number of skin cancers prior to enrollment had the highest relative reduction in skin cancers with nicotinamide. Importantly, the benefit was with nicotinamide, not nicotinic acid [95]. Larger randomized controlled trials are needed to further understand the nicotinamide's benefit in reducing skin cancers.

Skin screening examinations theoretically are an important aspect of detecting and reducing the burden of skin cancers. A recent literature review evaluating screening examinations and skin cancers, most notably melanoma, by the US Preventive Services Task Force did not demonstrate a clear benefit with regard to mortality and screening; however, few studies were incorporated due to the inclusion criteria, and few were specific to the United States, illustrating the need for further research [96]. The skin exam includes examination of the skin and provides counseling to patients on the signs and symptoms of skin cancer and to perform their own skin self-examination monthly. A non-healing, bleeding, or changing skin lesion needs evaluation by a trained dermatologist.

References

1. Madan V, Lear JT, Szeimies RM. Non-melanoma skin cancer. Lancet. 2010;375(9715):673–85.
2. Society AC. Cancer facts & figures 2016. Atlanta: American Cancer Society; 2016.
3. El Ghissassi F, Baan R, Straif K, Grosse Y, Secretan B, Bouvard V, et al. A review of human carcinogens--part D: radiation. Lancet Oncol. 2009;10(8):751–2.
4. Vitasa BC, Taylor HR, Strickland PT, Rosenthal FS, West S, Abbey H, et al. Association of nonmelanoma skin cancer and actinic keratosis with cumulative solar ultraviolet exposure in Maryland watermen. Cancer. 1990;65(12):2811–7.
5. Wehner MR, Shive ML, Chren MM, Han J, Qureshi AA, Linos E. Indoor tanning and non-melanoma skin cancer: systematic review and meta-analysis. BMJ. 2012;345:e5909.
6. Hearn RM, Kerr AC, Rahim KF, Ferguson J, Dawe RS. Incidence of skin cancers in 3867 patients treated with narrow-band ultraviolet B phototherapy. Br J Dermatol. 2008;159(4):931–5.
7. Stern RS, Study PF-U. The risk of squamous cell and basal cell cancer associated with psoralen and ultraviolet A therapy: a 30-year prospective study. J Am Acad Dermatol. 2012;66(4):553–62.
8. Lichter MD, Karagas MR, Mott LA, Spencer SK, Stukel TA, Greenberg ER. Therapeutic ionizing radiation and the incidence of basal cell carcinoma and squamous cell carcinoma. The New Hampshire Skin Cancer Study Group. Arch Dermatol. 2000;136(8):1007–11.

9. Perkins JL, Liu Y, Mitby PA, Neglia JP, Hammond S, Stovall M, et al. Nonmelanoma skin cancer in survivors of childhood and adolescent cancer: a report from the childhood cancer survivor study. J Clin Oncol. 2005;23(16):3733–41.
10. Cowen EW, Nguyen JC, Miller DD, McShane D, Arron ST, Prose NS, et al. Chronic phototoxicity and aggressive squamous cell carcinoma of the skin in children and adults during treatment with voriconazole. J Am Acad Dermatol. 2010;62(1):31–7.
11. Kolaitis NA, Duffy E, Zhang A, Lo M, Barba DT, Chen M, et al. Voriconazole increases the risk for cutaneous squamous cell carcinoma after lung transplantation. Transpl Int. 2017;30(1):41–8.
12. Su F, Viros A, Milagre C, Trunzer K, Bollag G, Spleiss O, et al. RAS mutations in cutaneous squamous-cell carcinomas in patients treated with BRAF inhibitors. N Engl J Med. 2012;366(3):207–15.
13. Cheng PS, Weng SF, Chiang CH, Lai FJ. Relationship between arsenic-containing drinking water and skin cancers in the arseniasis endemic areas in Taiwan. J Dermatol. 2016;43(2):181–6.
14. Mayer JE, Goldman RH. Arsenic and skin cancer in the USA: the current evidence regarding arsenic-contaminated drinking water. Int J Dermatol. 2016;55(11):e585–e91.
15. Gawkrodger DJ. Occupational skin cancers. Occup Med (Lond). 2004;54(7):458–63.
16. Copcu E, Aktas A, Sişman N, Oztan Y. Thirty-one cases of Marjolin's ulcer. Clin Exp Dermatol. 2003;28(2):138–41.
17. Tao J, Zhang X, Guo N, Chen S, Huang C, Zheng L, et al. Squamous cell carcinoma complicating discoid lupus erythematosus in Chinese patients: review of the literature, 1964–2010. J Am Acad Dermatol. 2012;66(4):695–6.
18. Au J, Patel D, Campbell JH. Oral lichen planus. Oral Maxillofac Surg Clin North Am. 2013;25(1):93–100. vii
19. Bleeker MC, Visser PJ, Overbeek LI, van Beurden M, Berkhof J. Lichen sclerosus: incidence and risk of vulvar squamous cell carcinoma. Cancer Epidemiol Biomarkers Prev. 2016;25(8):1224–30.
20. Sasson M, Krain AD. Porokeratosis and cutaneous malignancy. A review. Dermatol Surg. 1996;22(4):339–42.
21. Cribier B, Scrivener Y, Grosshans E. Tumors arising in nevus sebaceus: a study of 596 cases. J Am Acad Dermatol. 2000;42(2 Pt 1):263–8.
22. Marcil I, Stern RS. Risk of developing a subsequent nonmelanoma skin cancer in patients with a history of nonmelanoma skin cancer: a critical review of the literature and meta-analysis. Arch Dermatol. 2000;136(12):1524–30.
23. Bradford PT. Skin cancer in skin of color. Dermatol Nurs. 2009;21(4):170–7. 206; quiz 178
24. Kim GK, Del Rosso JQ, Bellew S. Skin cancer in asians: part 1: nonmelanoma skin cancer. J Clin Aesthet Dermatol. 2009;2(8):39–42.
25. Byrd-Miles K, Toombs EL, Peck GL. Skin cancer in individuals of African, Asian, Latin-American, and American-Indian descent: differences in incidence, clinical presentation, and survival compared to Caucasians. J Drugs Dermatol. 2007;6(1):10–6.
26. Garrett GL, Blanc PD, Boscardin J, Lloyd AA, Ahmed RL, Anthony T, et al. Incidence of and risk factors for skin cancer in organ transplant recipients in the United States. JAMA Dermatol. 2017;153(3):296–303.
27. Coghill AE, Johnson LG, Berg D, Resler AJ, Leca N, Madeleine MM. Immunosuppressive medications and squamous cell skin carcinoma: nested case-control study within the Skin Cancer after Organ Transplant (SCOT) Cohort. Am J Transplant. 2016;16(2):565–73.
28. Knoll GA, Kokolo MB, Mallick R, Beck A, Buenaventura CD, Ducharme R, et al. Effect of sirolimus on malignancy and survival after kidney transplantation: systematic review and meta-analysis of individual patient data. BMJ. 2014;349:g6679.
29. Scott FI, Mamtani R, Brensinger CM, Haynes K, Chiesa-Fuxench ZC, Zhang J, et al. Risk of nonmelanoma skin cancer associated with the use of immunosuppressant and biologic agents in patients with a history of autoimmune disease and nonmelanoma skin cancer. JAMA Dermatol. 2016;152(2):164–72.

30. Greene MH, Hoover RN, Fraumeni JF. Subsequent cancer in patients with chronic lymphocytic leukemia--a possible immunologic mechanism. J Natl Cancer Inst. 1978;61(2):337–40.
31. Mehrany K, Weenig RH, Pittelkow MR, Roenigk RK, Otley CC. High recurrence rates of basal cell carcinoma after mohs surgery in patients with chronic lymphocytic leukemia. Arch Dermatol. 2004;140(8):985–8.
32. Mehrany K, Weenig RH, Pittelkow MR, Roenigk RK, Otley CC. High recurrence rates of squamous cell carcinoma after Mohs' surgery in patients with chronic lymphocytic leukemia. Dermatol Surg. 2005;31(1):38–42. discussion
33. Zhao H, Shu G, Wang S. The risk of non-melanoma skin cancer in HIV-infected patients: new data and meta-analysis. Int J STD AIDS. 2016;27(7):568–75.
34. Kimonis VE, Goldstein AM, Pastakia B, Yang ML, Kase R, DiGiovanna JJ, et al. Clinical manifestations in 105 persons with nevoid basal cell carcinoma syndrome. Am J Med Genet. 1997;69(3):299–308.
35. Abuzahra F, Parren LJ, Frank J. Multiple familial and pigmented basal cell carcinomas in early childhood – Bazex-Dupré-Christol syndrome. J Eur Acad Dermatol Venereol. 2012;26(1):117–21.
36. Michaëlsson G, Olsson E, Westermark P. The Rombo syndrome: a familial disorder with vermiculate atrophoderma, milia, hypotrichosis, trichoepitheliomas, basal cell carcinomas and peripheral vasodilation with cyanosis. Acta Derm Venereol. 1981;61(6):497–503.
37. Lehmann AR, McGibbon D, Stefanini M. Xeroderma pigmentosum. Orphanet J Rare Dis. 2011;6:70.
38. Kraemer KH, Lee MM, Scotto J. Xeroderma pigmentosum. Cutaneous, ocular, and neurologic abnormalities in 830 published cases. Arch Dermatol. 1987;123(2):241–50.
39. Luande J, Henschke CI, Mohammed N. The Tanzanian human albino skin. Natural history. Cancer. 1985;55(8):1823–8.
40. Burger B, Itin PH. Epidermodysplasia verruciformis. Curr Probl Dermatol. 2014;45:123–31.
41. Group USCSW. United States cancer statistics: 1999–2013 incidence and mortality web-based report. Atlanta: U.S. Departments of Health and Human Services, Centers for Disease Control and Prevention and National Cancer Institute; 2016.
42. Kohler BA, Sherman RL, Howlader N, Jemal A, Ryerson AB, Henry KA, et al. Annual report to the Nation on the Status of Cancer, 1975–2011, featuring incidence of breast cancer subtypes by race/ethnicity, poverty, and state. J Natl Cancer Inst. 2015;107(6):djv048.
43. Nikolaou V, Stratigos AJ. Emerging trends in the epidemiology of melanoma. Br J Dermatol. 2014;170(1):11–9.
44. Jemal A, Saraiya M, Patel P, Cherala SS, Barnholtz-Sloan J, Kim J, et al. Recent trends in cutaneous melanoma incidence and death rates in the United States, 1992–2006. J Am Acad Dermatol. 2011;65(5 Suppl 1):S17–25. e1–3
45. Cormier JN, Xing Y, Ding M, Lee JE, Mansfield PF, Gershenwald JE, et al. Ethnic differences among patients with cutaneous melanoma. Arch Intern Med. 2006;166(17):1907–14.
46. (CDC) CfDCaP. Use of indoor tanning devices by adults--United States, 2010. MMWR Morb Mortal Wkly Rep. 2012;61(18):323–6.
47. Gandini S, Sera F, Cattaruzza MS, Pasquini P, Abeni D, Boyle P, et al. Meta-analysis of risk factors for cutaneous melanoma: I. Common and atypical naevi. Eur J Cancer. 2005;41(1):28–44.
48. Nelemans PJ, Groenendal H, Kiemeney LA, Rampen FH, Ruiter DJ, Verbeek AL. Effect of intermittent exposure to sunlight on melanoma risk among indoor workers and sun-sensitive individuals. Environ Health Perspect. 1993;101(3):252–5.
49. Wu S, Han J, Laden F, Qureshi AA. Long-term ultraviolet flux, other potential risk factors, and skin cancer risk: a cohort study. Cancer Epidemiol Biomarkers Prev. 2014;23(6):1080–9.
50. De Fabo EC, Noonan FP, Fears T, Merlino G. Ultraviolet B but not ultraviolet A radiation initiates melanoma. Cancer Res. 2004;64(18):6372–6.
51. Herman JR. Global increase in UV irradiance during the past 30 years (1979–2008) estimated from satellite data. J Geophys Res Atmos. 2010;115(D4):2156–202.

52. Lazovich D, Isaksson Vogel R, Weinstock MA, Nelson HH, Ahmed RL, Berwick M. Association between indoor tanning and melanoma in younger men and women. JAMA Dermatol. 2016;152(3):268–75.
53. Stern RS, Study PFu. The risk of melanoma in association with long-term exposure to PUVA. J Am Acad Dermatol. 2001;44(5):755–61.
54. Stern RS, Nichols KT, Väkevä LH. Malignant melanoma in patients treated for psoriasis with methoxsalen (psoralen) and ultraviolet A radiation (PUVA). The PUVA follow-up study. N Engl J Med. 1997;336(15):1041–5.
55. Geller AC, Mayer JE, Sober AJ, Miller DR, Argenziano G, Johnson TM, et al. Total nevi, atypical nevi, and melanoma thickness: an analysis of 566 patients at 2 US Centers. JAMA Dermatol. 2016;152(4):413–8.
56. Vourc'h-Jourdain M, Martin L, Barbarot S, aRED. Large congenital melanocytic nevi: therapeutic management and melanoma risk: a systematic review. J Am Acad Dermatol. 2013;68(3):493–8. e1-14
57. Alikhan A, Ibrahimi OA, Eisen DB. Congenital melanocytic nevi: where are we now? Part I. Clinical presentation, epidemiology, pathogenesis, histology, malignant transformation, and neurocutaneous melanosis. J Am Acad Dermatol. 2012;67(4):495.e1–17. quiz 512–4
58. Gandini S, Sera F, Cattaruzza MS, Pasquini P, Picconi O, Boyle P, et al. Meta-analysis of risk factors for cutaneous melanoma: II. Sun exposure. Eur J Cancer. 2005;41(1):45–60.
59. Disse M, Reich H, Lee PK, Schram SS. A review of the association between parkinson disease and malignant melanoma. Dermatol Surg. 2016;42(2):141–6.
60. Hemminki K, Zhang H, Czene K. Familial and attributable risks in cutaneous melanoma: effects of proband and age. J Invest Dermatol. 2003;120(2):217–23.
61. Olsen JH, Friis S, Frederiksen K, McLaughlin JK, Mellemkjaer L, Møller H. Atypical cancer pattern in patients with Parkinson's disease. Br J Cancer. 2005;92(1):201–5.
62. Robbins HA, Clarke CA, Arron ST, Tatalovich Z, Kahn AR, Hernandez BY, et al. Melanoma risk and survival among organ transplant recipients. J Invest Dermatol. 2015;135(11):2657–65.
63. Brewer JD, Shanafelt TD, Call TG, Cerhan JR, Roenigk RK, Weaver AL, et al. Increased incidence of malignant melanoma and other rare cutaneous cancers in the setting of chronic lymphocytic leukemia. Int J Dermatol. 2015;54(8):e287–93.
64. Olsen CM, Knight LL, Green AC. Risk of melanoma in people with HIV/AIDS in the pre- and post-HAART eras: a systematic review and meta-analysis of cohort studies. PLoS One. 2014;9(4):e95096.
65. Stam-Posthuma JJ, van Duinen C, Scheffer E, Vink J, Bergman W. Multiple primary melanomas. J Am Acad Dermatol. 2001;44(1):22–7.
66. Pomerantz H, Huang D, Weinstock MA. Risk of subsequent melanoma after melanoma in situ and invasive melanoma: a population-based study from 1973 to 2011. J Am Acad Dermatol. 2015;72(5):794–800.
67. Marghoob AA, Slade J, Salopek TG, Kopf AW, Bart RS, Rigel DS. Basal cell and squamous cell carcinomas are important risk factors for cutaneous malignant melanoma. Screening implications. Cancer. 1995;75(2 Suppl):707–14.
68. Kahn HS, Tatham LM, Patel AV, Thun MJ, Heath CW. Increased cancer mortality following a history of nonmelanoma skin cancer. JAMA. 1998;280(10):910–2.
69. Manson JE, Rexrode KM, Garland FC, Garland CF, Weinstock MA. The case for a comprehensive national campaign to prevent melanoma and associated mortality. Epidemiology. 2000;11(6):728–34.
70. Ransohoff KJ, Jaju PD, Tang JY, Carbone M, Leachman S, Sarin KY. Familial skin cancer syndromes: increased melanoma risk. J Am Acad Dermatol. 2016;74(3):423–34. quiz 35-6
71. Begg CB, Hummer A, Mujumdar U, Armstrong BK, Kricker A, Marrett LD, et al. Familial aggregation of melanoma risks in a large population-based sample of melanoma cases. Cancer Causes Control. 2004;15(9):957–65.
72. Goldstein AM. Familial melanoma, pancreatic cancer and germline CDKN2A mutations. Hum Mutat. 2004;23(6):630.

73. Vogelstein B, Kinzler KW. Cancer genes and the pathways they control. Nat Med. 2004;10(8):789–99.
74. Leachman SA, Carucci J, Kohlmann W, Banks KC, Asgari MM, Bergman W, et al. Selection criteria for genetic assessment of patients with familial melanoma. J Am Acad Dermatol. 2009;61(4):677.e1–14.
75. Njauw CN, Kim I, Piris A, Gabree M, Taylor M, Lane AM, et al. Germline BAP1 inactivation is preferentially associated with metastatic ocular melanoma and cutaneous-ocular melanoma families. PLoS One. 2012;7(4):e35295.
76. Bertolotto C, Lesueur F, Giuliano S, Strub T, de Lichy M, Bille K, et al. A SUMOylation-defective MITF germline mutation predisposes to melanoma and renal carcinoma. Nature. 2011;480(7375):94–8.
77. Valverde P, Healy E, Jackson I, Rees JL, Thody AJ. Variants of the melanocyte-stimulating hormone receptor gene are associated with red hair and fair skin in humans. Nat Genet. 1995;11(3):328–30.
78. Gorlin RJ, Cohen MM, Condon LM, Burke BA. Bannayan-Riley-Ruvalcaba syndrome. Am J Med Genet. 1992;44(3):307–14.
79. Tan MH, Mester JL, Ngeow J, Rybicki LA, Orloff MS, Eng C. Lifetime cancer risks in individuals with germline PTEN mutations. Clin Cancer Res. 2012;18(2):400–7. https://doi.org/10.1158/1078-0432.CCR-11-2283.
80. Hawkes JE, Cassidy PB, Manga P, Boissy RE, Goldgar D, Cannon-Albright L, et al. Report of a novel OCA2 gene mutation and an investigation of OCA2 variants on melanoma risk in a familial melanoma pedigree. J Dermatol Sci. 2013;69(1):30–7.
81. De Luca DA, Bollea Garlatti LA, Galimberti GN, Galimberti RL. Amelanotic melanoma in albinism: the power of dermatoscopy. J Eur Acad Dermatol Venereol. 2016;30(8):1422–3.
82. Thompson SC, Jolley D, Marks R. Reduction of solar keratoses by regular sunscreen use. N Engl J Med. 1993;329(16):1147–51.
83. Naylor MF, Boyd A, Smith DW, Cameron GS, Hubbard D, Neldner KH. High sun protection factor sunscreens in the suppression of actinic neoplasia. Arch Dermatol. 1995;131(2):170–5.
84. Green A, Williams G, Neale R, Hart V, Leslie D, Parsons P, et al. Daily sunscreen application and betacarotene supplementation in prevention of basal-cell and squamous-cell carcinomas of the skin: a randomised controlled trial. Lancet. 1999;354(9180):723–9.
85. Curiel-Lewandrowski C, Chen SC, Swetter SM, Sub-Committee MPWG-PSL. Screening and prevention measures for melanoma: is there a survival advantage? Curr Oncol Rep. 2012;14(5):458–67.
86. Otley CC, Maragh SL. Reduction of immunosuppression for transplant-associated skin cancer: rationale and evidence of efficacy. Dermatol Surg. 2005;31:163.
87. Kauffman HM, Cherikh WS, Cheng Y, et al. Maintenance immunosuppression with target-of-rapamycin inhibitors is associated with a reduced incidence of de novo malignancies. Transplantation. 2005;80:883.
88. Schena FP, Pascoe MD, Alberu J, et al. Conversion from calcineurin inhbitors to sirolimus maintenance therapy in renal allograft recipients: 24 month efficacy and safety results from the CONVERT trial. Transplantation. 2009;87:233.
89. Fisher GJ, Voorhees JJ. Molecular mechanisms of retinoid actions in skin. FASEB J. 1996;10:1002–13.
90. George R, Weightman W, Russ GR, Bannister KM, Mathew TH. Acitretin for chemoprevention of non-melanoma skin cancers in renal transplant recipients. Australas J Dermatol. 2002;43(4):269–73.
91. de Sévaux RG, Smit JV, de Jong EM, van de Kerkhof PC, Hoitsma AJ. Acitretin treatment of premalignant and malignant skin disorders in renal transplant recipients: clinical effects of a randomized trial comparing two doses of acitretin. J Am Acad Dermatol. 2003;49(3):407–12.
92. Harwood CA, Leedham-Green M, Leigh IM, Proby CM. Low-dose retinoids in the prevention of cutaneous squamous cell carcinomas in organ transplant recipients: a 16-year retrospective study. Arch Dermatol. 2005;141(4):456–64.

93. Weinstock MA, Bingham SF, Digiovanna JJ, Rizzo AE, et al. Tretinoin and the prevention of keratinocyte carcinoma (Basal and squamous cell carcinoma of the skin): a veterans affairs randomized chemoprevention trial. J Invest Dermatol. 2012;132(6):1583–90.
94. Surjana D, Halliday GM, Damian DL. Nicotinamide enhances repair of ultraviolet radiation-induced DNA damage in human keratinocytes and ex vivo skin. Carcinogen. 2013;34:1144–9.
95. Chen AC, Martin AJ, Choy B, et al. A phase 3 randomized trial of nicotinamide for skin cancer chemoprevention. N Engl J Med. 2015;373:1618–26.
96. Wernli KJ, Henrikson NB, Morrison CC, Nguyen M, Pocobelli G, Blasi PR. Screening for skin cancer in adults: updated evidence report and systematic review for the US Preventive Services Task Force. JAMA. 2016;316(4):436–47.

Chapter 2
Actinic Keratosis

Allison Pye, Daniel Wallis, and Vineet Mishra

Abstract Actinic keratosis (AK) is the most common precancerous skin lesion. AKs present on sun-damaged skin as pink to red gritty macules or papules. Patients with numerous AKs are at increased risk of developing skin cancer. AK development represents the initial step in keratinocytes' progression to squamous cell carcinoma. Patients with numerous AKs are at increased risk of developing skin cancer. Treatment options for AKs include cryosurgery, topical chemotherapies, chemical peels, and laser surgery. Prevention is of utmost importance, including photoprotection such as sun protective clothing and sunscreens.

Keywords Actinic keratosis · Solar keratosis · Photodamage · Precancerous · Cryosurgery · Topical chemotherapy · Sun protection

Epidemiology of Actinic Keratosis

Actinic keratosis (AK), also known as solar or senile keratosis, is defined as epidermal dysplasia that occurs on the skin chronically exposed to the sun, most commonly on the forehead, bald head, face, neck, or arms, and represents the most common precancerous lesion of the skin [1, 2]. AK signals the potential for progression to invasive squamous cell carcinoma and represents an increased risk for all skin cancers [1]. Risk factors include older age, male gender, sun exposure, and Fitzpatrick type I or II skin—most affected patients have at least two lesions and often more [1]. Lesions can be discrete with clearly defined borders or diffuse

A. Pye (✉)
Dermatology, McGovern Medical School, UT Houston, Houston, TX, USA
e-mail: Allisonpye@gmail.com

D. Wallis
Dermatology, Texas Tech University Health Sciences Center, Lubbock, TX, USA

V. Mishra
Department of Medicine, University of Texas Health Science Center – San Antonio, San Antonio, TX, USA

© Springer International Publishing AG, part of Springer Nature 2018   21
A. Hanlon (ed.), *A Practical Guide to Skin Cancer*,
https://doi.org/10.1007/978-3-319-74903-7_2

Fig. 2.1 Diffusely
actinically damaged scalp
with scattered actinic
keratoses

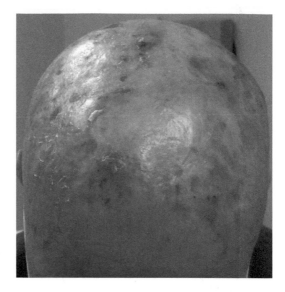

and multiple in the setting of "field damage." Lesions are usually red or pink hyper-keratotic papules or plaques that are rough in nature with overlying adherent scale. Sizes range from 1 to 3 millimeters in diameter (Fig. 2.1) [1, 2].

Prevalence is difficult to assess, as many AKs are either underdiagnosed or generally treated due to their ease of identification. AKs are most commonly present on sun-exposed skin of fair patients. Although future studies are necessary to determine more updated and specific information regarding incidence and prevalence of AK, these precancerous epidermal lesions clearly have a significant effect on our population.

The development of an actinic keratosis is thought to be the initial step within a disease spectrum that can ultimately lead to invasive squamous cell carcinoma, and AKs are associated with a greater than sixfold increased risk of developing skin cancer [1, 3]. The probability of a specific AK progressing to skin cancer is unpredictable; however, Dodson and colleagues determined that the risk of developing more invasive disease in a patient with seven to eight AKs was between 6.1% and 10.2% over 10 years [4].

Pathogenesis of Actinic Keratosis

Actinic keratoses more commonly affect those with lighter skin in chronically sun-exposed areas, and frequency of the lesions corresponds to an individual's cumulative UV exposure. UVB radiation from the sun at a wavelength of 290–320 nm plays the most important role in the formation of AKs, as it causes thymidine dimer formation in DNA and RNA, generating mutations in the telomerase and p53 genes [5].

Pathology of Actinic Keratosis

Histologic evaluation of an actinic keratosis reveals loss of orderly maturation, and atypical, dyskeratotic, or necrotic keratinocytes within the epidermis [5] (Fig. 2.2). There is often overlying parakeratosis, or retained nuclei within the stratum corneum, to suggest rapid turnover of cells. Atypical keratinocytes show loss of polarity; their nuclei are large, crowded, pleomorphic, and hyperchromatic with cytologic atypia [5]. Cytoplasm is eosinophilic and can appear pale or vacuolated [5].

There are six histologic types of AKs: hypertrophic, atrophic, Bowenoid, acantholytic, lichenoid, and pigmented (Table 2.1)—some types overlap, and several of these types correspond to their clinical variants.

There are multiple variations in the appearance of actinic keratoses: cutaneous horn, hypertrophic AK, pigmented AK, atrophic AK, Bowenoid AK, and lichenoid AK (Table 2.2).

Fig. 2.2 Hypertrophic actinic keratosis with focal parakeratosis over areas of atypical keratinocytes along the lower portion of the epidermis and lichenoid infiltrate with plasma cells in the dermis below the lesion (Image and description courtesy of Dr. Valerie Shiu, UT Health San Antonio Dermatology)

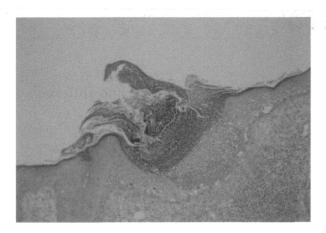

Table 2.1 Histology of actinic keratosis

Histologic type of AK	Histologic features
Hypertrophic	Hyperkeratosis and acanthosis
Atrophic	Thinned epidermis, missing rete ridges, only three to four layers of keratinocytes
Bowenoid	Full-thickness atypia, often indistinguishable from Bowen's disease
Acantholytic	Focal acantholysis, often accompanied by clefts
Lichenoid	Dense, band-like infiltrate of lymphocytes in papillary dermis, vacuolar alteration at dermoepidermal junction
Pigmented	Increased melanin within dermis

Adapted from Roewert et al. [5]

Table 2.2 Clinical variants of actinic keratosis

Clinical variant	Clinical description
Cutaneous horn	Conical projection of cohesive keratin protruding out of the skin. Can also arise from other skin pathologies such as keratoacanthoma, squamous cell carcinoma, verruca, and seborrheic keratosis [6]
Hyperkeratotic actinic keratosis (also known as hypertrophic actinic keratosis) (Fig. 2.3)	Rough papule or plaque with scale thicker than common actinic keratosis. The scale may become white or yellow-brown over time [7]
Atrophic actinic keratosis (Fig. 2.4)	Pink to red macule lacking overlying scale [7]
Pigmented actinic keratosis (Fig. 2.5)	Macules, papules, or plaques that are tan to brown in color, usually lacking associated erythema [8]
Bowenoid actinic keratosis (Fig. 2.6)	Solitary, erythematous, scaly patch or plaque with well-defined borders. Differentiated from Bowen's disease by the degree of epithelial dysplasia on histopathologic examination [9]
Lichenoid actinic keratosis	Similar to the common AK but more erythematous at the base of the lesion. Patients may report pruritus of the lesion. On histopathology, there is a dense band-like inflammatory infiltrate [7]

Diagnosis, Physical Exam, and Differential Diagnosis

AKs are most commonly a clinical diagnosis, although the clinical appearance of AKs varies (see Table 2.2 under "Clinical Variants of Actinic Keratosis"). Actinic keratoses appear most commonly as scaly macules, patches, papules, or plaques on a pink or erythematous base distributed on sun-exposed areas of the skin (commonly the head, neck, extremities, and upper trunk) [10] (Fig. 2.7). The variations in the appearance of actinic keratoses include cutaneous horn, hypertrophic AK, pigmented AK, atrophic AK, Bowenoid AK, and lichenoid AK (Table 2.2). The amount of scale present can differ; atrophic AKs lack scale, while hypertrophic AKs have very thick scale. The color also varies; some AKs can have the same color as surrounding skin, while other AKs, such as pigmented AKs, appear tan or brown in color. The overlying scale gives AKs their rough texture, similar to sandpaper [10]. The surrounding skin commonly exhibits signs of chronic sun damage, including telangiectasias, elastosis, and wrinkles [11]. Actinic keratoses are generally clinical diagnoses; however, biopsy for histologic exam may be necessary to rule out squamous cell carcinoma or melanoma when atypical lesions such as cutaneous horns, hypertrophic AKs, or pigmented AKs are present.

Fig. 2.3 Hypertrophic actinic keratosis between the second and third metacarpophalangeal joints of the left hand. Note the thicker scale (Image courtesy of Dr. Vineet Mishra, UT Health San Antonio Dermatology)

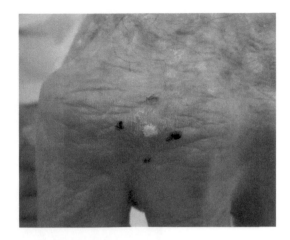

Fig. 2.4 Atrophic actinic keratosis on the right temple just anterior to the hairline. Note the lacking scale (Image courtesy of Dr. Vineet Mishra, UT Health San Antonio Dermatology)

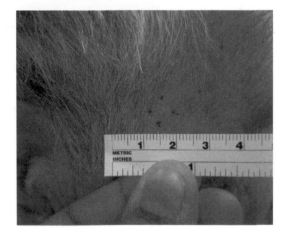

Fig. 2.5 Pigmented actinic keratosis on the right maxillary cheek. Note the brown, hyperpigmented color (Image courtesy of Dr. Vineet Mishra, UT Health San Antonio Dermatology)

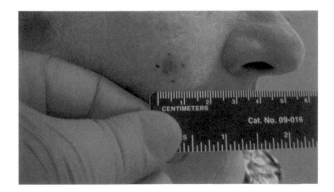

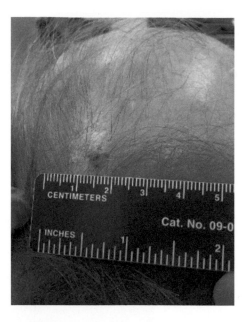

Fig. 2.6 Bowenoid actinic keratosis (Image courtesy of Dr. Vineet Mishra, UT Health San Antonio Dermatology

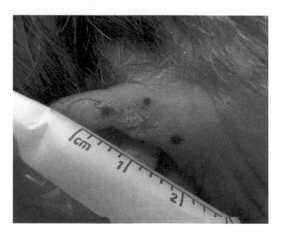

Fig. 2.7 Typical appearing actinic keratosis on the anterosuperior aspect of helix of the right area. Image courtesy of Dr. Vineet Mishra, UT Health San Antonio

Differential Diagnosis

- Squamous cell carcinoma (SCC)—Although invasive squamous cell carcinoma commonly has a higher degree of hyperkeratosis than AK, it can be difficult to differentiate from AK. SCCs usually present as erythematous keratotic papules or nodules that arise within a background of sun-damaged skin and are frequently accompanied by a history of tenderness as the lesion enlarges and becomes more nodular [7].

- Bowen's disease (squamous cell carcinoma in situ)—Usually presenting as an erythematous scaly patch or slightly elevated plaque on sun-damaged skin of elderly patients, Bowen's disease can be difficult to distinguish from AK. Generally, AKs tend to be smaller lesions. Bowen's disease may result from a preexisting AK but can also arise de novo [7].
- Superficial basal cell carcinoma (BCC)—Superficial BCCs can also resemble the clinical appearance of AKs. Superficial BCCs often present as erythematous macules or thin plaques. They frequently have slight elevation of the leading edge and more translucence, which can help distinguish them from AKs [7].
- Psoriasis—The scaling plaques of psoriasis may sometimes resemble AKs; however, psoriatic plaques are usually large and distributed on extensor surfaces in younger patients.
- Mechanical trauma—Superficial skin injuries such as healing erosions and lacerations may resemble AKs depending on the timing of presence. Clinical history usually reveals the inciting trauma, and superficial skin injuries heal while AKs remain present over time.
- Melanoma—Pigmented actinic keratoses can sometimes be difficult to distinguish from the pigment associated with melanoma. Lesions suspicious for melanoma must be biopsied.

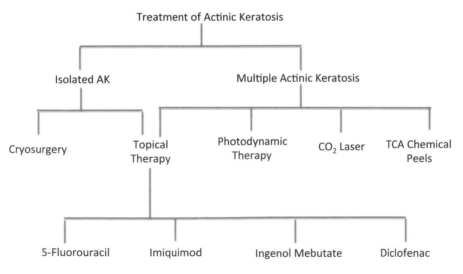

Fig. 2.8 Treatments for actinic keratoses

Management and Treatment of Actinic Keratosis

Management strategies for AKs are broad and varied, but the most common include local destruction by cryotherapy/cryosurgery or other methods, topical agents including topical chemotherapies, photodynamic therapy (PDT), chemical peels, and laser therapy (Fig. 2.8).

Cryotherapy/Cryosurgery

Cryosurgery is the application of liquid nitrogen to the skin resulting in local tissue destruction [12]. Cryosurgery causes injury by forming ice crystals within cells, leading to vascular thrombosis during freezing and vascular stasis after thawing; ischemic necrosis and failure of local microcirculation are the end results of these changes in the vasculature [12, 13].

The freeze time, or length of time for cooling, is brief for benign lesions when compared to malignancy, and 5–7 s of the "open-spray" technique is sufficient for elimination of an actinic keratosis [14]. The "open-spray" technique involves a fine spray of liquid nitrogen from a unit with spray tip attachments at a distance of 1–2 cm at a 90° angle from the lesion [12, 13]. One freeze-thaw cycle with freezing time of less than 60 s at a tissue temperature of −10° Celsius yields a 98.8% cure rate of actinic keratosis [12]. Cryosurgery side effects include pain, blistering, skin discoloration, and scar. Cryosurgery sites heal by second intention over 1–2 weeks following treatment.

Topical Therapy

"Field therapy" involves treating large areas of the skin and is frequently used when multiple lesions suspicious for AK are present across a large surface area [14]. Topical modalities include fluorouracil, imiquimod, diclofenac, and ingenol mebutate. Before initiating topical chemotherapy for AK, lesions suspicious for NMSC should be biopsied.

Topical 5-fluorouracil (Efudex, Carac, Fluoroplex, Adrucil), or 5-FU, is an antineoplastic thymidylate synthase inhibitor that interferes with DNA and RNA synthesis by blocking the synthesis of pyrimidine thymidine, a nucleoside required for DNA replication [15]. The frequency and duration of treatment depend on how well the patient tolerates the medication's side effects and the location treated. Concentrations of 5-FU range from 0.05% to 1–5%, and duration of treatment depends on concentration used [2]. The treatment duration can range from 2 to 6 weeks depending upon clinical response [2]. Treatment yields an erythematous reaction and is discontinued when a "peak response" occurs, demonstrated by reepithelialization and crust formation [2]. Healing usually occurs over the next few weeks. A low potency topical steroid or white petrolatum can be applied to facilitate healing. 5-FU is contraindicated in pregnant women. Dihydropyrimidine dehydrogenase (DPD), the enzyme required for 5-FU metabolism, is absent in 5% of the population and impaired in 3%–5% of the population. Patients with a partial or deficient DPD activity will not metabolize 5-FU leading to systemic symptoms of malaise, diarrhea, mouth sores, and anemia.

Topical 5-FU can be applied under occlusion with an Unna boot to treat lower extremity AKs in high-risk populations [16]. Ritchie and colleagues recommend using 20 grams of 5-FU per leg, followed by an Unna boot, kerlix, and coban. The "chemowrap" is applied in a physician office and removed 5–7 days later [16]. Patients usually tolerate one leg at a time rather than both, and the process can be repeated for 4–6 weeks [16]. Debridement may be necessary prior to subsequent applications, and any remaining lesions after 3 months warrant biopsy [16].

Imiquimod (Aldara or Zyclara) is a toll-like receptor 7 agonist that activates both the innate and acquired immune responses for AK treatment [7, 17]. Varying protocols exist for imiquimod topical application depending upon the medicine concentration [18]. Recent studies by Stockfleth et al. have described a new standard for AK management that includes daily use of 3.75% imiquimod (Zyclara) cream for two 2-week cycles, applied at bedtime, separated by a 2-week interval without treatment [17, 18]. This treatment protocol was thought to result in a 92% median percentage reduction in AK lesions [17, 18]. Imiquimod 5% (Aldara) can be used twice a week at bedtime for 16 weeks. Small studies have shown efficacy and safety in immunocompromised patients. Solid organ transplant recipients tolerated the medication when applied to areas with less than 100 cm^2 surface area [19].

Diclofenac, a nonsteroidal anti-inflammatory drug, can be used twice daily for 60–90 days to treat AK as a 3% topical gel mixed with 2.5% hyaluronate sodium (Solaraze). The treatment is well tolerated but less efficacious than aforementioned methods [20]. Common side effects include itching, contact dermatitis, and xerosis [20].

Ingenol mebutate (Picato) is a macrocyclic diterpene ester that comes from the sap of the *Euphorbia peplus* plant. Picato works by activating protein kinase C and neutrophils in the oxidative burst pathway and by initiating keratinocyte cell death. Two strengths are available: 0.015% for the face and scalp and 0.05% for the trunk and extremities [2, 20].

Topical retinoids (tretinoin, adapalene, and tazarotene) are used off label for the treatment of AK. Retinoids can normalize abnormal keratinocyte growth and maturation. Tretinoin can be tolerated for prolonged periods with varying concentrations. Topical retinoids are not as effective in AK treatment as other FDA-approved topical therapies. Importantly, topical retinoids do not prevent the development of NMSC [2, 20].

Photodynamic Therapy

Photodynamic therapy involves using the combination of a photosensitizer, a light source within the spectrum of the photosensitizer, and molecular oxygen to destroy a target tissue when stimulated [21]. The photosensitizer approved for actinic keratosis in the United States is 20% 5-aminolevulinic acid (ALA, Levulan), an intermediate naturally formed in cells during porphyrin synthesis. 5-ALA penetrates the stratum corneum to be absorbed by cancerous cells [21]. The "kerastick," a dermatologic applicator containing a 20% weight/volume ALA solution with 48% ethanol, is used to apply the solution, which incubates on the skin for a selected period of time. After incubation, the patient is exposed to a blue light (Blu-U) for 16 min and 40 s [21]. Side effects include pain, stinging sensation, erythema, and peeling. Handheld fans can be used to minimize patient discomfort. The treatment can be stopped if the patient cannot tolerate side effects. Strict photoprotection is needed for 48 h following treatment due to increased photosensitivity. A second treatment can be repeated in 8 weeks. Many patients prefer PDT due to the short treatments and minimal side effects. PDT is effective in treating AKs and may have sustained benefits with 69% of AKs remaining clear 4 years after treatment and only a 9% recurrence rate in one study [21].

Chemical Peels

Trichloroacetic acid (TCA) chemical peel is an effective field treatment of AKs. Trichloroacetic acid coagulates proteins in the skin, thereby serving as a chemical cauterant in a safe manner that is associated with limited morbidity [22]. Low concentration peels (<35%) applied to the face have been associated with increased efficacy similar to that of topical chemotherapies, and other peels have been used with various depths of penetration [22]. This treatment modality can peel the whole skin surface evenly, resulting in faster healing time, less pain, and a better cosmetic result; however, it can be difficult to assess the depth of destruction, and peeling too deeply can result in scarring [23].

Laser Therapy

Laser resurfacing involves concentrated beams of light that remove skin layer by layer [23]. High-energy short-pulsed lasers (CO2, Er:YAG) can be used in the treatment of actinic keratoses [22]. These lasers were originally used for cosmetic treatment of wrinkles, but improvement in photodamage and fewer precancerous and malignant lesions in treated areas were noted [23]. Iyer and colleagues conducted a retrospective study of patients with widespread AKs who were treated with full facial CO2 and/or Er:YAG laser therapy, finding that approximately 88% of patients were lesion-free 1 year after treatment [23]. The side effects include pain, swelling, infection, pigment changes, and permanent scarring.

Prognosis and Prophylaxis

AKs generally have a good prognosis; although they can progress to squamous cell carcinoma, the rate of transformation is low and AKs can resolve on their own. One study found that 55% of AKs followed clinically were not present at 1-year follow-up, and 70% were not present at 5-year follow-up [24]. This study referred to individual AKs; other studies have revealed regression rates for individual lesions between 20% and 30% and spontaneous regression of complete fields of AKs to be only 0–7% [11]. Reliable data regarding progression of AK to SCC is relatively scarce, and the actual risk of progression of a single AK lesion to invasive SCC is unclear. Multiple sources have found progression rates that range from 0% to 0.6% per AK lesion per year, demonstrating that while the risk of a single lesion over a short time frame may be less serious, the risk of innumerable lesions over time may be significant [11].

Certain characteristics of AKs that portend a poor prognosis and higher rate of transformation into SCC include bleeding, erythema, enlarging diameter, induration, and ulceration [25]. Although additional research is needed to better determine the degree to which these qualities are associated with higher progression rates to SCC, these findings can be helpful for guiding physicians and patients to more closely monitor certain lesions.

Because the pathogenesis of AKs involves UV damage to the skin, sun exposure is the most significant risk factor for development of AK. Other sources of UV exposure, including tanning beds, also contribute to skin damage and the subsequent development of AKs, melanoma, and nonmelanoma skin cancers [26]. Patients with fair skin, a compromised immune system, a family history of skin cancers, or predisposing genetic conditions (e.g., basal cell nevus syndrome, xeroderma pigmentosum, oculocutaneous albinism, etc.) are especially at risk for the development of AKs and other skin cancers [27]. Proper skin care, self skin exams, and regular visits to a dermatologist for screening exams are essential to the management of these patients who are at an increased risk.

The most important and effective prophylaxis measure is protection of the skin from the sun's harmful rays. There are three components to proper sun protection:

1. Avoiding sunlight during peak UVB hours (10:00 am–2:00 pm)
2. Wearing a photoprotective outfit: long sleeved clothing, wide brimmed hat, and sunglasses
3. Use of broad-spectrum sunscreen with SPF $\geq$ 30 [11]
4. Reapplication of sunscreen every 2–3 h, after swimming or sweating

The daily application of broad-spectrum sunscreen has been shown to reduce the incidence of new AKs and to reduce the overall AK lesion count in patients [11]. There have been multiple publications showing these reductions [28–30]. In one of these randomized control trials, the overall AK lesion count decreased by 24% over a 2-year time frame in patients randomized to use daily sunscreen [29]. Reducing the incidence and number of AKs also implicates reduction in the risk of developing skin cancers that arise from AKs in the long term [30].

References

1. Rosen T, Lebwohl MG. Prevalence and awareness of actinic keratosis: barriers and opportunities. J Am Acad Dermatol. 2013;68(1):S2–9.
2. James WD, Elston DM, Berger TG, Elston DM. Epidermal nevi, neoplasms, and cysts. In: James WD, Berger TG, Elston DM, editors. Andrews' diseases of the skin. 12th ed. Philadelphia: Elsevier; 2016.
3. Chen GJ, Feldman SR, Williford PM, Hester EJ, Kiang S-H, Gill I, et al. Clinical diagnosis of actinic keratosis identifies an elderly population at high risk of developing skin cancer. Dermatol Surg. 2005;31(1):43–7.
4. Dodson JM. Malignant potential of actinic keratoses and the controversy over treatment. A patient-oriented perspective. AMA Dermatol. 1991;127(7):1029–31.
5. Roewert-Huber J, Stockfleth E, Kerl H. Pathology and pathobiology of actinic (solar) keratosis - an update. Br J Dermatol. 2007;157(s2):18–20.
6. Nair PA, Chaudhary AH, Mehta MJ. Actinic keratosis underlying cutaneous horn at an unusual site— a case report. E Cancer Med Sci. 2013;7:376.
7. Soyer HP, Rigel DS, Wurm EMT. Actinic keratosis, basal cell carcinoma and squamous cell carcinoma. In: Bolognia J, Jorizzo JL, Schaffer JV, editors. Dermatology. 3rd ed. Philadelphia: Elsevier; 2012.
8. Zalaudek I, Ferrara G, Leinweber B, Mercogliano A, D'Ambrosio A, Argenziano G. Pitfalls in the clinical and dermoscopic diagnosis of pigmented actinic keratosis. J Am Acad Dermatol. 2005 Dec;53(6):1071–4.
9. Bagazgoitia L, Cuevas J, Expression JA. Of p53 and p16 in actinic keratosis, bowenoid actinic keratosis and Bowen's disease. J Eur Acad Dermatol Venereol. 2005;24(2):228–30.
10. Rowert-Huber J, Patel MJ, Forschner T, Ulrich C, Eberle J, Kerl H, et al. Actinic keratosis is an early in situ squamous cell carcinoma: a proposal for reclassification. Br J Dermatol. 2007;156(3):8–12.
11. Werner RN, Stockfleth E, Connolly SM, Correia O, Erdmann R, Foley P, et al. Evidence- and consensus-based (S3) guidelines for the treatment of actinic keratosis - international league of dermatological societies in cooperation with the European dermatology forum - short version. J Eur Acad Dermatol Venereol. 2015;29(11):2069–79.
12. Trost LB, Bailin PL. Cryosurgery. In: Vidimos AT, Ammirati CT, Poblete-Lopez C, editors. Dermatologic surgery. Philadelphia: Elsevier; 2009.
13. Kuflik EG, Kuflik JH. Cryosurgery. In: Bolognia JL, Jorizzo JL, Schaffer JV, editors. Dermatology. 3rd ed. Philadelphia: Elsevier; 2012.
14. Pomerantz H, Hogan D, Eilers D. Long-term efficacy of topical fluorouracil cream, 5%, for treating actinic keratosis. JAMA Dermatol. 2015;151(9):952–60.
15. Askew DA, Mickan SM, Soyer HP, Wilkinson D. Effectiveness of 5-fluorouracil treatment for actinic keratosis – a systemic review of randomized controlled trials. Int J Dermatol. 2009;48(5):453–63.

16. Ritchie SA, Patel MJ, Miller SJ. Therapeutic options to decrease actinic keratosis and squamous cell carcinoma incidence and progression in solid organ transplant recipients: a practical approach. Dermatol Surg. 2012 May;38(10):1604–21.
17. Hanna E, Abadi R, Abbas O. Imiquimod in dermatology: an overview. Int J Dermatol. 2016;55(8):831–44.
18. Stockfleth E. Lmax and imiquimod 3.75%: the new standard in AK management. J Eur Acad Dermatol Venereol. 2015;29(Supp.1):9–14.
19. Ulrich C, Bichel J, Euvrard S, Guidi B, Proby CM, et al. Topical immunomodulation under systemic immunosuppression: results of a multicentre, randomized, placebo-controlled safety and efficacy study of imiquimod 5% cream for the treatment of actinic keratosis in kidney, heart, and liver transplant patients. Br J Dermatol. 2007;157(Suppl 2):25–31.
20. Jenkins SN, Speck K, Actinic CSC. Keratosis and bowen's disease. In: Bigby M, Herxheimer A, editors. Evidence based dermatology. 3rd ed. Chichester, England: Wiley-Blackwell; 2014.
21. Gold MH. Lasers, photodynamic therapy, and the treatment of medical dermatological conditions. In: Goldberg DJ, editor. Laser dermatology. New York: Springer Publishing; 2005.
22. Hantash BM, Stewart DB, Cooper ZA. Facial resurfacing for nonmelanoma skin cancer prophylaxis. Arch Dermatol. 2006;142(8):976–82.
23. Iyer SS, Friedli A, Bowes L, Kricorian G. Full face laser resurfacing: therapy and prophylaxis for actinic keratosis and non-melanoma skin cancer. Lasers Surg Med. 2004;34(2):114–9.
24. Criscione VD, Weinstock MA, Naylor MF, Luque C, Eide MJ, Bingham SF, Department of Veterans Affairs Topical Tretinoin Chemoprevention Trial Group. Natural history and risk of malignant transformation in the veterans affairs topical Tretinoin chemoprevention trial. Cancer. 2009;115(11):2523–30.
25. Quaedvlieg PJ, Tirsi E, Thissen MR, Krekels GA. Actinic keratosis: how to differentiate the good from the bad ones? Eur J Dermatol. 2006;16(4):335–9.
26. Madigan LM, Lim HW. Tanning beds: impact on health, and recent regulations. Clin Dermatol. 2016;34(5):640–8.
27. Nikolaou V, Stratigos AJ, Tsao H. Hereditary nonmelanoma skin cancer. Semin Cutan Med Surg. 2012;31(4):204–10.
28. Naylor MF, Boyd A, Smith DW, Cameron GS, Hubbard D, Neldner KH. High sun protection factor sunscreens in the suppression of actinic neoplasia. Arch Dermatol. 1995;131(2):170–5.
29. Darlington S, Williams G, Neale R, Frost C, Green A. A randomized controlled trial to assess sunscreen application and beta carotene supplementation in the prevention of solar keratoses. Arch Dermatol. 2003;139(4):451–5.
30. Thompson SC, Jolley D, Marks R. Reduction of solar keratoses by regular sunscreen use. N Engl J Med. 1993;329(16):1147–51.

Chapter 3
Basal Cell Carcinoma

Shauna Higgins, Maggie Chow, and Ashley Wysong

Abstract Basal cell carcinoma (BCC) is the most common cancer in the United States. BCC is categorized by its clinical appearance and histology. The tumor subtype, anatomical location and patient's health are factored into the treatment choice. Multiple treatment options exist with varying efficacy. Post-treatment, patient monitoring is important for possible recurrence and for the development of new skin cancers.

Keywords Basal cell carcinoma · Nonmelanoma skin cancer · Nodular BCC · Superficial BCC · Morpheaform BCC · Cystic BCC · Basosquamous · Micronodular BCC · Infiltrative BCC · Pigmented BCC · Adenoid BCC · Radiation · Mohs micrographic surgery · Cryosurgery · Laser therapy · Photodynamic therapy · Chemotherapy · Retinoids · Interferon

Introduction

Basal cell carcinoma (BCC) is the most common cancer in the United States, constituting 25% of all cancers, which translates to over 2,000,000 cases diagnosed annually [1]. Although BCCs rarely metastasize, they can be locally destructive and highly morbid and therefore require conscientious work-up and management [2]. There are a number of clinical and histologic BCC variants with disparate clinical behavior. Thus, a complete knowledge of the BCC subtypes and treatment options is crucial to appropriate management. BCC subtypes can be described via clinical appearance, histologic appearance, or a combination of the two. Treatment options

S. Higgins · M. Chow · A. Wysong (✉)
Department of Dermatology, University of Southern California, Los Angeles, CA, USA
e-mail: awysong@usc.edu

are multitudinous, although the appropriate treatment is dependent upon the BCC subtype. The treatment modality most often utilized in BCC is electrodessication and curettage (ED&C), although high-risk subtypes may warrant therapies such as Mohs micrographic surgery (MMS). As treatment of BCC is under active research, there are also a number of additional therapies utilized with increasing amounts of data supporting their use.

Risk Factors

The development of BCC is the result of a dynamic interplay between genetic, clinical, and environmental risk factors (Table 3.1). Genetic risk factors include single nucleotide polymorphisms (SNPs) and sporadic mutations. Mutations in tumor suppressors such as protein patched homolog 1 (PTCH1) and tumor protein p53 (TP53) have also been associated with the development of BCC and BCC-associated syndromes [1]. Clinical factors that predispose individuals to developing BCCs include increased age, male sex, fair skin type, low ability to tan, childhood sunburns, signs of actinic damage, systemic immunosuppression, and personal or family history of skin cancer. Recent reports have also suggested an inverse relationship between BMI and early-onset BCC (under age 40) [3]. Some authors have hypothesized that estrogen exerts a potentially protective effect in obese individuals [3].

Human papillomaviruses (HPV) is another clinical factor reported to play a role in early-onset BCC [1, 3]. Several observational studies have reported a significant positive association between HPV DNA or seropositivity and BCC, though most case-control studies have failed to demonstrate a clear association [1]. Environmental risk factors include indoor tanning, history of PUVA/UVB therapy, and intense intermittent ultraviolet radiation (UVR) with UVB (290–320 nm) radiation playing the primary role in BCC development [1]. Cumulative exposure is believed to confer higher risk for BCC development when compared to short bursts of intense UVB exposure. However, the risk of BCC development derived from intermittent exposure remains significant [4]. UV exposure exerts its carcinogenic effects by inducing mutations in tumor suppressor genes and by predisposing individuals to tumor development by creating an immune-tolerant state in the skin [4].

Additional risk factors for the development of BCC include exposure to ionizing radiation, arsenic exposure, and iatrogenic immunosuppression after solid organ transplant. Ionizing doses as low as 450 rads have been associated with BCC development. The latency period for tumor development is long, and no clinical evidence of radiation damage is required. In the case of arsenic exposure, BCCs typically present on the trunk. Sources of arsenic include well water, pesticides (i.e., Paris green), medications (Fowler's solution, herbal remedies), and industry (min-

Table 3.1 BCC causes and associations [1, 6–11]

Sun exposure	Primarily UVB, 290–320 nm
Gene mutations	P53, PTCH1, PTCH2, BAP1, SUFU, CYLD
Exposure to artificial UV light	Tanning booths, UV light therapy, PUVA
Ionizing radiation exposure	Radiation therapy
Arsenic exposure	Fowler's solution of potassium and contaminated water source are most common sources of arsenic ingestion
Immunosuppression	Transplant recipients
Xeroderma pigmentosum	Inability to repair UV-induced DNA damage
Personal and family history of previous nonmelanoma skin cancer (NMSC)	The risk of developing new NMSC is 35% at 3 years and 50% at 5 years after an initial skin cancer diagnosis. Individuals with a first-degree relative diagnosed with skin cancer prior to age 50 are suggested to be at highest risk for BCC (OR 4.79, 95% CI 2.90–7.90).
Skin type	Skin types 1 and 2 are especially susceptible

Table 3.2 BCC genetic syndromes [5]

Syndrome	Associations
Nevoid basal cell carcinoma syndrome	PTCH or SUFU gene mutation Medulloblastomas, meningioma, fetal rhabdomyosarcoma, and ameloblastoma
Bazex syndrome	Atrophoderma ("ice pick marks," especially on dorsal hands), multiple basal cell carcinomas, and local anhidrosis (decreased or absent sweating)
Rombo syndrome	Vermiculate atrophoderma, milia, hypertrichosis, trichoepitheliomas, BCCs, and peripheral vasodilation
Brooke-Spiegler syndrome	CYLD mutation Multiple trichoepitheliomas, cylindromas, spiradenomas, and variably, multiple BCCs

ing, smelting, sheep dippings to control lice, and blowfly infestation). In regard to iatrogenic immunosuppression after solid organ transplantation, there is a significantly increased risk for SCC development and a modestly increased risk for BCC development. These patients typically develop BCCs on the trunk and arms at a rate of tenfold that of their immunocompetent counterparts [5].

There are also several genetic syndromes that have been associated with the development of numerous BCCs (Table 3.2). These syndromes include nevoid basal cell carcinoma syndrome (NBCCS, also known as Gorlin syndrome), Bazex syndrome, Rombo syndrome, and Brooke-Spiegler syndrome. NBCCS is an autosomal dominant disorder that predisposes individuals to as many as hundreds of BCCs. Additional clinical features include a broad nasal root, frontal bossing, borderline intelligence, jaw cysts, palmar pits, and multiple skeletal abnormalities. Bazex syndrome is an X-linked dominant disorder manifesting as multiple BCCs, follicular atrophoderma, dilated follicular ostia with ice pick scars, hypotrichosis, and hypohidrosis. Rombo syndrome is an autosomal dominant disorder that presents with vermiculate atrophoderma, milia, hypertrichosis, trichoepitheliomas, BCCs, and peripheral vasodilation [3]. Brooke-Spiegler syndrome is characterized by multiple trichoepitheliomas, cylindromas, spiradenomas and, variably, multiple BCCs [10].

Clinical Presentation

Consistent with its association with UV exposure, BCC traditionally presents in older individuals with high levels of cumulative sun exposure and is predominantly found on photo-exposed parts of the body. However, the incidence of BCCs in young individuals is rising. This may be due at least in part to increases in natural and artificial tanning behaviors [12].

BCCs are primarily found on the head, with these constituting 70% of all BCCs. The main area of involvement on the head is the face, with 30% appearing on the nose. After the head, the next most common sites for BCCs include the trunk and extremities [1, 3, 4]. The association between tumor incidence and UV exposure is not as consistent in BCC as in squamous cell carcinoma (SCC) as BCCs can also more rarely present in photo-protected areas such as the dorsal foot, nipple-areola complex, vulva, penis and scrotum, umbilicus, and mucosal lip [13–20].

BCCs classically present as pearly papules with colors ranging from white to skin-colored to brown or black [21] (Fig. 3.1). They can be flat, slightly raised, or circumscribed nodular lesions with visible and irregular blood vessels. They may develop ulceration as tumors outgrow their blood supply and become locally destructive or may have subtle central depressions in certain subtypes. They are typically slow-growing tumors with a propensity for local invasion rather than metastasis [2]. When neglected or misdiagnosed, however, there is increased potential for local tissue destruction and metastasis [22]. BCCs metastasize at a rate of 0.00285–0.55%, most commonly to the lymph nodes, lungs, bones, or skin [2, 23].

At presentation, patients may complain of a non-healing lesion that bleeds, oozes, or crusts [24]. They may present with a lesion that appears scar-like without prior trauma [25, 26]. BCC should generally be considered in the differential diagnosis of any non-healing lesion of greater than 3–4-week duration on sun-exposed skin. Additional variations in clinical presentation are dependent upon the specific BCC subtype, which will be described below [5].

Fig. 3.1 Basal cell
carcinoma. A well-defined,
pink to yellowish papule
with telangiectasias

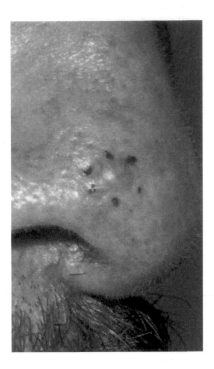

Nodular BCC

Nodular BCC, also known as the noduloulcerative variant or the "rodent ulcer," comprises half of all BCCs (Fig. 3.2). It can present as a circumscribed nodule with central ulceration and a raised, pearly border with telangiectasia. Melanin pigment may be present in variable amounts: flecks of brown may be present or the entire lesion may be black or blue-black (Fig. 3.3). Common dermoscopic features include irregular or arborizing vascularity, focal ulceration, and translucency [27]. If untreated, these tumors grow to be very large in size and can extend deeply, causing local destruction of tissue. This propensity for local destruction has led to the nickname "rodent ulcer," as the lesion is said to resemble tissue gnawed by a rat.

Histologically, nodular BCCs have several variants that include solid, keratotic (pilar), cystic, and adenoid subtypes [5]. Many also demonstrate unique secondary features. One such feature is squamous differentiation, which correlates with more aggressive behavior. Sclerosis of the stroma may also be found in recurrent lesions, which makes them particularly difficult to treat [5]. A rare subtype of nodular BCC with amyloid deposition has also been reported, with amyloid bodies appearing as whitish globules on dermoscopy (Fig. 3.4) [27].

Fig. 3.2 Nodular basal cell carcinoma. A well-defined, pink pearly papule with telangiectasias and central ulceration consistent with a "rodent ulcer"

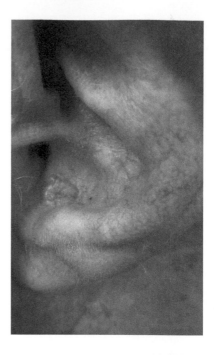

Fig. 3.3 Pigmented basal cell carcinoma. A well-defined, violaceous plaque with central pigmentation

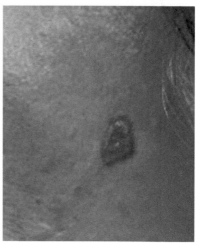

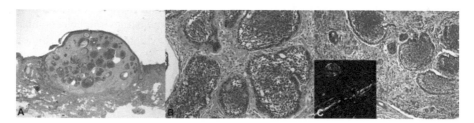

Fig. 3.4 Histopathologic features of nodular BCC. (**a**) Large clusters of basaloid cells. (**b**) Tumor nodules of basaloid cells with peripheral palisading. (**c**) Reddish deposits of amyloid in the stroma between tumor cells and center of tumor nodules, which demonstrate apple green birefringence under polarized light [27] (With permission: Park et al. [27], courtesy of Elsevier)

Fig. 3.5 Superficial basal cell carcinoma: An ill-defined, pink scaling patch with a crusted papule at the medial border

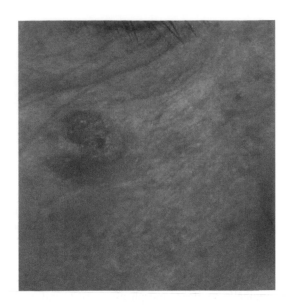

Superficial BCC

Superficial or multicentric BCCs are more frequently found on the trunk and extremities but can also be found on the head and neck (Fig. 3.5). Their size can range from a few millimeters to several centimeters. They are typically flat pink or red lesions with scale. They may have a small, translucent elevated border. There may be areas of spontaneous regression characterized by atrophy and hypopigmentation. There may also be variable amounts of pigment.

Dermoscopic features of nonpigmented superficial BCCs include a scattered vascular pattern, arborizing microvessels, telangiectatic or atypical vessels, milky-pink background, multiple small erosions, and shiny white or red structureless areas [28]. In pigmented superficial BCCs, dermoscopy reveals maple leaf-like areas, wheel-like structures, and multiple small blue-gray dots or globules (Fig. 3.6) [28, 29].

Initially, the growth pattern of superficial BCCs is primarily horizontal. With time, these tumors can become deeply invasive with induration, ulceration, and nodule formation. Extensive subclinical lateral spread accounts for the high recurrence rates after routine excision [5].

Morpheaform BCC

Morpheaform BCC acquired its name from its clinical resemblance to morphea [31]. Typically, these lesions are indurated, ivory in color, with occasional overlying telangiectasia. The clinical presentation can be subtle, often leading to a delay in

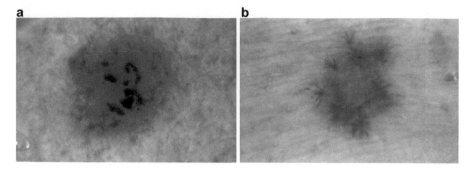

Fig. 3.6 Dermoscopic features of superficial BCC. (**a**) Dermoscopy of a black and brown-colored patch on lateral neck demonstrating typical maple leaf-like areas. (**b**) Dermoscopy of an erythematous and brown-colored patch of the anterior chest demonstrating typical spoke wheel areas [30] (Source: Copyright © 2011 Akiko Hirofuji et al. via Creative Commons Attribution License)

diagnosis. Of note, metastatic carcinoma to the skin can appear clinically and histologically similar to morpheaform BCC and, thus, should always be in the differential when considering a diagnosis of morpheaform BCC. This subtype is also characterized by extensive subclinical spread; the potential for invasion of the muscle, nerve, and bone; and a high rate of recurrence after treatment [5].

Cystic BCC

Cystic BCC may often appear clinically similar to nodular BCC. Histologically, however, these tumors possess cystic changes as the name implies. Clinically, they may have a blue-gray cystic appearance and can exude a clear fluid if punctured or cut. In the periorbital area, they may be confused with hidrocystomas (Fig. 3.7) [5].

Basosquamous BCC

BCC with squamous metaplasia is also called basosquamous (BSC) or metatypical carcinoma. Histologically, these tumors are characterized by areas of BCC and areas of SCC, sometimes with a transition zone in between [33]. The presence of stroma helps distinguish these lesions from SCC, which is not associated with stromal proliferation [5].

BSC was considered a primarily histologic variant until recent reports of distinct clinical findings [5]. In 36 histopathologically proven basosquamous BCCs, Akay et al. reported distinct dermoscopic features [34]. These included keratin mass (97.7% of the 36 BSCs), surface scaling (77.8%), ulceration (69.4%), white structureless areas (69.4%), white clods (66.7%), blood spots on keratin mass (66.7%),

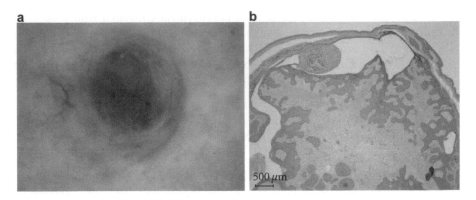

Fig. 3.7 Cystic BCC. (**a**) Dermatoscopic examination demonstrating a homogenous blue/black area and arborizing telangiectasia. (**b**) Histology demonstrates tumor mass predominantly in the dermis with continuation from the epidermis in some parts. The tumor contains cystic spaces [32] (Source: Copyright © 2011 Akihiro Yoneta et al. via Creative Commons Attribution License)

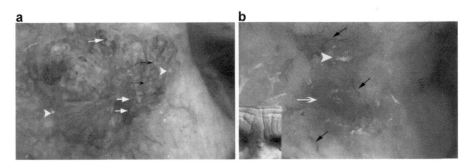

Fig. 3.8 Unique clinical features of basosquamous carcinoma. (**a**) This BCC-dominant BSC demonstrates white circles (white arrows), white clods (arrowhead), and four dots in a square (black arrow). (**b**) Focused serpentine vessel and out-of-focus straight vessels (black arrows), keratin (white arrow), and superficial squamatization (white arrowhead) [34] (With permission: Akay et al. [34], Figs. 1H and 2C, courtesy of John Wiley and Sons)

and polymorphous vascular patterns consisting of varied combinations of branched, serpentine, straight, coiled, or looped vessels (61%) (Fig. 3.8) [34].

Though BSC comprises only 1–2.3% of all NMSC, they are more aggressive and destructive relative to other BCC subtypes. They are more likely to metastasize and are more likely to recur after treatment [5]. The local recurrence rate of BSC is reported to be as high as 45% after wide local excision, which is almost double that seen in BCC and SCC alone [35]. Factors predictive of recurrence include male gender, positive surgical resection margins, lymphatic invasion, and perineural invasion [35]. The most common pattern of recurrence is local recurrence only, followed by local recurrence plus regional lymph node metastasis [35]. The use of Mohs micrographic surgery (MMS) has been reported to reduce recurrence rates to 4–9%

[35]. Although this recurrence rate is an improvement compared with wide local excision, it remains elevated relative to recurrence rates reported for BCC (0.64%) and SCC (1.2%) after MMS [35]. The estimated BSC metastatic rate has been reported to be as high as 9.7%, compared with less than 0.1% for other BCCs although this increases to approximately 2% in BCCs larger than 3 cm [5, 36].

Infiltrative and Micronodular BCCs

In 1951, Thackray coined the term "infiltrative" to distinguish a histologic subtype that he believed was more difficult to eradicate than nodular BCC [37]. Infiltrative and micronodular tumors are associated with an aggressive growth pattern and are reported to have wider and deeper tumor extensions when compared to nodular BCC. Thus, they are more likely (26.5%) to have positive tumor margins after simple surgical excision when compared to nodular BCC (6.4%) [37]. Mohs micrographic surgery is therefore the most appropriate treatment option for patients diagnosed with these tumors. Clinically, they appear as flat or slightly elevated plaques with ill-defined borders. If there is a sclerosing component (called sclerosing BCC), it may present as a firm plaque with some clinical features of morphea.

Pigmented BCC

Pigmented BCC is an uncommon variant most common in darker-skinned patients [38]. Clinically, it is commonly mistaken as melanoma due to its often dark and irregular pigmentation. A pearly, raised border with telangiectasia may help in distinguishing the tumor. Additional clinical features of the pigmented BCC include a firm consistency, translucence, and occasional surface ulceration [38]. Approximately 6.7–8.5% of all BCCs contain pigment [39].

Linear BCC is another rare BCC variant that can also appear pigmented. It primarily appears on the periocular skin and on the neck (37% and 34% of reported cases, respectively) [40]. Thirty-two percent of these possess aggressive histologic characteristics. They can be classified as having micronodular, infiltrative, or morpheaform histologic patterns. Mohs micrographic surgery is first-line therapy for these variants [39].

Giant BCC

Giant BCCs are defined as tumors greater than 5 cm. They have unique clinical and often psychosocial implications [41]. These BCCs comprise approximately 1% of all BCCs and often result from patient negligence [42]. They are most commonly

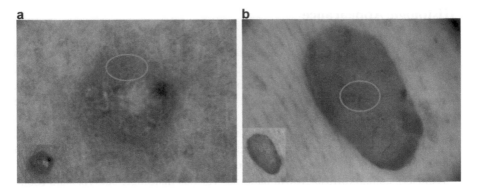

Fig. 3.9 Fibroepithelioma of Pinkus. (**a**) Dermatoscopic image of a fibroepithelioma of Pinkus demonstrating honeycomb white networks with variable-sized holes (gray circle). Larger-caliber vessels coursing parallel to the surface and short shiny white streaks are present in the central portion of the lesion. (**b**) Dermatoscopic image of a fibroepithelioma of Pinkus demonstrating a white network over a large area of the lesion (gray circle) accentuated by polymorphous vessels within the holes and semitranslucent area with arborizing vessels and thick short white streaks in the lower third area of the lesions [43] (With permission: Kornreich and Lee [40], Figs. 1 and 3, courtesy of Elsevier)

found in patients who live alone, are indifferent toward or lack concern for their disease, and suffer from alcoholism or other forms of addiction [41]. Patients with these lesions may exhibit significantly higher beta-endorphin and serotonin levels relative to patients with smaller (<5 cm) BCCs [41]. Histologically, adenoid, infiltrative, or morpheaform subtypes are common among giant BCCs. These BCCs are also more likely to metastasize, exhibit perineural invasion, ulcerate, and exhibit faster growth when compared to smaller, non-giant (<5 cm) BCCs [42].

Fibroepithelioma of Pinkus

Fibroepithelioma of Pinkus was first described by Herman Pinkus in 1953 as a premalignant neoplasm that may give rise to BCC [43]. These are most commonly found on the lumbosacral region. They often appear as solitary flesh-colored papules with occasional pigment, and they are often mistaken for a fibroma, dermal nevus, seborrheic keratosis, nevus lipomatosus superficialis, or an acrochordon [43, 44]. Dermatoscopic structures observed in fibroepithelioma of Pinkus include shiny white structures (*chrysalis* or *crystalline structures*), fine arborizing vessels, milia-like cysts, and ulceration (Fig. 3.9). Histologically, they are characterized by anastomosing strands of basaloid epithelial cells embedded within a fibrous stroma [43]. There has also been a case report of histology demonstrating a rare case of coexistence of fibroepithelioma of Pinkus and nodular BCC in a single lesion [45].

Histologic Appearance

The two major factors that influence histologic appearance are the cells from which the BCC originates and the stromal response to the epithelial growth [5]. BCCs occasionally show differentiation toward epithelial adnexal structures, although recent evidence suggests that the pattern of differentiation should be recognized primarily for the purpose of diagnosing BCC and creating a differential diagnosis [46]. The growth pattern is reported as the only proven histologic prognosticator of biologic behavior and is therefore more relevant to treatment planning [46]. The two main histologic umbrellas for BCC categorization include circumscribed and diffuse growth patterns. Various histologic subtypes are found under each category [5].

Circumscribed

Circumscribed BCCs clinically present as dome-shaped lesions with well-defined borders often corresponding with nodular or noduloulcerative subtypes. Histologically, these circumscribed tumors are often comprised of irregularly sized and shaped islands of basaloid cells bound by fibrovascular stroma. They comprise the vast majority of BCCs and include variants such as nodular, adenoid, keratinized, follicular, and pigmented BCCs in addition to the fibroepitheliomas of Pinkus [5].

Nodular BCCs

BCCs of the nodular or solid subtype are comprised of large aggregates of basal cells with no differentiation toward adnexal structures (Fig. 3.10) [46]. The cells at the periphery of the basaloid islands align in parallel. The base contacts the basement membrane, and the apex points inward toward the center of the island. This picket fence arrangement is referred to as palisading. The stroma often contains abundant mucin, especially adjacent to the island of epithelial cells. Because the glycosaminoglycans in the stroma are removed during tissue processing, the stroma pulls away from the island, producing artifactual clefts. These clefts appear so consistently that they have taken on diagnostic significance.

Large islands of epithelial cells may demonstrate central necrosis, leading to the formation of microcysts [5]. BCCs undergoing central necrosis thus develop characteristics of the cystic histologic subtype. These tumors are uncommon and consist of one or a few exceptionally large islands of basal cells with large central lacuna [5].

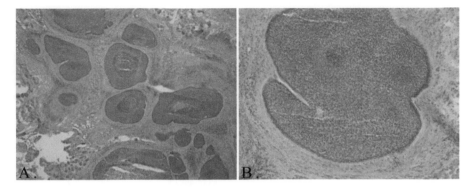

Fig. 3.10 Nodular basal cell carcinoma. (**a**) Note the symmetry and circumscription of the tumor. (H&E, original magnification ×4). (**b**) Tumor is composed primarily of large islands of uniform cells (H&E, original magnification ×10).

Adenoid BCCs

The adenoid subtype is a rare histopathological subtype with an incidence of approximately 1.3% [47]. It is characterized by interweaving cords and varying-sized islands of basal cells surrounded by mucinous stroma [47].The entrapment of stroma by anastomosing cords produces the appearance of gland-like structures. If these lesions demonstrate cystic changes, they are sometimes denoted as the adenoid cystic subtype [5]. However, some authors have advocated for avoiding the term adenoid cystic as it may be confused with adenoid cystic carcinoma, which is an entirely different entity [5]. Adenoid BCC is associated with low potential for recurrence or metastasis [48].

BCCs with Keratinization

Rarely, BCCs demonstrate the ability to cornify or create keratin, which usually occurs at the center of the basaloid islands (Fig. 3.11) [33]. The keratin may be orthokeratotic or parakeratotic. These lesions can be distinguished from trichoepithelioma by the absence of abortive hair papilla formation, the unusual presence of stromal retraction, and the predominance of the epithelial component over the stromal component [5].

Fig. 3.11 Cornifying basal cell carcinoma. There are central cystic structures containing masses of orthokeratin and a granular zone adjacent to the keratin. The structures resemble aberrant follicular units (H&E, ×10) [5] (With permission: Cockerell et al. [5], courtesy of Elsevier)

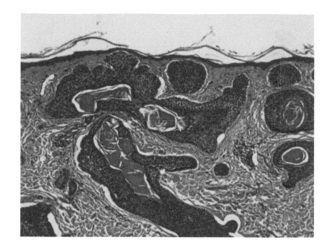

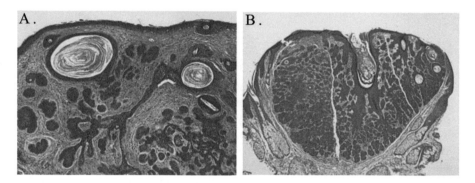

Fig. 3.12 Follicular basal cell carcinoma. (**a**) This tumor is typically, small, well-circumscribed, symmetric, and superficial. Many of the aggregates of basaloid cells resemble telogen follicles. Microcysts are present (H&E, ×40). (**b**) This lesion shows occasional small horn cysts and fissures in the stroma (H&E, ×80) [5] (With permission: Cockerell et al. [5], courtesy of Elsevier)

Follicular BCCs

Follicular BCCs (infundibulocystic BCC) usually appear on the face and are characterized histologically by small aggregates of basal cells containing microcysts and shadow cells adjacent to the islands of proliferating basaloid cells [46, 49]. The microcysts contain laminated orthokeratotic material and are often surrounded by squamoid metaplasia. Some basaloid islands may resemble hair follicles in telogen (Fig. 3.12). They are distinguished from trichoepithelioma in that the cell aggregates are usually continuous with the epidermis, the stroma comprises the minority of the tumor, there are no foreign body reactions to keratin, and hair papillae are not present [5].

Fibroepithelioma of Pinkus

The fibroepithelioma of Pinkus is composed of lace-like branches of basaloid cells that anastomose in an edematous-appearing fibrous stroma [50]. The strands of basal cells originate in the basal layer of the epidermis. More typical islands of basaloid cells with peripheral palisading may also be present [5].

Pigmented BCC

Melanin pigmentation can occur in all BCC types with the exception of the morpheaform type, and most pigmented BCCs are of the nodular type [5, 51]. In pigmented BCCs, there are nodular sheets of cells, peripheral palisading, an abundance of melanin, and increased mitotic activity (Fig. 3.12) [52]. The melanocytes are typically interspersed among the basal cells. There may also be numerous macrophages with melanin pigment in the stroma [5].

BCCs with Diffuse Growth Pattern

In contrast to circumscribed BCCs that present with generally well-defined borders, those with a diffuse growth pattern present as plaque-like or flat lesions that spread horizontally with poorly defined margins. As a result, these lesions tend to have a high recurrence rate. BCCs with diffuse growth pattern are classified into superficial, morpheaform, infiltrating, and micronodular subtypes [5].

Superficial BCC

Histologically, superficial BCCs appear as horizontally arranged lobules of atypical basal cells in the papillary dermis that have broad-based connections with the epidermis and demonstrate slit-like retraction of the palisaded basal cells [46]. A thin, fibrovascular stroma underlies the tumor nests [5]. All islands of basal cells contact the epidermis, and there is no downward extension (Fig. 3.13). Tumor cells may colonize the hair follicle and, rarely, the eccrine adnexal structures. Mitoses are infrequent and apoptotic cells are rare. A band-like lymphoid infiltrate is also characteristic [46].

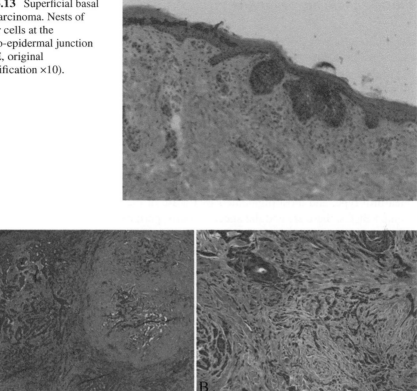

Fig. 3.13 Superficial basal cell carcinoma. Nests of tumor cells at the dermo-epidermal junction (H&E, original magnification ×10).

Fig. 3.14 Morpheaform basal cell carcinoma. (**a**) The epithelial component is made up of small, angulated nests, cords, and strands of basal cells. These are surrounded by a dense collagenous stroma. Inflammation is characteristically sparse or absent and palisading is not present. There is typically no connection of the tumor islands with the epidermis, although the lesion does have some epidermal connection (H&E, ×40). (**b**) Strands of hyperchromatic basal cells in the abundant fibrotic stroma. It resembles metastatic carcinoma of the breast (H&E, ×80) [5] (With permission: Cockerell et al. [5], courtesy of Elsevier)

Morpheaform BCC

Morpheaform BCCs are notoriously difficult to treat due to their extensions (averaging 7 mm) that make margin assessment by clinical inspection extremely difficult [26] . The dense fibrous stroma comprises the majority of the tumor and deems treatment with curettage inappropriate [5]. These tumors often show no connection with the epidermis, and the epithelial structures are completely effaced. Mucin is minimal to absent. Stromal retraction and palisading are usually absent, except in the case of occasional small islands (Fig. 3.14) [5].

Morpheaform BCCs must be distinguished histologically from syringoma, desmoplastic trichoepithelioma, and metastatic adenocarcinoma. Syringomas are characterized by small tubular epithelial structures embedded in a sclerotic stroma. Desmoplastic trichoepitheliomas possess microcysts containing keratin, which are not found in morpheaform BCCs. Metastatic adenocarcinoma is also on the histo-pathologic differential for morpheaform BCCs. Metastatic breast carcinoma is the most important histopathological mimic, as it can induce a scirrhous tissue reaction similar to that seen in morpheaform BCCs. In these cases, careful examination of the tissue may reveal areas of glandular differentiation in metastatic adenocarci-noma. Some metastatic adenocarcinoma will also show presence of carcinoembry-onic antigen (CEA) on staining by the immunoperoxidase method [5].

Infiltrating BCC

Infiltrating BCCs are particularly aggressive with a propensity for local tissue destruction [37]. This subtype lacks a central cohesive mass of basal cell islands. They are instead comprised of elongated islands and cords of widely spaced atypi-cal basal cells. The nests of tumor cells are often angulated and may be oriented perpendicular to the skin surface. Palisading may be present, but not well devel-oped. These tumors tend to exhibit both lateral and deep expansion [5].

Micronodular BCC

The micronodular subtype is characterized by small nests of basal cells (Fig. 3.15). The islands are typically the size of hair bulbs and palisading is often present. The island borders are often flat, indistinct, and poorly defined. These tumors have the

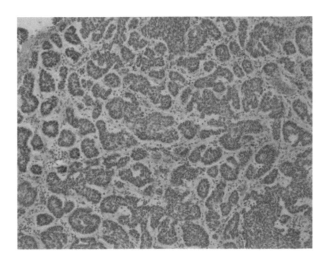

Fig. 3.15 Micronodular basal cell carcinoma. Small nests of basal cells located in skin dermis (H&E, original magnification ×10) [53]

ability to invade deeply. Nest cells at the deep aspect of the tumor can appear as cells lying free in tissue without surrounding stroma [5].

Diagnosis and Staging

Traditionally, BCCs are diagnosed clinically with or without the help of dermoscopy and confirmed with a shave, punch, or incisional biopsy. Histopathology of biopsy specimens can lead to the identification of additional risk factors for recurrence, which then guides further management. Recurrence risk factors identified by the National Comprehensive Cancer Network (NCCN) include:

- Diameter greater than 20 mm on the trunk and extremities
- Diameter greater than 10 mm on cheeks, forehead, scalp, or neck
- Diameter greater than 6 mm on genitalia, hands, feet, or face (except cheeks and forehead)
- Poorly defined borders
- Immunosuppression
- Area of prior radiation therapy
- Morpheaform, sclerosing, mixed infiltrative, or micronodular histologic features
- Perineural involvement

Additional high-risk features of the primary tumor may be identified via adjunctive imaging such as high-frequency ultrasound (HFUS) [54]. High-frequency sonography corresponds to a frequency of at least 20 MHz and can rapidly image and differentiate between the epidermal, dermal, and subcutaneous tissues [54]. The basic modes of ultrasound include the A-mode, B-mode, and Doppler method [55]. Tumor depth is ascertained in B-mode with a frequency of 20 MHz providing tissue penetration of approximately 6–7 mm [55]. The depth of evaluation is reported to have a 99% histopathologic correlation [54, 56]. Although most BCC lesions appear as well-defined, oval, echo-poor masses, lesions that may have higher aggressive potential may also appear as hyperechoic spots [54]. Three-dimensional Doppler flow technologies can also measure tumor neovascularity and map vascular structures and adjacent nerves [54]. Nodal basin lymphadenopathy and in-transit and nonpalpable locoregional metastases can be detected as well [54, 57]. Of note, the accuracy of ultrasonography is operator, site, and equipment dependent [54]. Transducer size is matched to the scan areas with three-dimensional imaging of ear and nose cartilage available with specialized probes [54]. An additional limitation includes the requirement of an acoustic window, which limits the depth of evaluation because of air or bone. Thus, sonography cannot reliably visualize retropharyngeal or nodes deeper in the head and neck, which may require computed tomography (CT) or magnetic resonance imaging (MRI) [57].

Radiographic imaging may be indicated for work-up and evaluation of high-risk tumors [58, 59]. Locally advanced tumors may be characterized by bony involvement, perineural invasion, or orbital infiltration with reports of penetration of the calvarium, dura, and, more rarely, the brain [58]. Clinical clues suggestive of orbital invasion include painful, fixed tumors involving the orbital rim or medial canthus, reduced range of motion of the extraocular muscles, or displacement of the globe [59]. Additional risk factors include infiltrative or sclerosing histology and multiple recurrent tumors in the periorbital area [59]. Computed tomography (CT) is the initial imaging for preoperative evaluation in the majority of periorbital and other head and neck tumors. MRI scans are generally more useful than CT in evaluation for subtle intracranial disease, central nervous system involvement, or perineural invasion [59]. PET/CT scans are ideal for the evaluation of distant metastases and potentially for postoperative surveillance although data in the context of BCC are sparse because metastatic disease is exceedingly rare [59, 60].

Surveillance After Initial Diagnosis

Patients with a single BCC have a 17-fold increased risk of subsequent BCC relative to the general population, a 3-fold increased risk of subsequent SCC, and a 2-fold increased risk of melanoma [1]. Thus, appropriate surveillance is imperative. Specific follow-up schedules depend on the number and severity of BCCs treated and the amount of background sun-damage present [5]. Although recurrent BCCs usually recur within the first 5 years after the initial tumor, they may also occur later.

Treatment

Few randomized controlled trials are available exploring optimal treatment strategies for BCC. The most current recommendations are periodically updated by a group of clinical experts as part of the NCCN. Based on NCCN guidelines, if the BCC has none of the above risk factors, treatment generally starts with standard excision or electrodessication and curettage (ED&C). If the BCC possesses one or more risk factors, treatment generally begins with Mohs surgery. Occasionally, excision is utilized if the only risk factor is a diameter greater than 20 mm on the trunk or extremities [5].

Electrodessication and Curettage (ED&C)

Electrodessication and curettage is the most commonly used modality for treating BCC [61]. When performed correctly on appropriate lesions, cure rates have been reported to be as high as 98% [5]. ED&C is most useful for well-defined, exophytic, nodular BCCs under 1 cm located in areas that are at low risk for recurrence. There is currently no standardization in regard to the number of cycles used. Some clinicians use a fixed number of cycles (generally three), while others continue ED&C until a healthy base is revealed.

Curettage is ineffective when the BCC is enmeshed in a sclerotic stroma and/or has an aggressive histologic growth pattern (i.e., recurrent, morpheaform, sclerosing, or micronodular BCC). It is also thought to be inappropriate when the BCC buds off or is concealed between pilosebaceous units (i.e., nose, scalp), is deeply invasive (i.e., perineural, deep dermis, subcutaneous fat, perichondrium, periosteum), or cannot be immobilized (i.e., lips, eyelids) [5].

In a review of 862 cases of BCC treated with ED&C, histopathological examination of curettage fragments with immunohistochemistry testing aided in predicting which patients were likely to experience recurrence [62]. Of the patients with no residual BCC seen in their curettage fragments, zero recurrences were noted. In those with residual BCC in the curettage fragments, 38% experienced recurrence [62].

Adverse side effects include occasional hypopigmentation, hypertrophic scarring (particularly in young adults and on the trunk and extremities), and notching and ectropion when performed near a free margin such as the eyelids or lips [5]. For improved cosmesis, the electrodessication component is occasionally omitted by some clinicians [5].

Surgical Excision

Surgical excision may be used for all types of BCCs in all locations. Benefits of this modality include histologic margin control, rapid healing, and optimal cosmetic result. However, the histologic margin control it offers in the context of recurrent BCC, morpheaform BCC, BCCs with an aggressive histology, and BCCs in high-risk areas is inferior to that achieved with Mohs micrographic surgery. The rate of positive margins after excision at one center was noted to be approximately 12.18% (49 of 402 tumors treated surgically) [63].

The recommended margins for excision are variable and range from 3–5 mm for small primary BCCs to 1.5–3 cm for recurrent BCCs [5, 64]. One study reports that a 3 mm surgical margin can safely be used for non-morpheaform BCC to achieve 95% cure rates for lesions 2 cm or smaller [65]. Another prospective study performed on 150 skin lesions excised over a 9-month period in an outpatient facility reported that a 4 mm surgical margin is optimal for skin lesions clinically diagnosed as basal cell or squamous cell carcinoma that are suitable for excision at an outpatient facility. Well-demarcated lesions, such as nodular basal cell carcinoma, may be excised with a 3 mm margin according to the same study [66]. Excision to the level of the fat is generally adequate for small primary BCCs. However, larger and more aggressive tumors may penetrate more deeply requiring larger excisions [5].

Of note, the number of lesions present on a patient should be considered in the decision to proceed with surgical excision. Patients with numerous BCCs may not be amenable to individual surgical excisions. In these cases, their BCCs may be more amenable to topical chemotherapy, cryosurgery, or curettage [5].

Mohs Micrographic Surgery

MMS allows for complete histologic margin evaluation, maximum tissue preservation, and complete cure for nearly any form of BCC. It is therefore the treatment of choice for any high-risk BCC [67]. As previously discussed, histologic high-risk BCCs include ill-defined, large, invasive, and/or recurrent lesions, those characterized by morpheaform or aggressive histologic features, and those with perineural spread [63]. MMS is also the treatment of choice for BCCs on high-risk areas, such as areas of previous irradiation, and in areas where tissue preservation is important [5]. Most elderly individuals can also tolerate both local anesthesia and the removal of large BCCs. Thus, the vast majority of patients are good surgical candidates.

Radiation Therapy

Radiation therapy (RT) is another option for the treatment of BCC. Currently available modalities include megavoltage electron beam RT, orthovoltage RT, electronic brachytherapy, and superficial/soft RT (Table 3.3) [68]. Megavoltage electron therapy is used by radiation oncologists in the hospital setting and consists of a concentrated stream of electrons generated by a linear accelerator [68]. The photon-emitting modalities vary with the kilovoltage and distance of the radiation source from the skin surface [68]. Orthovoltage RT is used to treat skin cancer in the 250 kV range. Electronic brachytherapy systems use a miniaturized X-ray tube to emit photon radiation between 2.5 and 6 cm from the skin's surface. Superficial radiation

Table 3.3 Comparison of common radiotherapy modalities used to treat nonmelanoma skin cancer [68]

Type	Synonyms	Type of generator	kV	Source to surface distance (cm)	Radiation emitted
Megavoltage electron therapy	Electron beam radiation	Linear accelerator	6000–9000 (6–9MV)	80	Electrons
Orthovoltage therapy	Deep X-ray	X-ray machine cathode	200–400	50–80	Photons
Contact therapy	Ultrashort distance X-ray	X-ray machine cathode	50–60	1.5–3.0	Photons
Electronic brachytherapy		Miniaturized X-ray cathode	50	2.5–6.0	Photons
Superficial X-ray therapy	Pyrex (glass) window (older units)	X-ray machine cathode	60–100	15–30	Photons
Soft X-ray therapy	Beryllium window (modern units)	X-ray machine cathode	20–100	10–30	Photons

Table 3.4 Cost comparison of radiotherapy modalities

Treatment method	2015 CPT/APC codes	Total cost to treat one lesion in US$
Dermatologic office-based superficial radiation (5 fractions)	77,261,77,300, 77,332, 77,427, 77,401 ×5	512.38
Dermatologic office-based superficial radiation (12 fractions)	77,261,77,300, 77,332, 77,427 ×2, 77,401 ×12	844.20
Outpatient high-dose rate electronic brachytherapy (8 fractions)	77,261, 77,290, 77,316, 77,334, 77,470, 77,789 ×8, 0182 T ×8	7871.86
Radiation oncologist hospital-based orthovoltage radiation (20 fractions)	77,261, 77,300, 77,332, 77,427 x 4, 77,401 ×20 (CPT + APC)	3714.80
Radiation oncologist hospital-based megavoltage electron beam radiation (20 fractions)	77,261, 77,306, 77,332, 77,280, 77,336, 77,427 ×4, 77,402/G6003 ×20 (CPT + APC)	7106.79

From Wolfe and Cognetta [68], Table 2, courtesy of Elsevier

therapy (SRT) utilizes X-rays to deliver low energy kilovoltage photons in the range of 50–150 kVp [69, 70]. These SRT machines spare the deeper structures and specifically target the skin [69]. There are few randomized, controlled trials regarding the use of SRT in NMSC treatment. However, retrospective analyses and case reports support its use in the treatment of BCC and its ability to cure BCCs with low rates of recurrence and good cosmetic endpoints [69].

Recent reports suggest SRT with orthovoltage X-rays is an alternative for re-excision of incompletely resected or recurrent BCC that are at risk of serious functional and cosmetic impairments after re-excision [70]. This method reports a 5-year control rate of 85% and a low toxicity profile [70]. Disadvantages of RT for BCC include a high failure rate for high-risk areas and for recurrent, large, deep, and/or aggressive BCC subtypes.

When considering RT, careful patient selection is needed. Appropriate cases include BCCs of the nose and the ear and periocular area in patients that are not good surgical candidates. Lesions in these locations can be treated with radiation to minimize damage to delicate structures such as the lacrimal collecting system. Radiation may also be appropriate for those who desire debulking and/or palliation [71]. Radiation therapy is also preferred in the elderly due to small risk of future malignancy in younger patients and may be helpful in relapsing cases [72]. Of note, a randomized controlled trial of surgery versus RT for BCC on the face found a higher 4-year recurrence rate (0.7% in surgery versus 7.5% with RT) and lower cosmetic results by blinded judges and patient assessment [73]. Additional considerations for radiation therapy include the cost and inconvenience of numerous treatments. The cost of treatment has been reported to be highly variable dependent upon the type of RT chosen (Table 3.4) [68]. Radiation therapy should be avoided in patients with NBCCS due to the possibility of stimulating additional BCCs. Thus, it becomes clear that appropriate selection of patients and tumors is essential when considering radiation therapy.

Cryosurgery

Cryosurgery is a tissue-sparing therapy that is useful for treating BCCs in patients with poor health, including those taking anticoagulants, those with pacemakers, and those with the appropriate tumors [5]. During cryosurgery, a cryoprobe with a liquid nitrogen spray unit is used. Adequate tumor destruction requires a rapid freezing and slow thawing, minimum tissue temperature of −25–60 °C, and, in malignant lesions, repetition of the freeze-thaw cycle [74]. Double freeze-thaw cycles are also recommended for the treatment of facial BCC [75]. A freeze rim of approximately 5 mm is regarded as acceptable [75]. Tumors overlying cartilage or bone should be treated until the tissue becomes fixed to the underlying structure, indicating sufficient depth. Treatment of a margin of "clinically normal" skin may compensate for subclinical involvement [5].

Although there are no current consensus guidelines, cryosurgery should generally not be utilized for BCCs with aggressive histologic features, recurrent BCCs, morpheaform BCCs, metatypical BCCs, and BCCs located in high-risk areas. Sclerosing BCCs may also be poorly responsive to cryosurgery as they are very poorly defined. Further, the sclerotic tissue may insulate against the thermal damage [5]. Cryosurgery on the leg has been reported to result in slow healing, poor cosmetic outcomes, and increased risk of infection. However, a recent study reports that intralesional cryotherapy using a cryosurgery needle can completely eradicate BCCs on the lower limb in elderly patients in a single session [76]. It has been reported to work well on lesions beyond the leg as well [77]. The technique has been associated with relatively minor complications and is well-tolerated by patients [76].

Cure rates as high as 97% have been achieved for nodular BCCs less than 1 cm and primary BCCs 2 cm or less [5]. A study comparing cryosurgery (20 s freeze, 60 s thaw ×2 cycles) to standard surgical excision for head and neck superficial BCCs and small nodular BCCs found no significant difference in recurrence rates at 1 year [75]. Cure rates are lower for BCCs greater than 2 cm and recurrent BCCs, morpheaform BCCs, or those in high-risk areas or with aggressive histologic growth patterns [5]. BCC tumors greater than 3 cm are generally poor candidates for cryosurgery.

The primary disadvantage of cryosurgery is suboptimal cosmesis [5]. A lasting depression may follow, particularly on the nose, forehead, back, chest, and ear. Cryosurgery near the vermilion of the upper lip or cartilage of the ear may result in notching. Hypertrophic scars, when they occur, are generally visible by 6 weeks [3]. Combination therapy such as immunocryosurgery (mild cryosurgery with constant imiquimod application) may be an option to minimize the adverse effects of conventional cryosurgical approaches [78].

Laser Therapy

Laser therapy is not FDA-approved for the treatment of BCC, but there has been some reported success with laser as an off-label therapy for BCC [79]. Lasers can be selected to target specific tumor components such as hemoglobin in the vasculature or for local tissue destruction targeting water [80]. Importantly, laser treatment does not have the histologic margin control that surgical excision does. Close clinical follow-up is advised for patients with BCC treated with this off-label therapy.

By targeting hemoglobin, lasers have been used to selectively destroy the tumor's vascular supply. A reported advantage of this selective approach is its preservation of the normal surrounding tissue. The pulsed dye laser (PDL) is one example of lasers that target hemoglobin. In a recent pilot study by Ortiz et al. examining the use of PDL for BCC, response rates were dependent on tumor size [81]. Nearly 92% of BCCs <1.5 cm in diameter demonstrated complete response to PDL treatment, whereas only 25% of BCC >1.5 cm in diameter demonstrated complete response [80]. Tumor histologic types with complete responses included superficial, nodular, micronodular, and keratinizing BCCs. In the incomplete response group, there was an estimated 71–99% reduction in tumor size after PDL.

Another study by Konnikov et al. evaluated longer-term outcomes of BCCs treated with PDL lasers [82]. Complete clinical response was seen in 95% of patients at first follow-up visit (3–7 months after last PDL treatment) regardless of tumor size (ranging from 8 to 17 mm) or histologic subtype. The authors reported that after a median follow-up of 18 months, 94.7% of the treated BCCs with complete initial response demonstrated no evidence of recurrence or residual tumor. Furthermore, nearly 90% of patients remained tumor-free up to 21 months after treatment [80]. Of note, the 595 nm wavelength demonstrates greater clinical efficacy for small, superficial BCC tumors as compared to 585 nm lasers [80]. This is likely due to the deeper maximum coagulation in a 595 nm laser relative to a 585 nm laser [80].

Ablative lasers such as the carbon dioxide (CO_2) and erbium yttrium aluminum garnet (Er:YAG) lasers work by vaporizing tissue water and have also been shown to be effective for treating BCC [80]. A prospective investigational trial demonstrated excellent clinical response of the CO_2 laser with a reported 100% cure rate and 0% recurrence at 3 years for superficial or nodular BCCs <1.5 cm [80]. Diameter and tumor depth, which may be inferred by BCC subtype, were important in determining appropriateness of laser treatment [80]. Superficial tumors were reported to have the highest cure rate at 86%, while nodular tumors were completely cured in approximately 50% of cases [80]. Data on the Er:YAG laser in the treatment of BCCs are far more limited [80]. Disadvantages of laser therapy include hypopigmentation, erythema, mild edema, dusky purpura, and scarring [80].

Photodynamic Therapy

Photodynamic therapy (PDT) is a noninvasive treatment that has been utilized in BCC by employing light-catalyzed chemical reactions to generate reactive oxygen species for tumor cell destruction [83]. The photosensitizing agent concentrates in the tumor. When the light source is directed toward the skin, the photosensitizer is activated. This process leads to necrosis of the tumor, selectively affecting cancer cells without damaging the surrounding tissue [83]. Treatment is used for superficial, low-risk tumors due to the reduced penetration of light for deeper tumors [83]. PDT can also be used in combination with PDL lasers as a light source with good effect [83].

The response rates are variable and reported in one study to range from 62% to 91% for superficial BCCs and 50–92% for nodular BCCs [83]. Another study reported clearance rates of 89.9% at 12-month follow-up for superficial BCCs [84]. Factors responsible for variations in PDT effectiveness include fluence (energy density), fluence rate, light source, illumination scheme, the photosensitizer incubation time, and the use of penetration enhancers [83]. PDT therapy may also be used successfully for patients with Gorlin syndrome [5].

Topical Therapies

Topical therapies are numerous and continuously expanding. They are typically utilized in more superficial lesions and are also particularly helpful in areas of multiple tumors or "field cancerization." The specific therapy choice, however, is patient specific.

Imiquimod

Topical imiquimod cream binds to toll-like receptor 7 on antigen-presenting cells to produce interferon-alpha, tumor necrosis factor-alpha, and other cytokines [5]. This results in the stimulation of both the innate and cell-mediated immunity resulting in apoptosis of tumor cells [85]. Imiquimod may also inhibit the Hedgehog signaling pathway to prevent tumor proliferation [86].

Imiquimod 5% is currently FDA-approved for treatment of immunocompetent adults with biopsy-proven, primary superficial BCCs less than 2 cm in diameter on the trunk, neck, or extremities (excluding hands and feet) [79]. Since its approval, imiquimod has been reported to be most useful as an adjunct therapy in the management of large and multiple superficial BCCs [87]. The 3-year success rates were noted to be 83.6% (178/213) and 98.4% (185/188) for imiquimod and surgical excision, respectively [87, 88]. Five-year success rates for imiquimod were 82.5% compared with 97.7% for surgery. Most of the imiquimod treatment failures occurred in year 1. Thus, although surgery is clearly superior, this recent study demonstrates sustained benefit for lesions that respond early to topical imiquimod [87].

Dermatoscopic ulceration has been reported to be a predictor of BCC response to imiquimod [89]. Specifically, the presence of a solitary small erosion infers a sevenfold increased probability for complete response (OR 7.0, 95% CI: 1.25–39.15). The presence of multiple small erosions poses a 38-fold higher odd for complete response (OR 38.89, 95% CI: 7.52–201.04). The presence of large ulcerations was associated with an eightfold increased probability for complete response (OR 8.17, 95% CI: 1.63–40.85) [89].

5-Fluorouracil

Topical 5-fluorouracil (5-FU) is a pyrimidine analogue that preferentially affects DNA synthesis in neoplastic cells via inhibition of thymidylate synthase [79]. Due to its variable penetration, it should be used at a concentration of at least 5% and is only approved for treatment of superficial BCCs [79].

5-FU should be applied twice a day for at least 6 weeks. It may be used up to 3 months in areas of deep disease foci. It may also be used prophylactically for patients at risk of developing multiple and recurrent BCCs. It is not effective for invasive BCC or those with follicular involvement [5]. Treatment is associated with significant pain and discomfort.

Although there are no direct head-to-head studies comparing 5-FU and imiquimod, current evidence suggests the two topical therapies are equally efficacious for short-term treatment of superficial BCC [79]. 5-FU is a teratogen and is used with caution in women of child-bearing age.

Additional Therapies

Ingenol Mebutate

Ingenol mebutate is FDA-approved for the treatment of actinic keratosis but more recently has been studied in the context of treating BCC [90, 91]. It is a diterpene ester derived from the plant *Euphorbia peplus*. The treatment induces cell necrosis within a few hours of application, followed by an inflammatory response in subsequent days [79].

In a small case series by Diluvio et al., patients applied ingenol mebutate 0.015% to superficial BCCs on the face and scalp and 0.05% for the trunk and extremities. Three of the four patients achieved complete remission after a single course of therapy. One healed after a second cycle, with dermoscopy demonstrating rapid disappearance 1 month after treatment. The dermoscopic diagnostic criteria included arborizing vessels, ulceration, maple leaf-like areas, and spoke-wheel areas [28].

Another small case series of seven patients demonstrated efficacy of ingenol mebutate gel 0.05% on superficial BCC lesions on the trunk [92]. Patients were treated for 10–14 days after shave biopsy. The lesions were occluded in six patients and not occluded in three patients. All patients completed a 7-day regimen. All patients experienced local skin reactions that began on day 1 or 2 of treatment, peaked on day 2–7, and were largely resolved at 2 weeks. These included mild erythema, crusting, flaking, discomfort, pruritus, or burning. All BCCs were clinically resolved at the 2–4-week follow-up [92].

In another phase 2 randomized study of 60 patients with superficial BCC treated with varying doses of ingenol mebutate, significant histologic clearance at 85 days posttreatment was shown in 63% of lesions with application of 0.05% gel for 2 consecutive days [92]. Ingenol mebutate was thought to be a safe therapy with a low incidence of adverse events. Long-term studies with larger sample sizes are indicated to determine recurrence rates [79].

Tranexamic Acid

Tranexamic acid (TXA) is another option for patients with large, locally advanced tumors who seek palliative care [93]. TXA is a synthetic derivative of the amino acid lysine that reduces bleeding via inhibition of local fibrinolysis. Specifically, it blocks plasminogen-binding sites, preventing the conversion of plasminogen into plasmin.

Locally advanced tumors commonly result in bleeding secondary to local vessel damage or invasion by the tumor. This may be distressing to the patient and is typically managed with dressings, cauterization, and radiotherapy. Topical TXA appears to be a viable alternative for this bleeding.

A recent meta-analysis of 29 trials involving 26 using topical TXA to treat BCC demonstrated a decrease in blood loss by 29% with no risk of thromboembolic events such as myocardial infarction, stroke, pulmonary embolism, or deep vein thrombosis [93, 94]. Clearance and recurrence rates were not assessed [94].

Retinoids

Retinoids interfere with cell proliferation and differentiation via their interaction with specific cellular and nuclear receptors. They include a variety of vitamin A (retinol) derivatives including tretinoin, isotretinoin, adapalene, and tazarotene and are used off-label in the treatment of skin cancer [95]. Available topical formulations used in the treatment of cancerous lesions including BCCs include tretinoin 0.05% and 0.1% cream, isotretinoin 0.1% cream (not commercially available in the United States), adapalene 0.1% and 0.3% gel, and tazarotene 0.1% gel [95]. Side effects include erythema, peeling, dryness, burning, and pruritus. Ultraviolet light may exacerbate these effects [95].

Tazarotene is a retinoid used for the treatment of plaque psoriasis, acne, and photodamaged skin. It has been recently reported to inhibit growth of BCC through activation of caspase-dependent apoptosis [79]. In an open-label clinical trial, tazarotene 0.1% gel applied once a day for up to 8 months produced complete clinical response in 53% of cases of superficial and nodular BCCs [79]. In another follow-up study, tazarotene 0.1% gel was applied daily for 24 weeks. At 3-year follow-up, 30.5% of total treated lesions healed without recurrence. Reported adverse effects included application site reactions including erythema, erosions, pruritus, and burning [79].

Systemic etretinate, isotretinoin, and acitretin may be used in the management of BCCs in patients with NBCCS and likely other patients at high risk for developing multiple BCCs [5, 92, 95]. Doses of 4.5 mg/kg per day of isotretinoin and 1 mg/kg per day of etretinate are necessary to induce partial regression of the BCCs. As a result of many side effects, this regimen may be poorly tolerated by some patients. Cessation of therapy has been associated with relapse of disease [5]. Of note, systemic retinoids are pregnancy category X and use during pregnancy is therefore not recommended [95].

Systemic Chemotherapy

Systemic chemotherapy regimens have not been well studied given the rarity of metastatic BCC. However, a recent review of metastatic BCC cases over 30 years at one institution reported that cisplatin-based regimens are most commonly used [79]. Platinum-based chemotherapy has also been used to treat metastatic giant BCC [42]. Additional agents utilized include cisplatin, bleomycin, cyclophosphamide, vinblastine, 5-FU, smoothened inhibitors, PD-1 inhibitors, and gefitinib [16, 96–101].

Vismodegib and sonidegib are two FDA-approved oral medications that work through inhibition of smoothened (SMO) in the Hedgehog pathway [102–107]. While vismodegib was approved by the FDA in 2012, sonidegib was more recently approved for locally advanced, unresectable, and metastatic BCC in 2015 [108, 109]. These two drugs have an overall reported response rate for locally advanced and metastatic BCC of 40–50% [110, 111]. Adverse effects are class specific, and thus, the side effects of sonidegib are similar to those of vismodegib [112, 113]. Common adverse side effects of vismodegib include taste disturbances, muscle cramps or spasms, weight loss, asthenia, and alopecia [100]. These effects limit compliance to therapy [100]. Treatment breaks or pulsed therapy may be considered if side effects are severe [103]. Extended therapy may be indicated in patients at risk for multiple BCCs.

Two vismodegib dosing regimens were recently evaluated in a randomized, regimen-controlled, double-blind phase 2 trial [114]. The first regimen consisted of 150 mg per day for 12 weeks and then three rounds of 8 weeks of placebo daily, followed by 12 weeks of 150 mg daily. Regimen two was comprised of 150 mg per day for 24 weeks and then three rounds of 8 weeks of placebo, followed by 8 weeks of 150 mg daily. Both intermittent dosing schedules demonstrated good efficacy. At the end of treatment, 66% (76 of 116) of patients in the first treatment group and 50% (57 of 113) of patients in the second group had at least 50% reductions in number of BCCs from baseline and no new lesions [114].

For unresectable metastatic disease, systemic chemotherapy (i.e., cisplatin and doxorubicin) alone or with radiation is generally well-tolerated and has provided long-term disease control [5]. If metastasis is confined to lymph nodes, however, surgery or surgery plus radiation is often the treatment of choice.

Interferon

Interferon may be utilized in patients for whom surgical therapy is not feasible or in combination with surgical excision [115]. Local injection with interferon-alpha-2b at doses of 5 million IU three times per week for 4–8 weeks are typically used [5]. Cure rates when used alone have been reported to be approximately 80% [5]. When used in combination with surgical excision, cure rates are reported to exceed those of excision alone [115].

A study by Wettstein et al. evaluated recurrence rates in 23 patients with facial nodular or solid BCC treated with surgery and perilesional interferon. Patients were randomized to receive surgical removal with frozen section control followed by a single perilesional infiltration of either interferon-alpha or Ringer's lactate. Recurrences were assessed at 1 year. One patient suffered from a recurrence in the control group (4%), and no recurrence was observed in the interferon group. Thus, the authors concluded that a single perilesional infiltration of interferon-alpha was safe with no incidence of recurrence, although larger studies are required [116].

Adverse events noted in this study included transient, mild to moderate flu-like symptoms in 95% of patients and asymptomatic leukopenia or neutropenia in 25%. Other less common adverse events include fever, malaise, rheumatic complaints, altered psyche, chills, transient leukopenia, and injection site pain and itching [116].

Conclusion

BCC is the most common cancer in the United States. Despite the high prevalence, there continues to be much to learn about this disease, including the complex interplay between genetics and environment in the development of BCCs. Refinement of diagnostic and therapeutic approaches continues to be under active investigation.

References

1. Verkouteren JA, et al. Epidemiology of basal cell carcinoma: scholarly review. Br J Dermatol. 2017;177:359.
2. Wysong A, Aasi SZ, Tang JY. Update on metastatic basal cell carcinoma: a summary of published cases from 1981 through 2011. JAMA Dermatol. 2013;149(5):615–6.
3. Zhang Y, et al. Body mass index, height and early-onset basal cell carcinoma in a case-control study. Cancer Epidemiol. 2017;46:66–72.
4. Wu S, et al. Cumulative ultraviolet radiation flux in adulthood and risk of incident skin cancers in women. Br J Cancer. 2014;110(7):1855–61.
5. Cockerell CJ, Tan KT, Carucci J, Tierney E, Lang P, Maize JC Sr, Rigel D. Basal cell carcinoma. In: Cancer of the skin. Edinburgh: Elsevier Inc; 2011. p. 99–123.
6. Wang GY, et al. Differing tumor-suppressor functions of Arf and p53 in murine basal cell carcinoma initiation and progression. Oncogene. 2017;36(26):3772–80.
7. Chaudhary SC, et al. Naproxen inhibits UVB-induced basal cell and squamous cell carcinoma development in Ptch1+/− /SKH-1 hairless mice. Photochem Photobiol. 2017;93:1016.
8. Fan Z, et al. A missense mutation in PTCH2 underlies dominantly inherited NBCCS in a Chinese family. J Med Genet. 2008;45(5):303–8.
9. Kijima C, et al. Two cases of nevoid basal cell carcinoma syndrome associated with meningioma caused by a PTCH1 or SUFU germline mutation. Familial Cancer. 2012;11(4):565–70.
10. Scheinfeld N, et al. Identification of a recurrent mutation in the CYLD gene in Brooke-Spiegler syndrome. Clin Exp Dermatol. 2003;28(5):539–41.
11. Berlin NL, et al. Family history of skin cancer is associated with early-onset basal cell carcinoma independent of MC1R genotype. Cancer Epidemiol. 2015;39(6):1078–83.
12. Levine JA, et al. The indoor UV tanning industry: a review of skin cancer risk, health benefit claims, and regulation. J Am Acad Dermatol. 2005;53(6):1038–44.
13. Narala S, Cohen PR. Basal cell carcinoma of the umbilicus: a comprehensive literature review. Cureus. 2016;8(9):e770.
14. Loh TY, Rubin AG, Jiang SI. Basal cell carcinoma of the dorsal foot: an update and comprehensive review of the literature. Dermatol Surg. 2017;43(1):32–9.
15. Alsaedi M, Shoimer I, Kurwa HA. Basal cell carcinoma of the nipple-areola complex. Dermatol Surg. 2017;43(1):142–6.
16. Watson GA, et al. An unusual case of basal cell carcinoma of the vulva with lung metastases. Gynecol Oncol Rep. 2016;18:32–5.
17. Loh T, Rubin AG, Brian Jiang SI. Management of mucosal basal cell carcinoma of the lip: an update and comprehensive review of the literature. Dermatol Surg. 2016;42(12):1313–9.
18. Hone NL, Grandhi R, Ingraffea AA. Basal cell carcinoma on the sole: an easily missed cancer. Case Rep Dermatol. 2016;8(3):283–6.
19. Hoashi T, et al. A case of penile basal cell carcinoma reconstructed by scrotal myofasciocutaneous flap. Dermatol Ther. 2016;29(5):349–52.
20. Hernandez-Aragues I, Baniandres-Rodriguez O. Basal cell carcinoma of the scrotum. Actas Urol Esp. 2016;40(9):592–3.
21. Buljan M, et al. Variations in clinical presentation of basal cell carcinoma. Acta Clin Croat. 2008;47(1):25–30.
22. Sarkar S, et al. Neglected basal cell carcinoma on scalp. Indian J Dermatol. 2016;61(1):85–7.
23. Mehta KS, et al. Metastatic Basal cell carcinoma: a biological continuum of Basal cell carcinoma? Case Rep Dermatol Med. 2012;2012:157187.
24. Brodell RT, Wagamon K. The persistent nonhealing ulcer. Could it be basal cell carcinoma? Postgrad Med. 2001;109(1):29–32.
25. Lim KR, et al. Basal cell carcinoma presenting as a hypertrophic scar. Arch Plast Surg. 2013;40(3):289–91.
26. Nadiminti U, Rakkhit T, Washington C. Morpheaform basal cell carcinoma in African Americans. Dermatol Surg. 2004;30(12 Pt 2):1550–2.

27. Park JY, et al. A rare dermoscopic pattern of nodular basal cell carcinoma with amyloid deposition. J Am Acad Dermatol. 2017;76(2s1):S55–6.
28. Diluvio L, Bavetta M, Di Prete M, Orlandi A, Bianchi L, and Campione E. Dermoscopic monitoring of efficacy of ingenol mebutate in the treatment of pigmented and non-pigmented basal cell carcinomas. Dermatologic Therapy 2017;30:e12438. doi:10.1111/dth.12438. (electronic publication)
29. Arpaia N, et al. Vascular patterns in cutaneous ulcerated basal cell carcinoma: a retrospective blinded study including dermoscopy. Acta Derm Venereol. 2017;97:612.
30. Hirofuji A, et al. Superficial type of multiple basal cell carcinomas: detailed comparative study of its dermoscopic and histopathological findings. J Skin Cancer. 2011;2011:385465.
31. Mary Nolen VB, King J, Bryn N, Morin LK. Nonmelanoma skin cancer: part 1. J Dermatol Nurses Assoc. 2011;3(5):260–81.
32. Yoneta A, et al. A case of cystic basal cell carcinoma which shows a homogenous blue/black area under Dermatoscopy. J Skin Cancer. 2011;2011:450472.
33. Lima NL, et al. Basosquamous carcinoma: histopathological features. Indian J Dermatol. 2012;57(5):382–3.
34. Akay BN, et al. Basosquamous carcinoma: dermoscopic clues to diagnosis. J Dermatol. 2016;44:127–134
35. Tan CZ, Rieger KE, Sarin KY. Basosquamous carcinoma: controversy, advances, and future directions. Dermatol Surg. 2017;43(1):23–31.
36. Tchernev G, et al. Multiple nonsyndromic acquired basal cell carcinomas : Uncommon clinical presentation in a Bulgarian patient. Wien Med Wochenschr. 2017;167:134.
37. Hendrix JD Jr, Parlette HL. Duplicitous growth of infiltrative basal cell carcinoma: analysis of clinically undetected tumor extent in a paired case-control study. Dermatol Surg. 1996;22(6):535–9.
38. Coleman CI, Wine-Lee L, James WD. Pigmented basal cell carcinoma: uncommon presentation in blue-eyed patients. JAMA Dermatol. 2013;149(8):995–6.
39. Alcantara-Reifs CM, et al. Linear basal cell carcinoma: report of three cases with dermoscopic findings. Indian J Dermatol Venereol Leprol. 2016;82(6):708–11.
40. Yamaguchi Y, et al. A case of linear basal cell carcinoma: evaluation of proliferative activity by immunohistochemical staining of PCTAIRE1 and p27. J Eur Acad Dermatol Venereol. 2017;31:e359.
41. Yazdani Abyaneh MA, et al. Giant basal cell carcinomas express neuroactive mediators and show a high growth rate: a case-control study and meta-analysis of etiopathogenic and prognostic factors. Am J Dermatopathol. 2017;39(3):189–94.
42. Bellahammou K, et al. Metastatic giant basal cell carcinoma: a case report. Pan Afr Med J. 2016;24:157.
43. Kornreich DA, Lee JB. White network in fibroepithelioma of Pinkus. JAAD Case Rep. 2016;2(5):400–2.
44. Gomez-Martin I, et al. Pigmented fibroepithelioma of Pinkus: a potential dermoscopic simulator of malignant melanoma. J Dermatol. 2017;44(5):542–3.
45. Dongre AM, et al. Fibroepithelioma of Pinkus in continuity with nodular basal cell carcinoma: a rare presentation. Indian Dermatol Online J. 2016;7(4):285–7.
46. Crowson AN. Basal cell carcinoma: biology, morphology and clinical implications. Mod Pathol. 2006;19(Suppl 2):S127–47.
47. Saxena K, et al. Adenoid basal cell carcinoma: a rare facet of basal cell carcinoma. BMJ Case Rep. 2016;2016. https://doi.org/10.1136/bcr-2015-214166.
48. Murkey N, et al. Adenoid variant of basal cell carcinoma: a case report with a glance at biological behavior of the tumor. Indian J Dermatol. 2017;62(1):103–5.
49. Anjum N, et al. Follicular proliferation or basal cell carcinoma? The first prospective UK study of this histological challenge during Mohs Surgery. Br J Dermatol. 2017;177(2):549–50.

50. Viera M, et al. A new look at fibroepithelioma of pinkus: features on confocal microscopy. J Clin Aesthet Dermatol. 2008;1(2):42–4.
51. Hasbun Acuna P, et al. Pigmented basal cell carcinoma mimicking a superficial spreading melanoma. Medwave. 2016;16(11):e6805.
52. Nagi R, Sahu S, Agarwal N. Unusual presentation of pigmented basal cell carcinoma of face: surgical challenge. J Clin Diagn Res. 2016;10(7):Zj06–7.
53. Christian MM, et al. A correlation of alpha-smooth muscle actin and invasion in micronodular basal cell carcinoma. Dermatol Surg. 2001;27(5):441–5.
54. Bard RL. High-frequency ultrasound examination in the diagnosis of skin cancer. Dermatol Clin. 2017;35(4):505–11.
55. Hong H, Sun J, Cai W. Anatomical and molecular imaging of skin cancer. Clin Cosmet Investig Dermatol. 2008;1:1–17.
56. Zeitouni NC, et al. Preoperative ultrasound and photoacoustic imaging of nonmelanoma skin cancers. Dermatol Surg. 2015;41(4):525–8.
57. MacFarlane D, et al. The role of imaging in the management of patients with nonmelanoma skin cancer: diagnostic modalities and applications. J Am Acad Dermatol. 2017;76(4):579–88.
58. Belkin DA, Wysong A. Radiographic imaging for skin cancer. Semin Cutan Med Surg. 2016;35(1):42–8.
59. Humphreys TR, et al. The role of imaging in the management of patients with nonmelanoma skin cancer: when is imaging necessary? J Am Acad Dermatol. 2017;76(4):591–607.
60. Duncan JR, Carr D, Kaffenberger BH. The utility of positron emission tomography with and without computed tomography in patients with nonmelanoma skin cancer. J Am Acad Dermatol. 2016;75(1):186–96.
61. Lubeek SF, Arnold WP. A retrospective study on the effectiveness of curettage and electrodesiccation for clinically suspected primary nodular basal cell carcinoma. Br J Dermatol. 2016;175(5):1097–8.
62. Woldow AB, Melvin ME. Early detection of desiccation and curettage failure in the treatment of basal cell carcinoma. Dermatology. 2016;232:696.
63. Lara F, Santamaria JR, Garbers LE. Recurrence rate of basal cell carcinoma with positive histopathological margins and related risk factors. An Bras Dermatol. 2017;92(1):58–62.
64. Sexton M, Jones DB, Maloney ME. Histologic pattern analysis of basal cell carcinoma. Study of a series of 1039 consecutive neoplasms. J Am Acad Dermatol. 1990;23(6 Pt 1):1118–26.
65. Gulleth Y, et al. What is the best surgical margin for a basal cell carcinoma: a meta-analysis of the literature. Plast Reconstr Surg. 2010;126(4):1222–31.
66. Thomas DJ, King AR, Peat BG. Excision margins for nonmelanotic skin cancer. Plast Reconstr Surg. 2003;112(1):57–63.
67. Sin CW, Barua A, Cook A. Recurrence rates of periocular basal cell carcinoma following Mohs micrographic surgery: a retrospective study. Int J Dermatol. 2016;55(9):1044–7.
68. Wolfe CM, Cognetta AB Jr. Radiation therapy (RT) for nonmelanoma skin cancer (NMSC), a cost comparison: clarifying misconceptions. J Am Acad Dermatol. 2016;75(3):654–5.
69. McGregor S, Minni J, Herold D. Superficial radiation therapy for the treatment of nonmelanoma skin cancers. J Clin Aesthet Dermatol. 2015;8(12):12–4.
70. Duinkerken CW, et al. Orthovoltage X-rays for postoperative treatment of resected basal cell carcinoma in the head and neck area. J Cutan Med Surg. 2017;21(3):243–9. https://doi.org/10.1177/1203475416687268.
71. Vuong W, Lin J, Wei RL. Palliative radiotherapy for skin malignancies. Ann Palliat Med. 2017;6(2):165–72.
72. Piccinno R, et al. Dermatologic radiotherapy in the treatment of extensive basal cell carcinomas: a retrospective study. J Dermatolog Treat. 2017;28(5):1–5.
73. Avril MF, et al. Basal cell carcinoma of the face: surgery or radiotherapy? Results of a randomized study. Br J Cancer. 1997;76(1):100–6.
74. Zouboulis CC. Cryosurgery in dermatology. Hautarzt. 2015;66(11):834–48.
75. Erratum. Could cryosurgery be an alternative treatment for basal cell carcinoma of the vulva?: Erratum. Indian Dermatol Online J. 2015;6(4):314.

76. Har-Shai Y, et al. Intralesional cryosurgery for the treatment of basal cell carcinoma of the lower extremities in elderly subjects: a feasibility study. Int J Dermatol. 2016;55(3):342–50.
77. Weshahy AH, et al. The efficacy of intralesional cryosurgery in the treatment of small- and medium-sized basal cell carcinoma: a pilot study. J Dermatolog Treat. 2015;26(2):147–50.
78. Gaitanis G, Kalogeropoulos CD, Bassukas ID. Cryosurgery during Imiquimod (Immunocryosurgery) for periocular basal cell carcinomas: an efficacious minimally invasive treatment alternative. Dermatology. 2016;232(1):17–21.
79. Lanoue J, Goldenberg G. Basal cell carcinoma: a comprehensive review of existing and emerging nonsurgical therapies. J Clin Aesthet Dermatol. 2016;9(5):26–36.
80. Soleymani T, Abrouk M, Kelly KM. An analysis of laser therapy for the treatment of non-melanoma skin cancer. Dermatol Surg. 2017;43(5):615–24.
81. Ortiz AE, Anderson RR, Avram MM. 1064 nm long-pulsed Nd:YAG laser treatment of basal cell carcinoma. Lasers Surg Med. 2015;47(2):106–10.
82. Konnikov N, et al. Pulsed dye laser as a novel non-surgical treatment for basal cell carcinomas: response and follow up 12-21 months after treatment. Lasers Surg Med. 2011;43(2):72–8.
83. Carija A, et al. Single treatment of low-risk basal cell carcinomas with pulsed dye laser-mediated photodynamic therapy (PDL-PDT) compared with photodynamic therapy (PDT): a controlled, investigator-blinded, intra-individual prospective study. Photodiagn Photodyn Ther. 2016;16:60–5.
84. Kessels JP, et al. Ambulatory photodynamic therapy for superficial basal cell carcinoma: an effective light source? Acta Derm Venereol. 2017;97:649.
85. Karabulut GO, et al. Imiquimod 5% cream for the treatment of large nodular basal cell carcinoma at the medial canthal area. Indian J Ophthalmol. 2017;65(1):48–51.
86. Yang X, Dinehart MS. Triple hedgehog pathway inhibition for basal cell carcinoma. J Clin Aesthet Dermatol. 2017;10(4):47–9.
87. Williams HC, et al. Surgery versus 5% Imiquimod for nodular and superficial basal cell carcinoma: 5-year results of the SINS randomized controlled trial. J Invest Dermatol. 2017;137(3):614–9.
88. Singal A, et al. Facial basal cell carcinoma treated with topical 5% Imiquimod cream with Dermoscopic evaluation. J Cutan Aesthet Surg. 2016;9(2):122–5.
89. Urech M, et al. Dermoscopic ulceration is a predictor of basal cell carcinoma response to Imiquimod: a retrospective study. Acta Derm Venereol. 2017;97(1):117–9.
90. Jung YS, et al. Superficial basal cell carcinoma treated with two cycles of ingenol mebutate gel 0.015. Ann Dermatol. 2016;28(6):796–7.
91. Izzi S, et al. Successfully treated superficial basal cell carcinomas with ingenol mebutate 0.05% gel: report of twenty cases. Dermatol Ther. 2016;29(6):470–2.
92. Bettencourt MS. Treatment of superficial basal cell carcinoma with ingenol mebutate gel, 0.05%. Clin Cosmet Investig Dermatol. 2016;9:205–9.
93. Wong Y, Low JA, Chio MT. Role of topical tranexamic acid in hemostasis of locally advanced basal cell carcinoma. JAAD Case Rep. 2016;2(2):162–3.
94. Ker K, Beecher D, Roberts I. Topical application of tranexamic acid for the reduction of bleeding. Cochrane Database Syst Rev. 2013;(7):CD010562.
95. Micali G, et al. Topical pharmacotherapy for skin cancer: part I. Pharmacology. J Am Acad Dermatol. 2014;70(6):965.e1–12; quiz 977–8.
96. Chang J, et al. Association between programmed death ligand 1 expression in patients with basal cell carcinomas and the number of treatment modalities. JAMA Dermatol. 2017;153:285.
97. Chen L, Silapunt S, Migden MR. Sonidegib for the treatment of advanced basal cell carcinoma: a comprehensive review of sonidegib and the BOLT trial with 12-month update. Future Oncol. 2016;12(18):2095–105.
98. Cox KF, Margo CE. Role of vismodegib in the management of advanced periocular basal cell carcinoma. Cancer Control. 2016;23(2):133–9.
99. Falchook GS, et al. Responses of metastatic basal cell and cutaneous squamous cell carcinomas to anti-PD1 monoclonal antibody REGN2810. J Immunother Cancer. 2016;4:70.

100. Lacouture ME, et al. Characterization and management of hedgehog pathway inhibitor-related adverse events in patients with advanced basal cell carcinoma. Oncologist. 2016;21(10):1218–29.
101. McGrane J, Carswell S, Talbot T. Metastatic spinal cord compression from basal cell carcinoma of the skin treated with surgical decompression and vismodegib: case report and review of hedgehog signalling pathway inhibition in advanced basal cell carcinoma. Clin Exp Dermatol. 2017;42(1):80–3.
102. Fife D, et al. Vismodegib therapy for basal cell carcinoma in an 8-year-old Chinese boy with xeroderma pigmentosum. Pediatr Dermatol. 2017;34(2):163–5.
103. Fife K, et al. Managing adverse events associated with vismodegib in the treatment of basal cell carcinoma. Future Oncol. 2017;13(2):175–84.
104. Guo D, Kossintseva I, Leitenberger J. Neoadjuvant vismodegib before Mohs: lack of tissue sparing and squamous differentiation of basal cell carcinoma in a patient with chronic lymphocytic leukemia. Dermatol Surg. 2016;42(6):780–3.
105. Kwon GP, et al. Update to an open-label clinical trial of vismodegib as neoadjuvant before surgery for high-risk basal cell carcinoma (BCC). J Am Acad Dermatol. 2016;75(1):213–5.
106. Lima JP. Statistical concerns on vismodegib for basal cell carcinoma meta-analysis. JAMA Dermatol. 2017;153:337.
107. Paulsen JF, et al. Vismodegib and surgery combined – effective treatment of locally advanced basal cell carcinoma. Acta Oncol. 2016;55(12):1492–4.
108. Casey D, et al. FDA approval summary: sonidegib for locally advanced basal cell carcinoma. Clin Cancer Res. 2017;23:2377.
109. Tibes R. Sonidegib phosphate: new approval for basal cell carcinoma. Drugs Today (Barc). 2016;52(5):295–303.
110. Yin VT, Esmaeli B. Targeting the hedgehog pathway for locally advanced and metastatic basal cell carcinoma. Curr Pharm Des. 2017;23(4):655–9.
111. Silapunt S, Chen L, Migden MR. Hedgehog pathway inhibition in advanced basal cell carcinoma: latest evidence and clinical usefulness. Ther Adv Med Oncol. 2016;8(5):375–82.
112. Ramelyte E, Amann VC, Dummer R. Sonidegib for the treatment of advanced basal cell carcinoma. Expert Opin Pharmacother. 2016;17(14):1963–8.
113. Collier NJ, Ali FR, Lear JT. The safety and efficacy of sonidegib for the treatment of locally advanced basal cell carcinoma. Expert Rev Anticancer Ther. 2016;16(10):1011–8.
114. Dreno B, et al. Two intermittent vismodegib dosing regimens in patients with multiple basal-cell carcinomas (MIKIE): a randomised, regimen-controlled, double-blind, phase 2 trial. Lancet Oncol. 2017;18(3):404–12.
115. Yonjan Lama I, Wharton S. Comment Re: 'Treatment of basal cell carcinoma with surgical excision and perilesional interferon-alpha'. J Plast Reconstr Aesthet Surg. 2015;68(6):877–8.
116. Wettstein R, et al. Treatment of basal cell carcinoma with surgical excision and perilesional interferon-alpha. J Plast Reconstr Aesthet Surg. 2013;66(7):912–6.

Chapter 4
Squamous Cell Carcinoma

Eileen Larkin Axibal and Mariah Ruth Brown

Abstract Cutaneous squamous cell carcinoma is an exceedingly common neoplasm with a rising incidence. It frequently affects individuals who are fair-skinned with high cumulative ultraviolet radiation exposure, are immunosuppressed, or have a genetic predisposition. Squamous cell carcinoma can be suspected clinically by an erythematous, hyperkeratotic, tender, infiltrated, or ulcerated papule or plaque. Biopsy with histopathologic examination is the gold standard diagnostic modality, but several noninvasive techniques for diagnosis are being developed. Features affecting tumor risk include location, clinical size, depth of extension, histologic subtype, degree of histologic differentiation, recurrence, and immunosuppressed status of patient. Aggressive, high-risk lesions have the potential to invade surrounding tissue, metastasize, and recur, resulting in significant morbidity and even death. Mohs micrographic surgery is the preferred treatment for high-risk tumors, as it affords the highest cure rates, preservation of normal tissue, and cosmetic outcome. The standard of treatment for low-risk tumors is conventional surgical excision. Other treatment options include electrodesiccation and curettage, cryosurgery, radiotherapy, photodynamic therapy, and topical agents. Due to the risk of tumor recurrence and additional skin cancers, patients with a history of SCC should undergo regular clinical follow-up with a frequency guided by risk assessment.

Keywords Squamous cell carcinoma · SCC · Non-melanoma skin cancer · Epidemiology · Risk factors · Prevention · High-risk · Treatment · Mohs micrographic surgery · Recurrence

Epidemiology

Squamous cell carcinoma (SCC) is the second most common cutaneous and overall malignancy in the United States, preceded only by basal cell carcinoma (BCC). It accounts for 20% of all skin cancers [1]. The actual rate of SCC is difficult to estimate

E. L. Axibal · M. R. Brown (✉)
Department of Dermatology, University of Colorado Denver, Aurora, CO, USA
e-mail: Mariah.brown@ucdenver.edu

© Springer International Publishing AG, part of Springer Nature 2018   69
A. Hanlon (ed.), *A Practical Guide to Skin Cancer*,
https://doi.org/10.1007/978-3-319-74903-7_4

because cases are not required to be reported to cancer registries. A systematic review found that, in the United States (US) in 2012, 186,157 to 419,543 Caucasians were given a diagnosis of cutaneous SCC, 5604 to 12,572 developed nodal metastasis, and 3932 to 8791 died from the disease [2]. The same study concluded that deaths from SCC may be as common as deaths from renal carcinomas, oropharyngeal carcinomas, and melanomas in the Central and Southern United States. A 2017 population-based study in Minnesota found that the overall incidence of SCC increased by 263% between 1984 and 2010 and that this increase was disproportionately higher than the increase in BCCs [3]. Epidemiologic evidence suggests that exposure to ultraviolet radiation (UVR) and the sensitivity of an individual's skin to UVR are important for the development of SCC. Thus, most SCCs occur in fair-skinned individuals on anatomic locations with maximum cumulative sun exposure, specifically the head, neck, and extremities. A 2012 worldwide systematic review by Lomas and colleagues found that SCC incidence is consistently higher in white populations than in dark-skinned populations and generally greater in geographic areas with high ambient UVR levels [4]. Despite being less common in dark-skinned populations, SCC is the most common skin cancer in African and Asian Indians and second most common (behind pigmented BCC) in Hispanics and East Asians (including Japanese and Chinese patients) [5]. The average age of onset of cutaneous SCC in the United States is the mid-sixth decade of life. SCC occurs more often in men than in women (ratio of 1.9:1), and its incidence increases markedly with age in both genders [6]. The discrepancy between genders is thought to potentially reflect traditional role differences whereby men were more likely to have outdoor occupations and leisure activities and use less sun protection than women, resulting in higher UVR exposure. Xiang and colleagues demonstrated a greater gender difference in older versus younger populations, suggesting that social changes may be leading to less marked differences in occupation, behavior, and SCC risk between sexes in younger individuals [6].

SCC is estimated to have a lifetime incidence of 7–11% in the United States, and numerous studies have demonstrated that the population incidence has been increasing for several decades [7–9]. Many factors may be contributing to the increase in SCC, including earlier detection, population shifts to sunny climates, increase in cutaneous UVR exposure through outdoor activities and tanning bed usage, depletion of the ozone layer, increase in immunosuppressive drug therapy, and an increasing life expectancy [8]. Despite the increasing incidence of SCC, studies have demonstrated that mortality is decreasing [10]. This may be due to improved detection and treatment modalities.

Risk Factors

UV Radiation

Cumulative lifetime exposure to solar UVR is the most important environmental cause of SCC [11]. Historically, individuals have been exposed to UVR largely through occupational exposure to sunlight. However, recreational UV exposure has increased significantly in recent years as a result of outdoor sport/leisure activities and sun tanning for aesthetic purposes. An individual's UV exposure is influenced by factors including latitude, altitude, cloud cover, time of day, and atmospheric pollution [12]. Ambient sunlight is a mixture of primarily UVA (320–400 nm) and UVB (290–320 nm) radiation. UVB is a potent stimulator of inflammation and causes the formation of mutagenic DNA thymidine dimers; it is felt to be the main driver of keratinocyte photocarcinogenesis. UVA is a potent driver of oxidative free radical damage to DNA and other macromolecules and also plays a role in carcinogenesis through different mechanisms [13]. The causality between UVR and SCC has been demonstrated in numerous ecological, migration, and analytical epidemiologic studies [14]. In addition, UVB-specific mutations in the p53 tumor suppressor gene have been identified in cutaneous SCCs [15]. Exposure to artificial UVR from indoor tanning is also associated with SCC development. In 2012, Wehrner and colleagues performed a systematic review and meta-analysis of 12 studies (9238 total cases of non-melanoma skin cancer (NMSC)) and concluded that indoor tanning increases the risk of SCC by 67% [16]. Studies evaluating patients with psoriasis treated with psoralen and ultraviolet A (PUVA) have also shown an increase in the incidence of cutaneous SCC. Stern demonstrated, in a 30-year prospective study, that the risk of developing one or more SCCs in a year was strongly associated with total number of PUVA treatments in a dose-related fashion [17]. Specifically, patients exposed to fewer than 150 treatments did not demonstrate a clinically important increase in risk, those with 151–350 treatments had a moderate increase in risk, and those with > 350 treatments had a substantial increase in risk (incidence rate ratio > 6). This potential complication should be considered and discussed with patients during treatment planning for medical light therapies. Exposure to solar UVR, indoor tanning, and phototherapy are major modifiable risk factors in the development of cutaneous SCC.

Immunosuppression

Although BCC is the most common type of skin cancer in the immunocompetent population, this ratio is reversed and SCC predominates in organ transplant recipients (OTRs). In OTRs, the risk of BCC development is increased tenfold, while the incidence of SCC is 65–250 times higher compared to the general population [18, 19]. The lifelong immunosuppressive regimens required to preserve graft function in OTRs place these individuals at an increased risk of skin cancer. Other constitutional risk factors for the development of posttransplant SCC include increased age; longer duration of immunosuppressive therapy; increased intensity of immunosuppressive therapy; history of increased UV exposure; infection with human papillomavirus (HPV) types 16, 18, and 31; the possession of certain human leukocyte antigen (HLA) and glutathione S-transferase polymorphisms; easily burned skin; CD4 lymphocytopenia; male sex; history of actinic keratosis and prior NMSC; blue or hazel eyes; and birth in a hot climate [20, 21]. A 2017 multicenter retrospective cohort study examining 10,649 adult OTRs at 26 centers across the United States demonstrated a SCC incidence rate (IR) of 1355 per 100,000 person-years. This is in contrast to the population age-adjusted IR of SCC, which is 38 per 100,000.

The authors also found that increased age, white race, male sex, and thoracic organ transplantation placed patients at higher risk of posttransplant skin cancer [22]. Specific immunosuppressive medications, such as azathioprine and cyclosporine, have been linked to the development of posttransplant SCC [23]. Azathioprine, an antimetabolite, results in the production of 6-thioguanine which photosensitizes skin to UVA radiation and accelerates photocarcinogenesis [24]. Cyclosporine, a calcineurin inhibitor, promotes tumor invasiveness and stimulates growth via VEGF-mediated angiogenesis and allows for keratinocyte survival under conditions of increased genotoxic stress [25]. Mammalian target of rapamycin (mTOR) inhibitors such as sirolimus and everolimus, in contrast, are associated with a reduced incidence of posttransplant malignancy [26]. The risk of cutaneous SCC increases with time since transplant, with the incidence ranging from 10% to 27% at 10 years and 40% to 60% at 20 years in the United States and Western Europe [19]. In Australia, the risk of cutaneous SCC at 20 years is as high as 80%. A 2017 study by Ducroux and colleagues demonstrated that, in OTRs with a history of posttransplant SCC undergoing kidney retransplantation, there is an increased risk of developing aggressive SCC [27].

Patients with HIV/AIDS and non-Hodgkin lymphoma, including chronic lymphocytic leukemia, have also demonstrated an increased incidence and recurrence rates of SCC (Fig. 4.1a) [28–30]. The risk of SCC may also be increased in rheumatoid arthritis patients being treated with TNF-alpha inhibitors compared to patients undergoing non-biologic therapies [31] and inflammatory bowel disease patients treated with thiopurines [32]. While it has been proposed that oral glucocorticoid therapy in the non-OTR population may be associated with increased risk of SCC [33], the results of one large prospective study did not support this finding [34]. Sun protection and avoidance, regular skin checks, and education are important in the immunosuppressed population. Additionally, any immunosuppressed patient with diagnosed skin cancer should be treated promptly and aggressively to decrease recurrence and metastases, as SCC in transplant patients tends to grow more rapidly and results in higher mortality [35].

Familial Syndromes

Several genodermatoses result in an elevated risk of SCC. Patients with xeroderma pigmentosum (XP) have a germline deficit in DNA repair leading to increased genomic instability, resulting in a 1000-fold increase in cutaneous malignancies including SCC. If a patient with XP is not protected from UVR, he or she will develop NMSC at a median age of 8.5 years [36]. Two subtypes of oculocutaneous albinism (OCA), OCA1 and OCA2, comprise 80% of OCA cases and are associated with skin cancer due to insufficient melanin synthesis and melanosome function, respectively. SCC is the number one skin tumor seen in patients with albinism [37]. Epidermodysplasia verruciformis (EV) is a rare autosomal recessive disease characterized by numerous non-resolving, verrucous skin lesions [38]. The condition is

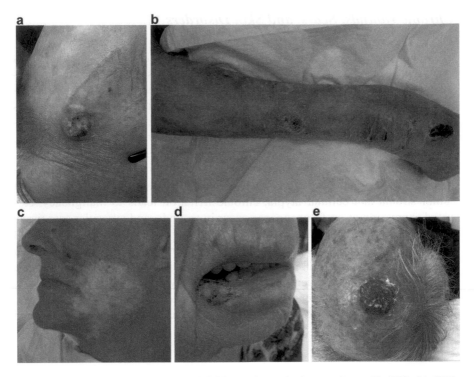

Fig. 4.1 (**a**) Moderately differentiated SCC on the scalp in a patient with HIV (**b**) Well-differentiated SCC of the arm in a patient with recessive dystrophic epidermolysis bullosa (**c**) Well-differentiated SCC in a burn scar (**d**) Well-differentiated SCC of the lower lip (**e**) Moderately differentiated SCC on the scalp

caused by mutations in the epidermodysplasia verruciformis 1 (EVER1) or EVER2 genes, which encode proteins that regulate zinc homeostasis [39]. These patients have an abnormal susceptibility to cutaneous HPV infections and an increased risk for the development of cutaneous SCC. About 30–50% of EV patients will develop SCC, most commonly in the fourth and fifth decades of life [40]. Some forms of epidermolysis bullosa (EB) are associated with the development of cutaneous or mucosal SCC. These SCCs tend to arise at sites of chronic skin blistering, wounds, and scarring (Fig. 4.1b). Multiple primary SCCs often occur, they generally behave more aggressively than conventional SCCs, and they carry a significant morbidity and mortality for patients [41]. SCC is the leading cause of death in individuals with recessive dystrophic EB (RDEB), especially the Hallopeau-Siemens subtype (RDEB-HS). A review of the National EB Registry from 1986 to 2006 revealed that the risk of a RDEB-HS patient having at least one SCC is 7.5% by age 20, 67.8% by age 35, 80.2% by age 45, and 90.1% by age 55 [42]. The same study demonstrated the cumulative risk of death from SCC as 38.7%, 70.0%, and 78.7% by ages 35, 45, and 55, respectively. Other genodermatoses that are associated with cutaneous SCC are dyskeratosis congenita, Rothmund-Thomson syndrome, Bloom syndrome, Werner syndrome, Muir-Torre syndrome, Huriez syndrome, and Fanconi anemia [36].

Chronic Wounds, Scars, and Skin Disorders

SCC may arise in sites of chronic wounds, inflammation, osteomyelitis, sinus tracts, ulcers, and scars (Fig. 4.1c) [43]. A Marjolin's ulcer is a rare and frequently aggressive cutaneous malignancy that arises within previously traumatized and chronically inflamed skin – especially after burns – and often presents 30–40 years after the injury [8]. To date, no concrete pathogenesis for the development of Marjolin's ulcers in burns or other wound types has been elucidated. Theories are numerous and include the idea that decreased vascularity combined with weakened epithelium creates a susceptibility of chronic wounds to carcinogens, prolonged attempts at wound healing parallel the generation of tumor stroma and cellular atypia, chronic irritation leads to malignancy, elevated expression of proto-oncogenes occur in wounds, and avascular scar tissue in chronic wounds interferes with lymphocyte mobility and results in impaired antitumor immune surveillance [44]. Chronic dermatoses associated with an increased risk for the development of SCC include porokeratosis, discoid lupus, lupus vulgaris, lichen sclerosus et atrophicus, lymphogranuloma venereum, granuloma inguinale, lichen planus, acne conglobata, hidradenitis suppurativa, dystrophic epidermolysis bullosa (EB), nevus sebaceous, erythema ab igne, and others [43].

Viruses

Human papillomavirus (HPV) may act as a cocarcinogen with other factors to increase the risk of cutaneous SCC. A 2014 meta-analysis by Wang and colleagues found that SCCs were more likely to carry HPV than normal-appearing skin and that SCCs in immunosuppressed patients have an increased prevalence of HPV compared to immunocompetent patients [45]. This association does not imply causality; however, the absence of detectable HPV in many SCCs may mean that the virus is implicated in initiation, but not promotion or maintenance, of carcinogenesis [46]. It has been hypothesized that HPV may inhibit cellular DNA repair or apoptosis mechanisms, making cells more susceptible to UVR damage. Conversely, UVR may have a temporary immunosuppressive effect on the skin, allowing HPV to evade the immune system [45]. HPV types 5 and 8 are associated with SCC in epidermodysplasia verruciformis [47]. HPV types 6, 11, 16, and 18 are commonly found in SCC of the anogenital region, and type 16 is associated with periungual SCC [8]. Verrucous carcinoma has been associated with both low-risk (types 6 and 11) and high-risk (types 16 and 18) types of HPV [40].

Ionizing Radiation

The carcinogenic effects of ionizing radiation are well documented; exposure results in a threefold increased risk of NMSC [48]. In the 1940s and 1950s, low-energy radiation became a popular therapy for several benign cutaneous diseases, including acne, dermatitis, hypertrichosis, tinea capitis, hemangioma, congenital nevus, and cysts. In addition to therapeutic exposure, occupational exposure to ionizing radiation occurs in healthcare professionals, technicians, and engineers [43]. The risk of radiation-induced SCC is proportional to cumulative dose. Exposure to UVR is considered an additive cocarcinogen. The average latency period for development of SCC is approximately 21 years but may be as long as 60 years [43]. X-rays pose the greatest risk, but more superficial penetrating Grenz rays and gamma rays also cause SCC [8]. Fair-skinned (Fitzpatrick skin types 1 and 2) individuals have a higher risk of radiation-induced skin cancers [49].

Other Medications

Cutaneous SCCs are common findings in melanoma patients treated with BRAF inhibitors. The discovery of frequent RAS mutations in cutaneous SCCs that develop in patients treated with BRAF inhibitors suggests that a paradoxical activation of the MAP kinase signaling pathway may lead to accelerated growth of these tumors [50]. Voriconazole is a widely prescribed antifungal medication used for prevention and treatment of invasive fungal infections, often in organ transplant recipients. Due to the frequent reports of SCC in patients on voriconazole, numerous cohort studies have established that voriconazole is an independent risk factor for the development of cutaneous malignancy. The mechanism by which voriconazole increases risk of skin cancer is not entirely clear, but the drug's phototoxic properties and the primary metabolite voriconazole N-oxide may be implicated [51].

Occupational/Chemical Exposures

Exposure to arsenic, polycyclic aromatic hydrocarbons, pesticides, and herbicides result in an increased risk of SCC [52–54]. Numerous cases of scrotal SCC have been reported in men due to exposure to occupational carcinogens including soot, lubricating oils, and cutting oils [55].

History of Non-melanoma Skin Cancer

Within 5 years after treatment of an index SCC, there is a 30–50% increased risk of developing another primary SCC [56, 57]. Marcil and Stern demonstrated that the 3-year cumulative risk of developing an SCC in patients with a prior BCC is low – 6% within 3 years [58].

Prevention

Sun Protection

Sun protection practices include wearing wide-brimmed hats and clothing cover, wearing sunscreen, staying out of the sun in the middle part of the day, and using shade [14]. The majority of behavioral interventions aiming to decrease sun exposure have been measured by reduction in frequency of sunburns or tanning response rather than development of actinic neoplasms. Evidence, in the form of randomized controlled trials, that has validated sun protection as safe and effective in preventing actinic keratoses (AKs) and SCC primarily relates to sunscreen use. An Australian randomized control trial evaluating regular application of a broad-spectrum sun protection factor (SPF) 15+ sunscreen compared with discretionary use sunscreen showed a 40% reduction in SCC in an 8-year follow-up period [59]. Another study estimated that 9.3% of Australians (14,192 people) who would otherwise have developed cutaneous SCC in 2008 had their cancers prevented through regular sunscreen use [60]. A 2003 study evaluating development of AKs demonstrated that, over a 2-year period, individuals randomized to daily sunscreen application had a 24% reduction in AKs compared to those with discretionary use [61]. Consensus from numerous reviews on sun protection outreach efforts is that patient-directed educational and behavioral interventions are effective in improving sun-protective behaviors. Thus, regular education and advice about primary prevention should be routine clinical practice with all patients but especially with parents of newborn children, primary school children, adolescents, young adults, and organ transplant recipients [14].

Nicotinamide, Difluoromethylornithine, and Retinoids

Nicotinamide (vitamin B3) is reported to have a range of photoprotective effects including enhancing DNA repair, reducing UVR-induced suppression of skin immune responses, modulating inflammatory cytokine production and skin barrier function, and restoring cellular energy levels after UV exposure [62]. The ONTRAC (Oral Nicotinamide to Reduce Actinic Cancer) phase III double-blinded randomized controlled trial assessed the safety and chemopreventive efficacy of oral nicotinamide in high-risk patients with a history of SCC. After 12 months, patients who took nicotinamide 500 mg twice daily had a 30% lower rate of new SCCs than placebo [63]. Another oral agent, difluoromethylornithine (DFMO), has also been studied for its potential to prevent non-melanoma skin cancer. Kreul and colleagues reported a retrospective review of long-term efficacy and toxicity for subjects participating in a phase III study of DFMO; they concluded that those treated with DFMO had a nonsignificant, persistent decrease in NMSC after completion of treatment and that treatment did not result in late toxicity after discontinuation [64]. Topical and systemic retinoids – derivatives of vitamin A – have also been investigated as a means of chemoprevention against the development of SCCs. The evidence on the effect of tropical tretinoin for prevention of NMSC has been debated [65]. The largest trial by Weinstock and colleagues demonstrated that, in 1131 high-risk patients randomized to topical 0.1% tretinoin or a matching vehicle for 1.5–5.5 years, there was no difference in any precancer or cancer-related end points [66]. Regarding oral therapy, Harwood and colleagues performed a retrospective evaluation of the efficacy of low-dose systemic retinoids (etretinate and acitretin) for chemoprevention of SCCs in a population of 32 OTRs with at least one histologically proven SCC; they found that those who received prophylactic systemic retinoids at dosages of 0.2–0.4 mg/kg/d developed significantly fewer SCCs in the first 3 years of treatment, the effect was sustained for at least 8 years, and there was a well-tolerated side-effect profile [67]. Similarly, George and colleagues demonstrated, in a prospective randomized crossover trial including 23 renal transplant patients, that the number of SCCs observed during acitretin therapy was 43% lower than during the drug-free control arm [68]. Systemic retinoids are teratogens and should be used with caution in women of childbearing age. Further studies on these, and other potential chemopreventive agents, are warranted.

Clinical Presentation and Differential Diagnosis

Squamous Cell Carcinoma In Situ

SCC in situ (SCCIS) – often called Bowen's disease – typically presents as an erythematous scaly patch or minimally elevated plaque on sun-exposed skin. Most commonly, SCCIS affects the head and neck, followed by the extremities and trunk. Because it is often related to HPV infection, SCCIS in the anogenital region (also called Bowenoid papulosis) may occur more prominently in young adults [69]. Bowenoid papulosis carries a 2.6% risk of transformation to invasive SCC [40]. SCCIS may arise from a preexisting actinic keratosis (AK) or de novo. SCCIS may be confused clinically with inflammatory conditions like psoriasis and nummular dermatitis, actinic keratosis, seborrheic keratosis, superficial BCC, amelanotic melanoma, and extramammary Paget's disease (Fig. 4.2a–d).

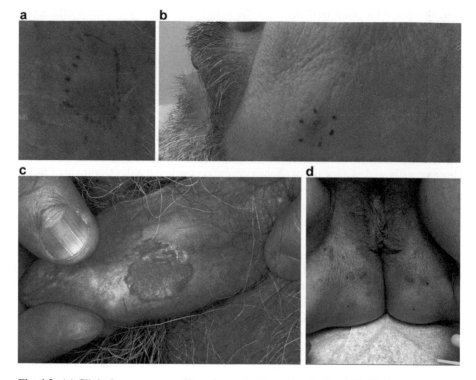

Fig. 4.2 (a) Clinical – squamous cell carcinoma in situ on the forehead (**b**) Clinical – squamous cell carcinoma in situ on the cheek (**c**) Clinical – squamous cell carcinoma in situ of the penis (**d**) Clinical – Bowenoid papulosis of the vulva and perineal area (Figures courtesy of the Fitzsimons Army Medical Center Collection (Public Domain))

Invasive Squamous Cell Carcinoma

Cutaneous SCC most often presents in sun-exposed areas – with lip and ear lesions being particularly aggressive – as a hyperkeratotic, tender, or ulcerated growth (Fig. 4.1d) [69]. Most SCCs arise within the context of a preexisting AK, but the rate of transformation of AK to SCC is low; a 2013 systematic review of 24 studies demonstrated that progression rates of AK to SCC ranged from 0% to 0.075% per lesion per year, with an increased risk of 0.53% in patients with prior history of non-melanoma skin cancer [70, 71]. One 1997 meta-analysis reported that up to 20% of individual AKs progress to SCC each year [72]. Rates of regression of single AKs range between 15% and 63% after 1 year [70]. The progression of AKs has been shown to be more common in lesions with persistent beta-HPV infections [73]. When a SCC arises de novo, it can present as an asymptomatic or tender papule, plaque, or nodule that enlarges over time and can become ulcerated or necrotic (Fig. 4.1e) [74]. SCCs may infiltrate beyond the visible borders of the lesion and can invade through the fascia, periosteum, perichondrium, and neural sheath in aggressive cases. The differential diagnosis of SCC often depends on tumor location and appearance. Invasive SCC may be confused clinically with hypertrophic actinic keratosis, inflamed seborrheic keratosis, verruca vulgaris, or any persistent nodule, plaque, or ulcer on sun-damaged skin, prior irradiated regions, old burns, scars, and on the lips and genitals [20] (Fig. 4.1).

Keratoacanthoma

Keratoacanthoma (KA) is considered a less-aggressive, potentially self-resolving squamous neoplasm that presents as a rapidly growing, well-circumscribed, dome-shaped nodule with central keratin plug and crateriform appearance (Fig. 4.3a). After resolution, a KA may leave an atrophic scar. KAs can be solitary, multiple, grouped, giant, constantly enlarging (KA centrifugum marginatum), multiple spontaneously regressing (Ferguson-Smith disease), and generalized eruptive (Grzybowski syndrome). They may be associated with sun exposure, immunosuppression, trauma, and genetic syndromes including Muir-Torre syndrome and XP [75]. Due to reports of cases of KAs behaving aggressively and metastasizing, the clinical perspective of this tumor has evolved in the last 30 years toward viewing it as a subtype of SCC (squamous cell carcinoma, keratoacanthoma type) rather than its own separate entity. The difficulty with clear histopathological differentiation between SCC and KA favors the current classification. KAs should be treated with the same modalities as well-differentiated SCCs, but overaggressive treatment resulting in functional impairment or aesthetic disfigurement should be avoided [75]. The differential diagnosis for a KA often includes verruca vulgaris, BCC, prurigo nodule, and others (Fig. 4.3).

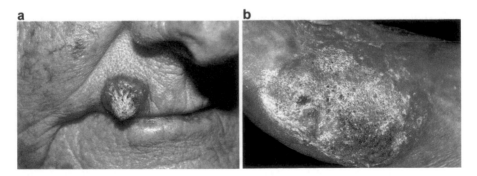

Fig. 4.3 Clinical keratoacanthoma and verrucous carcinoma (**a**) Keratoacanthoma of the upper cutaneous lip (**b**) Verrucous carcinoma of the foot (Figures courtesy of the Fitzsimons Army Medical Center Collection (Public Domain))

Verrucous Carcinoma

A verrucous carcinoma is rare variant of SCC characterized by a well-defined, exophytic, cauliflower-like growth affecting the penis, scrotum, or perianal region (Buschke-Loewenstein tumor), plantar foot (epithelioma cuniculatum), or oral mucosa (oral florid papillomatosis, Ackerman tumor) (Fig. 4.3b). These are commonly associated with HPV infection. While verrucous carcinomas often recur locally after removal and can cause extreme local tissue destruction, they have very low metastatic potential [76]. Verrucous carcinomas are often difficult to distinguish from a large verruca, condyloma acuminata, or seborrheic keratosis.

Diagnosis

The gold standard for diagnosis of any clinically suspicious cutaneous lesion is biopsy with histologic evaluation. Depending on the size, location, and anticipated treatment approach of the tumor, an incisional biopsy, punch biopsy, shave biopsy, or excisional biopsy of the entire lesion may be performed. Routine hematoxylin and eosin (H&E) stains are used to confirm the diagnosis in most instances. However, in cases of diagnostic uncertainty, immunohistochemical markers, such as AE1/AE3 (pancytokeratin), p53, and epithelial membrane antigen (EMA), can be used [77]. In addition to biopsy, any patient with suspected or confirmed SCC should undergo a full skin examination with palpation of regional lymph node basins for evidence of coexisting tumors and metastatic disease, respectively.

In recent years, noninvasive diagnostic aides have garnered attention. Dermoscopy is a technique whereby a practitioner uses a handheld, 10x magnification dermatoscope to noninvasively evaluate colors and microstructures of the epidermis and superficial dermis that are otherwise not visible to the naked eye. This diagnostic method may be helpful in identifying features of SCC, including keratin scale/crust, white circles, white structureless areas, ulceration, and glomerular or hairpin vessels [78]. Reflectance confocal microscopy (RCM) is a noninvasive optical imaging technique that allows high-resolution visualization images of the skin of the epidermis and papillary dermis (to an imaging depth of 200 μm) in real time, at near histologic resolution [79]. RCM relies on a low-power laser that emits near-infrared light (830 nm) and allows only light back-reflected from a desired focal point within the skin to enter the detector. Under RCM, SCC shows an atypical honeycomb or disarranged pattern of the spinous-granular layer of the epidermis, round nucleated bright cells in the epidermis, and round vessels in the dermis [80]. Optical coherence tomography (OCT) and high-frequency ultrasound (HFUS) are also emerging as potential tools in the evaluation of tumor size and characteristics in patients with suspected or confirmed SCC [81, 82].

Pathology

Histopathology of SCCIS (Bowen's disease) demonstrates a broad area of full-thickness atypia of the epidermis with nuclear pleomorphism, apoptosis, and mitoses (Fig. 4.4a). The atypical keratinocytes commonly extend down the adnexa but do not invade into the dermis. Invasive SCC is characterized by strands and lobules

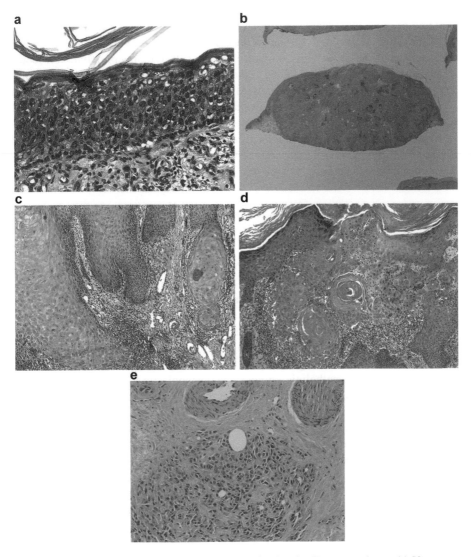

Fig. 4.4 Pathology (**a**) Squamous cell carcinoma in situ (**b**) Keratoacanthoma (**c**) Verrucous carcinoma (**d**) Well-differentiated squamous cell carcinoma (**e**) Poorly differentiated squamous cell carcinoma

of atypical, glassy, brightly eosinophilic keratinocytes infiltrating into the dermis. Keratoacanthomas are comprised of well-differentiated, minimally atypical, bright pink keratinocytes surrounding a core filed with cornified material (Fig. 4.4b). Often a lymphocytic and eosinophilic inflammatory infiltrate is present. Verrucous carcinomas show papillomatosis, keratinocyte proliferation invading the dermis in a "pushing" manner, and minimal cytologic atypia; the histologic appearance is surprisingly benign [40] (Fig. 4.4c).

SCCs range from well-differentiated (minimal pleomorphism, prominent keratinization, extracellular keratin pearls) (Fig. 4.4d) to poorly differentiated (pleomorphic nuclei with high degree of atypia, frequent mitoses, few or no keratin pearls) [74] (Fig. 4.4e). Histologic variants of SCC include acantholytic or adenoid, pagetoid, small cell, basosquamous, single cell, clear cell, lymphoepithelial, verrucous, adenosquamous (mucin-producing), desmoplastic, sclerosing, infiltrating, pigmented, sarcomatoid, and spindle cell [8]. In addition to grade of differentiation and histologic subtype, histopathologic evaluation should assess tumor depth; level of dermal invasion; presence of perineural, lymphatic, or vascular invasion; and margin status. Because there are no defined criteria for assigning histologic subtype and grade of differentiation for cutaneous SCC, there is expected interobserver variability in pathologic diagnoses.

High-Risk SCC

While the majority of patients with SCC have excellent outcomes, 3.7–5.2% of patients develop lymph node metastasis, and 1.5–2.1% die from their disease [83–85]. Approximately 85% of metastases involve regional lymph nodes, followed by metastases to the lungs, liver, brain, skin, and bone [74] (Fig. 4.5a, b). The following parameters have been established as high-risk prognostic factors in several studies: tumor location (ear, lip, and areas of long-lasting chronic ulcers or inflammation), clinical size (>2 cm), histological depth extension (beyond the subcutaneous tissue), histologic subtype (acantholytic, spindle, and desmoplastic subtypes), degree of differentiation (poorly differentiated or undifferentiated), recurrence, and immunosuppressed status [83, 86, 87] (Fig. 4.5c, d). In 2016, Thompson and colleagues completed the largest meta-analysis of SCC risk factors to date – including 36 studies with 17,248 patients and 23,421 SCCs – and their findings validated many of these previously reported high-risk features. They found that tumor depth >2 mm was associated with the highest increased risk of local recurrence and tumor size >20 mm was associated with the highest increase in disease-specific mortality [88]. They also found that tumor location on the temple was associated with an increased risk of metastasis; this location had not previously been acknowledged as high-risk (Fig. 4.5e, f).

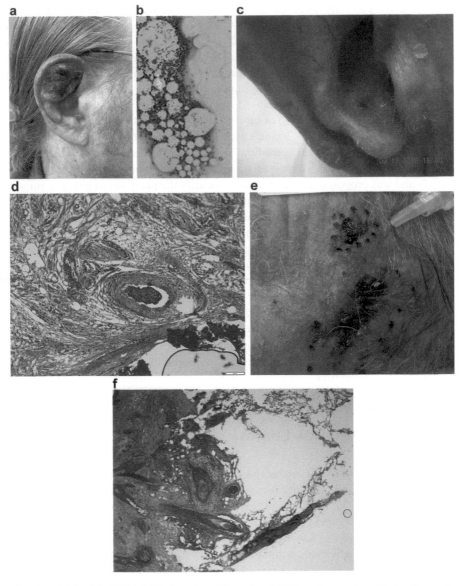

Fig. 4.5 High-risk SCC (**a**) Moderately differentiated SCC on the ear in-patient with a palpable lymph node in the neck (**b**) Fine-needle aspirate of lymph node of patient in image 5A with metastatic SCC visualized (**c**) Poorly differentiated SCC of the ear (**d**) Intravascularly invasive SCC seen on Mohs frozen section histology from case **c** (**e**) Moderately differentiated SCC of the left temple with perineural invasion (**f**) Perineurally invasive SCC on Mohs frozen sections from case **e**

There are currently three available staging systems for cutaneous SCC: the American Joint Committee on Cancer (AJCC) Cancer Staging Manual, the Union for International Cancer Control (UICC) system, and the Brigham and Women's Hospital (BWH) staging system [89–91]. The AJCC and UICC systems were developed based on expert consensus, and the BWH system was developed by a single institution as an alternative staging system in an attempt to more accurately stratify risk. In the AJCC and UICC systems, T2 defines high-risk tumors based on tumor width > 2 cm (AJCC and UICC) or tumor width ≤ 2 cm with 2–5 high-risk features including tumor thickness > 2 mm, Clark level IV or higher, perineural invasion, location on ear, location on vermilion lip, and poor differentiation (AJCC). The BWH system is based on a retrospective review of 256 primary high-risk cutaneous SCCs and was proposed in 2013 to further stratify the many heterogeneous tumors that fall under the T2 umbrella. The authors identified four factors that make tumors high-risk: poor differentiation, perineural invasion of at least 0.1 mm, tumor diameter >2 cm, and invasion beyond subcutaneous fat. The proposed stratification defines T1 tumors by 0 risk factors, T2a by 1 risk factor, T2b by 2–3 risk factors, and T3 by ≥ 4 risk factors or bone invasion. The authors of the BWH staging system found that T2b encompassed 19% of the tumors but 72% of nodal metastases and 83% of deaths from SCC [89]. A 2017 study by Gonzalez and colleagues compared the BWH and AJCC systems for staging SCCs in immunosuppressed patients and found that the BWH staging criteria was better at risk stratifying SCC in this population [92]. Another study by Stevenson and colleagues validated the staging system and identified hematologic malignancy as a comorbidity also associated with poor outcome [93] (Table 4.1).

Work-Up of High-Risk Lesions

Patients with high-risk SCC are at risk of developing nodal metastasis. The risk of tumor recurrence and mortality increases with nodal size and number of involved nodes [94] (Fig. 4.5a, b). In patients with lymph node metastasis, 5-year survival decreases to 46–70% [95]. It is possible that early detection of subclinical nodal metastasis could lead to fewer deaths from SCC [96]. Lymph node ultrasound is recommended in individuals with high-risk tumors [97]. If abnormal lymph nodes are identified on clinical exam or imaging studies, histologic confirmation should be obtained with a fine-needle aspiration (FNA) with ultrasound (US) guidance; US-guided FNA has been found to be more sensitive and specific than conventional FNA [98]. If the FNA is negative, repeat imaging, repeat FNA, or sentinel lymph node biopsy (SLNB) should be considered, especially because FNA can produce false-negative results in certain situations (i.e., in patients with a history of radiation) [8, 99]. Currently SLNB is not the standard of care for work-up of cutaneous SCC but is gaining interest due to its high negative predictive value, low false-negative rate, and low risk of complications [100]. Schmitt and colleagues found that

Table 4.1 Risk factors for cutaneous squamous cell carcinoma

Ultraviolet radiation
Immunosuppression
Organ transplant recipients
HIV/AIDS
Chronic lymphocyte leukemia
Non-Hodgkin lymphoma
Familial syndrome
Xeroderma pigmentosum
Oculocutaneous albinism
Epidermodysplasia verruciformis
Epidermolysis bullosa
Dyskeratosis congenital
Rothmund-Thomson syndrome
Bloom syndrome
Werner syndrome
Muir-Torre syndrome
Huriez syndrome
Fanconi anemia
Chronic wounds
Human papillomavirus
Radiation
Medications
BRAF inhibitors
Voriconazole
Azathioprine
Cyclosporine
History of non-melanoma skin cancer
Occupational chemical exposure
Arsenic
Polycyclic aromatic hydrocarbons
Pesticides
Herbicides

positive SLNB most often occurs in high-risk T2b tumors (BWH staging) [101]. A 2015 review by Navarrete-Dechent and colleagues concluded that SLNB can detect occult nodal metastases in patients at risk and, due to its higher precision than imaging studies and decreased invasiveness compared with lymph node dissection, it may gain utility for staging of high-risk SCC [94].

In patients with positive lymph node biopsies or large infiltrating tumors with signs of involvement of underlying structures, additional imaging studies may be required to assess for tumor extent and metastasis. A 2017 study of 108 high-risk (BWH T2a or T3) SCCs found that, of the 45 patients that underwent imaging

(58% for staging, 33% for evaluation of clinically suspicious or known disease), management was altered and disease-related outcomes were improved in 33% [102]. The majority (69%) received one type of study, and the remainder underwent two studies. The most common imaging modality used was computed tomography (CT) scan (79%) followed by positron-emission tomography (PET)/CT (21%) and magnetic resonance imaging (MRI) (19%). In terms of choosing imaging modality, CT and MRI can identify soft tissue infiltration, bony erosion, and lymph node involvement, while PET can detect metastases especially in areas of necrosis, dense fibrosis, or scarring from radiation therapy [8]. CT with contrast is typically the initial imaging study in the preoperative evaluation of head and neck SCCs, as it offers superior spatial resolution compared to MRI [103]. If the patient experiences neurological symptoms concerning for perineural invasion, MRI is preferred.

Treatment

The goals of treatment of cutaneous SCC include complete removal of the tumor, minimizing the risk of recurrence and metastasis, restoring normal function of the tissue, and achieving optimal cosmetic outcome. Cure rate should be the main consideration in choosing therapy in almost all cases [8]. In 1992, Rowe and colleagues published a 50-year review of outcomes based on numerous treatment modalities for primary and recurrent cutaneous SCC [87]. As a whole, treatment of primary tumors has a significantly higher success rate than treatment of persistent or recurrent tumors, highlighting the importance of selecting the most effective initial therapy. After recurrence, the risk that a SCC spreads to lymph nodes and/or metastasizes is 25–45%, depending on tumor location [104].

Low-Risk Tumors

Conventional surgical excision is the treatment of choice for any low-risk invasive SCC, as it allows confirmation of the tumor type and assessment of the margins on histopathology. A study by Brodland and Zitelli demonstrated a 95% cure rate for well-defined, low-risk tumors (<2 cm in size; not occurring on the ears, lips, eyelids, nose, or scalp; and not invading the fat) using a 4 mm surgical resection margin [105]. The European consensus-based interdisciplinary guidelines recommend a standardized minimal margin of 5 mm for low-risk tumors (<6 mm with no high-risk features) [74]. While many other destructive or topical options are available, they are not preferred because failure of these techniques often ultimately leads to surgery anyway. In situations when a patient is unable or refuses to undergo surgery, however, destructive (radiation therapy, cryosurgery, electrodessication and curettage

(ED&C), photodynamic therapy (PDT)) or topical (imiquimod, 5-fluorouracil, diclofenac, ingenol mebutate, chemical peel) modalities can be used [74]. These options may also be used in patients where the tumor is growing in a "field" of background actinic damage. Intralesional chemotherapy (methotrexate, 5-fluorouracil, or bleomycin) may also be considered in select patients and has often been used for the treatment of keratoacanthoma [75]. Importantly, both topical and destructive treatments do not allow for histological examination of the margin. Clinical follow-up is important to monitor for tumor recurrence.

External beam radiation has been reported to have an 80% 5-year cure rate of SCC [8]. Due to the poor quality of irradiated tissue and the chance for tumor induction 20–30 years posttreatment, radiation should be reserved for patients >50 years old with contraindications to surgery. Brachytherapy, a form of radiation therapy that places the radiation source close to the treated area, may have advantages relative to conventional external beam radiation in particular patients [106]. A 2016 review of the literature found that brachytherapy for the treatment of non-melanoma skin cancer was well tolerated with acceptable toxicity and a high local control rate of 97% (median); SCC control rates were not specified [107]. Cryosurgery should be considered only for small, low-risk tumors because of the low cure rates achieved when the technique is used for high-risk lesions [108]. ED&C should be used to treat only small, low-risk, well-circumscribed, non-recurrent SCCs on the trunk, arms, or legs; it should not be used to treat tumors on terminal hair-bearing skin because of the risk of tumor extension along follicular structures [109]. PDT using [1] 20% topical aminolevulinic acid (ALA) in combination with a blue light source or [2] the methyl ester of ALA (MAL) under occlusion in combination with a red light source is approved by the FDA for the treatment of AKs. While some studies show reasonable results using ALA-PDT and MAL-PDT for the treatment of SCCIS, a study of 6 invasive SCCs treated with a series of 4 ALA-PDT treatments every other day showed only 33% (2/6 cases) pathologic clearance at a median follow-up time of 29 months [110–112]. Cyclic PDT treatments may be beneficial for prevention of NMSC in organ transplant recipients [113].

The FDA has approved three topical medications for the treatment of AKs: 5-fluorouracil cream (Efudex; Valeant Pharmaceuticals International, Bridgewater, NJ), imiquimod cream (Aldara; Medicis Pharmaceuticals, Scottsdale, AZ), and ingenol mebutate gel (Picato; Leo Pharma, Parsippany, NJ). While these medications are not FDA approved for the treatment of SCC in the United States, they may be considered under limited circumstances. Two studies of the efficacy of 5-fluorouracil cream revealed a 48–69% SCCIS clearance rate 1 year after a 4-week treatment regimen [111, 114]. The daily application of imiquimod for 16 weeks has demonstrated a 73–87.5% cure rate for SCCIS [115, 116]. Ingenol mebutate is a newer medication that has demonstrated clinical benefit for the treatment of multiple actinic keratoses and field cancerization, but no human studies for the treatment of SCC have been done. Successful treatment of SCC tumors with ingenol mebutate has been demonstrated, however, in a mouse model [117].

High-Risk Tumors

Mohs micrographic surgery (MMS) is a technique that allows for the complete assessment of all deep and peripheral margins using intraoperative en face frozen sections – compared to standard vertical sectioning, where < 1% of the peripheral and deep margins is examined – with the added goal of sparing as much unaffected tissue as possible while still controlling disease. Rowe and colleagues found that MMS allows for the highest cure rates for both primary and recurrent SCCs of the skin, lip, and ear [87]. Due to the longer duration of therapy, higher costs, and need for specialized staff, MMS should be reserved for high-risk tumors or low-risk tumors in anatomic sites where conventional excision may result in significant functional impairment. To guide clinicians, the appropriate use criteria (AUC) for MMS was developed by national dermatology organizations in 2013 [118]. Based on the expert opinions of a 17-member panel regarding 270 clinical scenarios, the AUC is a tool that advises when MMS is an appropriate treatment option for a particular skin cancer. The document does recognize, however, that other acceptable approaches may also exist. Mohs surgery is a safe outpatient procedure with a low complication rate. A 2013 multicenter prospective cohort study by Alam and colleagues demonstrated only 149 adverse events (0.72%) among 20,821 MMS procedures [119]. Of the adverse events, 61.1% were infections, 20.1% were wound dehiscence or partial or full tissue necrosis, and 15.4% were related to bleeding or hematomas. There were four serious events (0.02%) and no deaths. If MMS is unavailable, the next best options for treatment of high-risk SCCs include excision with frozen section analysis of the complete peripheral and deep margins or "slow Mohs" utilizing rush paraffin sections for margin control and subsequent delayed closure [8] (Fig. 4.6a–c).

Adjuvant radiotherapy (ART) may benefit some patients with high-risk SCC. While there is no consensus as to when ART should be utilized, it may be beneficial in those with uncertain or positive surgical margins or with more advanced nerve involvement (involvement of named nerves, nerves 0.1 mm or greater in diameter, or with clinical or radiologic evidence of nerve invasion) [120].

Oral targeted therapies that aim to block the growth of SCC from a molecular standpoint are under active investigation. Prior studies have demonstrated that up to 80% of cutaneous SCCs and 100% of metastatic SCCs express epidermal growth

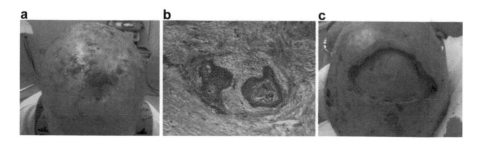

Fig. 4.6 Mohs surgery (**a**) Well- to moderately differentiated SCC on the scalp (**b**) Histologic appearance of tumor on Mohs frozen sections (**c**) Final Mohs defect with clear surgical margins

factor receptor (EGFR) [121]. Cetuximab, erlotinib, and gefitinib are small molecule tyrosine kinase inhibitors that target the intracellular portion of EGFR [122, 123]. Cetuximab has been used to treat a wide array of cancers and has been used off-label to treat advanced cutaneous SCC over the past 10 years. A 2017 study by Trodello and colleagues showed that, of nine patients with metastatic SCC treated between 1989 and 2014 with cetuximab, six (67%) obtained a complete response with a median disease-free survival of 25 (range 3–48) months and one (11%) obtained a partial response [124]. The combination of EGFR inhibitors with other immuno-modulators is also allowing for new therapeutic approaches [122]. Programmed cell death 1 protein (PD-1) inhibitors are recently being investigated for their potential role in managing advanced cutaneous SCC. When the PD-1 receptor is bound by its ligands, T-cell activation and proliferation, which is essential for antitumor activity, is suppressed. Blocking the receptor with an anti-PD-1 antibody (i.e., pembroli-zumab) allows for potent and durable T-cell responses. Stevenson and colleagues reported a case of locally advanced cutaneous squamous cell carcinoma that, after four cycles of pembrolizumab, achieved nearly complete tumor regression; there continued to be no evidence of disease after 11 months of maintenance therapy [125]. PD-1 inhibition for SCC is an active area of investigation and publication [126, 127]. Caution is advised in treating OTR patients with PD-1 inhibitors as there is a risk of transplant rejection. Cisplatin is a cytotoxic agent that acts by introducing cross-links into DNA, thereby interfering with mitosis and cell division. It has been used to treat cutaneous SCC. Of 60 SCC patients treated with cisplatin between 1989 and 2014, 13 (22%) achieved a complete response with median disease-free survival of 14.6 (range 3–112) months and 14 (23%) had a partial response [124]. There is some anecdotal evidence for adjuvant oral retinoids and oral capecitabine (an ana-logue of 5-FU) in the treatment of advanced SCC, but the data support more of a chemopreventive role for these agents in high-risk groups including OTRs on chronic immunosuppression [123].

Follow-Up

Patients who have had one SCC have a 30–50% risk of another non-melanoma skin cancer within 5 years. They are also at increased risk of melanoma [58, 128, 129]. For this reason, patients with a history of invasive or high-risk SCC should be fol-lowed regularly for full skin and lymph node examinations. The recommended fol-low-up period is every 3–6 months for the first 2 years, every 6–12 months for the next 3 years, and then annually thereafter. Patients with regional metastatic disease should be seen more frequently: every 1–3 months for the first year, every 2–4 months for the second year, every 4–6 months up to 5 years, and then every 6–12 months thereafter [8]. The first 2 years after diagnosis is the most critical follow-up period, since 75% of local recurrence and metastases occur within this time period [74]. High-risk patients with immunosuppression, genetic predisposition, and/or prior multiple SCC should be monitored with an increased frequency long term.

References

1. Alam M, Ratner D. Cutaneous squamous-cell carcinoma. N Engl J Med. 2001;344(13):975–83.
2. Karia PS, Han J, Schmults CD. Cutaneous squamous cell carcinoma: estimated incidence of disease, nodal metastasis, and deaths from disease in the United States, 2012. J Am Acad Dermatol. 2013;68(6):957–66.
3. Muzic JG, Schmitt AR, Wright AC, Alniemi DT, Zubair AS, Olazagasti Lourido JM, et al. Incidence and trends of basal cell carcinoma and cutaneous squamous cell carcinoma: a population-based study in Olmsted County, Minnesota, 2000 to 2010. Mayo Clin Proc. 2017;92(6):890–8.
4. Lomas A, Leonardi-Bee J, Bath-Hextall F. A systematic review of worldwide incidence of nonmelanoma skin cancer. Br J Dermatol. 2012;166(5):1069–80.
5. Agbai ON, Buster K, Sanchez M, Hernandez C, Kundu RV, Chiu M, et al. Skin cancer and photoprotection in people of color: a review and recommendations for physicians and the public. J Am Acad Dermatol. 2014;70(4):748–62.
6. Xiang F, Lucas R, Hales S, Neale R. Incidence of nonmelanoma skin cancer in relation to ambient UV radiation in white populations, 1978–2012: empirical relationships. JAMA Dermatol. 2014;150(10):1063–71.
7. Miller DL, Weinstock MA. Nonmelanoma skin cancer in the United States: incidence. J Am Acad Dermatol. 1994;30(5 Pt 1):774–8.
8. Kauvar AN, Arpey CJ, Hruza G, Olbricht SM, Bennett R, Mahmoud BH. Consensus for non-melanoma skin cancer treatment, part II: squamous cell carcinoma, including a cost analysis of treatment methods. Dermatol Surg. 2015;41(11):1214–40.
9. Donaldson MR, Coldiron BM. No end in sight: the skin cancer epidemic continues. Semin Cutan Med Surg. 2011;30(1):3–5.
10. Lewis KG, Weinstock MA. Nonmelanoma skin cancer mortality (1988–2000): the Rhode Island follow-back study. Arch Dermatol. 2004;140(7):837–42.
11. Armstrong BK, Kricker A. The epidemiology of UV induced skin cancer. J Photochem Photobiol B. 2001;63(1–3):8–18.
12. O'Sullivan NA, Tait CP. Tanning bed and nail lamp use and the risk of cutaneous malignancy: a review of the literature. Australas J Dermatol. 2014;55(2):99–106.
13. D'Orazio J, Jarrett S, Amaro-Ortiz A, Scott T. UV radiation and the skin. Int J Mol Sci. 2013;14(6):12222–48.
14. Green AC, Olsen CM. Cutaneous squamous cell carcinoma: an epidemiological review. Br J Dermatol. 2017;177(2):373–81.
15. Brash DE, Rudolph JA, Simon JA, Lin A, McKenna GJ, Baden HP, et al. A role for sunlight in skin cancer: UV-induced p53 mutations in squamous cell carcinoma. Proc Natl Acad Sci U S A. 1991;88(22):10124–8.
16. Wehner MR, Chren MM, Nameth D, Choudhry A, Gaskins M, Nead KT, et al. International prevalence of indoor tanning: a systematic review and meta-analysis. JAMA Dermatol. 2014;150(4):390–400.
17. Stern RS, Study PF-U. The risk of squamous cell and basal cell cancer associated with psoralen and ultraviolet A therapy: a 30-year prospective study. J Am Acad Dermatol. 2012;66(4):553–62.
18. Euvrard S, Kanitakis J, Claudy A. Skin cancers after organ transplantation. N Engl J Med. 2003;348(17):1681–91.
19. Zwald FO, Brown M. Skin cancer in solid organ transplant recipients: advances in therapy and management: part I. Epidemiology of skin cancer in solid organ transplant recipients. J Am Acad Dermatol. 2011;65(2):253–61. quiz 62
20. Kallini JR, Hamed N, Khachemoune A. Squamous cell carcinoma of the skin: epidemiology, classification, management, and novel trends. Int J Dermatol. 2015;54(2):130–40.

21. Otley CC, Cherikh WS, Salasche SJ, McBride MA, Christenson LJ, Kauffman HM. Skin cancer in organ transplant recipients: effect of pretransplant end-organ disease. J Am Acad Dermatol. 2005;53(5):783–90.
22. Garrett GL, Blanc PD, Boscardin J, Lloyd AA, Ahmed RL, Anthony T, et al. Incidence of and risk factors for skin cancer in organ transplant recipients in the United States. JAMA Dermatol. 2017;153(3):296–303.
23. Chockalingam R, Downing C, Tyring SK. Cutaneous squamous cell carcinomas in organ transplant recipients. J Clin Med. 2015;4(6):1229–39.
24. Perrett CM, Walker SL, O'Donovan P, Warwick J, Harwood CA, Karran P, et al. Azathioprine treatment photosensitizes human skin to ultraviolet A radiation. Br J Dermatol. 2008;159(1):198–204.
25. Norman KG, Canter JA, Shi M, Milne GL, Morrow JD, Sligh JE. Cyclosporine A suppresses keratinocyte cell death through MPTP inhibition in a model for skin cancer in organ transplant recipients. Mitochondrion. 2010;10(2):94–101.
26. Kauffman HM, Cherikh WS, Cheng Y, Hanto DW, Kahan BD. Maintenance immunosuppression with target-of-rapamycin inhibitors is associated with a reduced incidence of de novo malignancies. Transplantation. 2005;80(7):883–9.
27. Ducroux E, Martin C, Bouwes Bavinck JN, Decullier E, Brocard A, Westhuis-van Elsacker ME, et al. Risk of aggressive skin cancers after kidney retransplantation in patients with previous post-transplant cutaneous squamous cell carcinomas: a retrospective study of 53 cases. Transplantation. 2017;101(4):e133–e41.
28. Brewer JD, Shanafelt TD, Khezri F, Sosa Seda IM, Zubair AS, Baum CL, et al. Increased incidence and recurrence rates of nonmelanoma skin cancer in patients with non-Hodgkin lymphoma: a Rochester Epidemiology Project population-based study in Minnesota. J Am Acad Dermatol. 2015;72(2):302–9.
29. Zhao H, Shu G, Wang S. The risk of non-melanoma skin cancer in HIV-infected patients: new data and meta-analysis. Int J STD AIDS. 2016;27(7):568–75.
30. Hock BD, McIntosh ND, McKenzie JL, Pearson JF, Simcock JW, MacPherson SA. Incidence of cutaneous squamous cell carcinoma in a New Zealand population of chronic lymphocytic leukaemia patients. Intern Med J. 2016;46(12):1414–21.
31. Amari W, Zeringue AL, McDonald JR, Caplan L, Eisen SA, Ranganathan P. Risk of non-melanoma skin cancer in a national cohort of veterans with rheumatoid arthritis. Rheumatology (Oxford). 2011;50(8):1431–9.
32. Singh H, Nugent Z, Demers AA, Bernstein CN. Increased risk of nonmelanoma skin cancers among individuals with inflammatory bowel disease. Gastroenterology. 2011;141(5):1612–20.
33. Karagas MR, Cushing GL, Greenberg ER, Mott LA, Spencer SK, Nierenberg DW. Non-melanoma skin cancers and glucocorticoid therapy. Br J Cancer. 2001;85(5):683–6.
34. Baibergenova AT, Weinstock MA, Group VT. Oral prednisone use and risk of keratinocyte carcinoma in non-transplant population. The VATTC trial. J Eur Acad Dermatol Venereol. 2012;26(9):1109–15.
35. Veness MJ, Quinn DI, Ong CS, Keogh AM, Macdonald PS, Cooper SG, et al. Aggressive cutaneous malignancies following cardiothoracic transplantation: the Australian experience. Cancer. 1999;85(8):1758–64.
36. Jaju PD, Ransohoff KJ, Tang JY, Sarin KY. Familial skin cancer syndromes: increased risk of nonmelanotic skin cancers and extracutaneous tumors. J Am Acad Dermatol. 2016;74(3):437–51. quiz 52-4
37. Perry PK, Silverberg NB. Cutaneous malignancy in albinism. Cutis. 2001;67(5):427–30.
38. Burger B, Itin PH. Epidermodysplasia verruciformis. Curr Probl Dermatol. 2014;45:123–31.
39. Ramoz N, Rueda LA, Bouadjar B, Montoya LS, Orth G, Favre M. Mutations in two adjacent novel genes are associated with epidermodysplasia verruciformis. Nat Genet. 2002;32(4):579–81.
40. Dubina M, Goldenberg G. Viral-associated nonmelanoma skin cancers: a review. Am J Dermatopathol. 2009;31(6):561–73.

41. Mellerio JE, Robertson SJ, Bernardis C, Diem A, Fine JD, George R, et al. Management of cutaneous squamous cell carcinoma in patients with epidermolysis bullosa: best clinical practice guidelines. Br J Dermatol. 2016;174(1):56–67.
42. Fine JD, Johnson LB, Weiner M, Li KP, Suchindran C. Epidermolysis bullosa and the risk of life-threatening cancers: the National EB Registry experience, 1986–2006. J Am Acad Dermatol. 2009;60(2):203–11.
43. Johnson TM, Rowe DE, Nelson BR, Swanson NA. Squamous cell carcinoma of the skin (excluding lip and oral mucosa). J Am Acad Dermatol. 1992;26(3 Pt 2):467–84.
44. Kerr-Valentic MA, Samimi K, Rohlen BH, Agarwal JP, Rockwell WB. Marjolin's ulcer: modern analysis of an ancient problem. Plast Reconstr Surg. 2009;123(1):184–91.
45. Wang J, Aldabagh B, Yu J, Arron ST. Role of human papillomavirus in cutaneous squamous cell carcinoma: a meta-analysis. J Am Acad Dermatol. 2014;70(4):621–9.
46. Arron ST, Ruby JG, Dybbro E, Ganem D, Derisi JL. Transcriptome sequencing demonstrates that human papillomavirus is not active in cutaneous squamous cell carcinoma. J Invest Dermatol. 2011;131(8):1745–53.
47. Arron ST, Jennings L, Nindl I, Rosl F, Bouwes Bavinck JN, Seçkin D, et al. Viral oncogenesis and its role in nonmelanoma skin cancer. Br J Dermatol. 2011;164(6):1201–13.
48. Lichter MD, Karagas MR, Mott LA, Spencer SK, Stukel TA, Greenberg ER. Therapeutic ionizing radiation and the incidence of basal cell carcinoma and squamous cell carcinoma. The New Hampshire Skin Cancer Study Group. Arch Dermatol. 2000;136(8):1007–11.
49. Davis MM, Hanke CW, Zollinger TW, Montebello JF, Hornback NB, Norins AL. Skin cancer in patients with chronic radiation dermatitis. J Am Acad Dermatol. 1989;20(4):608–16.
50. Su F, Viros A, Milagre C, Trunzer K, Bollag G, Spleiss O, et al. RAS mutations in cutaneous squamous-cell carcinomas in patients treated with BRAF inhibitors. N Engl J Med. 2012;366(3):207–15.
51. Williams K, Mansh M, Chin-Hong P, Singer J, Arron ST. Voriconazole-associated cutaneous malignancy: a literature review on photocarcinogenesis in organ transplant recipients. Clin Infect Dis. 2014;58(7):997–1002.
52. Yu HS, Liao WT, Chai CY. Arsenic carcinogenesis in the skin. J Biomed Sci. 2006;13(5):657–66.
53. Gallagher RP, Bajdik CD, Fincham S, Hill GB, Keefe AR, Coldman A, et al. Chemical exposures, medical history, and risk of squamous and basal cell carcinoma of the skin. Cancer Epidemiol Biomarkers Prev. 1996;5(6):419–24.
54. Gawkrodger DJ. Occupational skin cancers. Occup Med (Lond). 2004;54(7):458–63.
55. Sorahan T, Cooke MA, Wilson S. Incidence of cancer of the scrotum, 1971–84. Br J Ind Med. 1989;46(6):430–1.
56. Karagas MR. Occurrence of cutaneous basal cell and squamous cell malignancies among those with a prior history of skin cancer. The Skin Cancer Prevention Study Group. J Invest Dermatol. 1994;102(6):10S–3S.
57. Dzubow LM, Rigel DS, Robins P. Risk factors for local recurrence of primary cutaneous squamous cell carcinomas. Treatment by microscopically controlled excision. Arch Dermatol. 1982;118(11):900–2.
58. Marcil I, Stern RS. Risk of developing a subsequent nonmelanoma skin cancer in patients with a history of nonmelanoma skin cancer: a critical review of the literature and meta-analysis. Arch Dermatol. 2000;136(12):1524–30.
59. van der Pols JC, Williams GM, Pandeya N, Logan V, Green AC. Prolonged prevention of squamous cell carcinoma of the skin by regular sunscreen use. Cancer Epidemiol Biomarkers Prev. 2006;15(12):2546–8.
60. Olsen CM, Wilson LF, Green AC, Bain CJ, Fritschi L, Neale RE, et al. Cancers in Australia attributable to exposure to solar ultraviolet radiation and prevented by regular sunscreen use. Aust N Z J Public Health. 2015;39(5):471–6.

61. Darlington S, Williams G, Neale R, Frost C, Green A. A randomized controlled trial to assess sunscreen application and beta carotene supplementation in the prevention of solar keratoses. Arch Dermatol. 2003;139(4):451–5.
62. Damian DL. Nicotinamide for skin cancer chemoprevention. Australas J Dermatol. 2017;58(3):174–80.
63. Chen AC, Martin AJ, Choy B, Fernández-Peñas P, Dalziell RA, McKenzie CA, et al. A phase 3 randomized trial of nicotinamide for skin-cancer chemoprevention. N Engl J Med. 2015;373(17):1618–26.
64. Kreul SM, Havighurst T, Kim K, Mendonça EA, Wood GS, Snow S, et al. A phase III skin cancer chemoprevention study of DFMO: long-term follow-up of skin cancer events and toxicity. Cancer Prev Res (Phila). 2012;5(12):1368–74.
65. Wu PA, Stern RS. Topical tretinoin, another failure in the pursuit of practical chemoprevention for non-melanoma skin cancer. J Invest Dermatol. 2012;132(6):1532–5.
66. Weinstock MA, Bingham SF, Digiovanna JJ, Rizzo AE, Marcolivio K, Hall R, et al. Tretinoin and the prevention of keratinocyte carcinoma (Basal and squamous cell carcinoma of the skin): a veterans affairs randomized chemoprevention trial. J Invest Dermatol. 2012;132(6):1583–90.
67. Harwood CA, Leedham-Green M, Leigh IM, Proby CM. Low-dose retinoids in the prevention of cutaneous squamous cell carcinomas in organ transplant recipients: a 16-year retrospective study. Arch Dermatol. 2005;141(4):456–64.
68. George R, Weightman W, Russ GR, Bannister KM, Mathew TH. Acitretin for chemoprevention of non-melanoma skin cancers in renal transplant recipients. Australas J Dermatol. 2002;43(4):269–73.
69. Prieto-Granada C, Rodriguez-Waitkus P. Cutaneous squamous cell carcinoma and related entities: epidemiology, clinical and histological features, and basic science overview. Curr Probl Cancer. 2015;39(4):206–15.
70. Werner RN, Sammain A, Erdmann R, Hartmann V, Stockfleth E, Nast A. The natural history of actinic keratosis: a systematic review. Br J Dermatol. 2013;169(3):502–18.
71. Marks R, Rennie G, Selwood TS. Malignant transformation of solar keratoses to squamous cell carcinoma. Lancet. 1988;1(8589):795–7.
72. Callen JP, Bickers DR, Moy RL. Actinic Keratoses. J Am Acad Dermatol. 1997 Apr; 36(4):650–3.
73. Plasmeijer EI, Neale RE, de Koning MN, Quint WG, McBride P, Feltkamp MC, et al. Persistence of betapapillomavirus infections as a risk factor for actinic keratoses, precursor to cutaneous squamous cell carcinoma. Cancer Res. 2009;69(23):8926–31.
74. Stratigos A, Garbe C, Lebbe C, Malvehy J, del Marmol V, Pehamberger H, et al. Diagnosis and treatment of invasive squamous cell carcinoma of the skin: European consensus-based interdisciplinary guideline. Eur J Cancer. 2015;51(14):1989–2007.
75. Kwiek B, Schwartz RA. Keratoacanthoma (KA): an update and review. J Am Acad Dermatol. 2016;74(6):1220–33.
76. Klima M, Kurtis B, Jordan PH. Verrucous carcinoma of skin. J Cutan Pathol. 1980;7(2):88–98.
77. Compton LA, Murphy GF, Lian CG. Diagnostic immunohistochemistry in cutaneous neoplasia: an update. Dermatopathology (Basel). 2015;2(1):15–42.
78. Warszawik-Hendzel O, Olszewska M, Maj M, Rakowska A, Czuwara J, Rudnicka L. Non-invasive diagnostic techniques in the diagnosis of squamous cell carcinoma. J Dermatol Case Rep. 2015;9(4):89–97.
79. Ulrich M, Lange-Asschenfeldt S. In vivo confocal microscopy in dermatology: from research to clinical application. J Biomed Opt. 2013;18(6):061212.
80. Rishpon A, Kim N, Scope A, Porges L, Oliviero MC, Braun RP, et al. Reflectance confocal microscopy criteria for squamous cell carcinomas and actinic keratoses. Arch Dermatol. 2009;145(7):766–72.
81. Wortsman X, Wortsman J. Clinical usefulness of variable-frequency ultrasound in localized lesions of the skin. J Am Acad Dermatol. 2010;62(2):247–56.

82. Boone MA, Suppa M, Marneffe A, Miyamoto M, Jemec GB, Del Marmol V. A new algorithm for the discrimination of actinic keratosis from normal skin and squamous cell carcinoma based on in vivo analysis of optical properties by high-definition optical coherence tomography. J Eur Acad Dermatol Venereol. 2016;30(10):1714–25.
83. Schmults CD, Karia PS, Carter JB, Han J, Qureshi AA. Factors predictive of recurrence and death from cutaneous squamous cell carcinoma: a 10-year, single-institution cohort study. JAMA Dermatol. 2013;149(5):541–7.
84. Mourouzis C, Boynton A, Grant J, Umar T, Wilson A, Macpheson D, et al. Cutaneous head and neck SCCs and risk of nodal metastasis – UK experience. J Craniomaxillofac Surg. 2009;37(8):443–7.
85. Brougham ND, Dennett ER, Cameron R, Tan ST. The incidence of metastasis from cutaneous squamous cell carcinoma and the impact of its risk factors. J Surg Oncol. 2012;106(7):811–5.
86. Miller SJ. The National Comprehensive Cancer Network (NCCN) guidelines of care for non-melanoma skin cancers. Dermatol Surg. 2000;26(3):289–92.
87. Rowe DE, Carroll RJ, Day CL. Prognostic factors for local recurrence, metastasis, and survival rates in squamous cell carcinoma of the skin, ear, and lip. Implications for treatment modality selection. J Am Acad Dermatol. 1992;26(6):976–90.
88. Thompson AK, Kelley BF, Prokop LJ, Murad MH, Baum CL. Risk factors for cutaneous squamous cell carcinoma recurrence, metastasis, and disease-specific death: a systematic review and meta-analysis. JAMA Dermatol. 2016;152(4):419–28.
89. Jambusaria-Pahlajani A, Kanetsky PA, Karia PS, Hwang WT, Gelfand JM, Whalen FM, et al. Evaluation of AJCC tumor staging for cutaneous squamous cell carcinoma and a proposed alternative tumor staging system. JAMA Dermatol. 2013;149(4):402–10.
90. Edge S, Byrd D, Comptom C, Fritz A, Greene F, Trotti A. AJCC cancer staging manual. 7th ed. New York: Springer; 2010.
91. Sobin L, Gospodarowicz M, Wittekind C. TNM classification of malignant tumours. 7th ed. Chichester: Wiley-Blackwell; 2010.
92. Gonzalez JL, Cunningham K, Silverman R, Madan E, Nguyen BM. Comparison of the American Joint Committee on Cancer Seventh Edition and Brigham and Women's Hospital cutaneous squamous cell carcinoma tumor staging in immunosuppressed patients. Dermatol Surg. 2017;43(6):784–91.
93. Stevenson ML, Kim R, Meehan SA, Pavlick AC, Carucci JA. Metastatic cutaneous squamous cell carcinoma: the importance of T2 stratification and hematologic malignancy in prognostication. Dermatol Surg. 2016;42(8):932–5.
94. Navarrete-Dechent C, Veness MJ, Droppelmann N, Uribe P. High-risk cutaneous squamous cell carcinoma and the emerging role of sentinel lymph node biopsy: a literature review. J Am Acad Dermatol. 2015;73(1):127–37.
95. Kelder W, Ebrahimi A, Forest VI, Gao K, Murali R, Clark JR. Cutaneous head and neck squamous cell carcinoma with regional metastases: the prognostic importance of soft tissue metastases and extranodal spread. Ann Surg Oncol. 2012;19(1):274–9.
96. Ross AS, Schmults CD. Sentinel lymph node biopsy in cutaneous squamous cell carcinoma: a systematic review of the English literature. Dermatol Surg. 2006;32(11):1309–21.
97. Jank S, Robatscher P, Emshoff R, Strobl H, Gojer G, Norer B. The diagnostic value of ultrasonography to detect occult lymph node involvement at different levels in patients with squamous cell carcinoma in the maxillofacial region. Int J Oral Maxillofac Surg. 2003;32(1):39–42.
98. Griffith JF, Chan AC, Ahuja AT, Leung SF, Chow LT, Chung SC, et al. Neck ultrasound in staging squamous oesophageal carcinoma – a high yield technique. Clin Radiol. 2000;55(9):696–701.
99. Chan JY, Chan RC, Chow VL, To VS, Wei WI. Efficacy of fine-needle aspiration in diagnosing cervical nodal metastasis from nasopharyngeal carcinoma after radiotherapy. Laryngoscope. 2013;123(1):134–9.

100. Allen JE, Stolle LB. Utility of sentinel node biopsy in patients with high-risk cutaneous squamous cell carcinoma. Eur J Surg Oncol. 2015;41(2):197–200.
101. Schmitt AR, Brewer JD, Bordeaux JS, Baum CL. Staging for cutaneous squamous cell carcinoma as a predictor of sentinel lymph node biopsy results: meta-analysis of American Joint Committee on Cancer criteria and a proposed alternative system. JAMA Dermatol. 2014;150(1):19–24.
102. Ruiz ES, Karia PS, Morgan FC, Schmults CD. The positive impact of radiologic imaging on high-stage cutaneous squamous cell carcinoma management. J Am Acad Dermatol. 2017;76(2):217–25.
103. MacFarlane D, Shah K, Wysong A, Wortsman X, Humphreys TR. The role of imaging in the management of patients with nonmelanoma skin cancer: diagnostic modalities and applications. J Am Acad Dermatol. 2017;76(4):579–88.
104. Cherpelis BS, Marcusen C, Lang PG. Prognostic factors for metastasis in squamous cell carcinoma of the skin. Dermatol Surg. 2002;28(3):268–73.
105. Brodland DG, Zitelli JA. Surgical margins for excision of primary cutaneous squamous cell carcinoma. J Am Acad Dermatol. 1992;27(2 Pt 1):241–8.
106. Alam M, Nanda S, Mittal BB, Kim NA, Yoo S. The use of brachytherapy in the treatment of nonmelanoma skin cancer: a review. J Am Acad Dermatol. 2011;65(2):377–88.
107. Delishaj D, Rembielak A, Manfredi B, Ursino S, Pasqualetti F, Laliscia C, et al. Nonmelanoma skin cancer treated with high-dose-rate brachytherapy: a review of literature. J Contemp Brachytherapy. 2016;8(6):533–40.
108. Nguyen TH, Ho DQ. Nonmelanoma skin cancer. Curr Treat Options Oncol. 2002;3(3):193–203.
109. Reschly MJ, Shenefelt PD. Controversies in skin surgery: electrodessication and curettage versus excision for low-risk, small, well-differentiated squamous cell carcinomas. J Drugs Dermatol. 2010;9(7):773–6.
110. Brightman L, Warycha M, Anolik R, Geronemus R. Do lasers or topicals really work for nonmelanoma skin cancers? Semin Cutan Med Surg. 2011;30(1):14–25.
111. Morton C, Horn M, Leman J, Tack B, Bedane C, Tjioe M, et al. Comparison of topical methyl aminolevulinate photodynamic therapy with cryotherapy or fluorouracil for treatment of squamous cell carcinoma in situ: results of a multicenter randomized trial. Arch Dermatol. 2006;142(6):729–35.
112. Calzavara-Pinton PG. Repetitive photodynamic therapy with topical delta-aminolaevulinic acid as an appropriate approach to the routine treatment of superficial non-melanoma skin tumours. J Photochem Photobiol B. 1995;29(1):53–7.
113. Willey A, Mehta S, Lee PK. Reduction in the incidence of squamous cell carcinoma in solid organ transplant recipients treated with cyclic photodynamic therapy. Dermatol Surg. 2010;36(5):652–8.
114. Salim A, Leman JA, McColl JH, Chapman R, Morton CA. Randomized comparison of photodynamic therapy with topical 5-fluorouracil in Bowen's disease. Br J Dermatol. 2003;148(3):539–43.
115. Patel GK, Goodwin R, Chawla M, Laidler P, Price PE, Finlay AY, et al. Imiquimod 5% cream monotherapy for cutaneous squamous cell carcinoma in situ (Bowen's disease): a randomized, double-blind, placebo-controlled trial. J Am Acad Dermatol. 2006;54(6):1025–32.
116. Mackenzie-Wood A, Kossard S, de Launey J, Wilkinson B, Owens ML. Imiquimod 5% cream in the treatment of Bowen's disease. J Am Acad Dermatol. 2001;44(3):462–70.
117. Cozzi SJ, Le TT, Ogbourne SM, James C, Suhrbier A. Effective treatment of squamous cell carcinomas with ingenol mebutate gel in immunologically intact SKH1 mice. Arch Dermatol Res. 2013;305(1):79–83.
118. Connolly SM, Baker DR, Coldiron BM, Fazio MJ, Storrs PA, Vidimos AT, et al. AAD/ACMS/ASDSA/ASMS 2012 appropriate use criteria for Mohs micrographic surgery: a report of the American Academy of Dermatology, American College of Mohs Surgery, American Society for Dermatologic Surgery Association, and the American Society for Mohs Surgery. Dermatol Surg. 2012;38(10):1582–603.

119. Alam M, Kakar R, Nodzenski M, Ibrahim O, Disphanurat W, Bolotin D, et al. Multicenter prospective cohort study of the incidence of adverse events associated with cosmetic dermatologic procedures: lasers, energy devices, and injectable neurotoxins and fillers. JAMA Dermatol. 2015;151(3):271–7.
120. Jambusaria-Pahlajani A, Miller CJ, Quon H, Smith N, Klein RQ, Schmults CD. Surgical monotherapy versus surgery plus adjuvant radiotherapy in high-risk cutaneous squamous cell carcinoma: a systematic review of outcomes. Dermatol Surg. 2009;35(4):574–85.
121. Galer CE, Corey CL, Wang Z, Younes MN, Gomez-Rivera F, Jasser SA, et al. Dual inhibition of epidermal growth factor receptor and insulin-like growth factor receptor I: reduction of angiogenesis and tumor growth in cutaneous squamous cell carcinoma. Head Neck. 2011;33(2):189–98.
122. Bejar C, Maubec E. Therapy of advanced squamous cell carcinoma of the skin. Curr Treat Options Oncol. 2014;15(2):302–20.
123. Rudnick EW, Thareja S, Cherpelis B. Oral therapy for nonmelanoma skin cancer in patients with advanced disease and large tumor burden: a review of the literature with focus on a new generation of targeted therapies. Int J Dermatol. 2016;55(3):249–58. quiz 56, 58.
124. Trodello C, Pepper JP, Wong M, Wysong A. Cisplatin and cetuximab treatment for metastatic cutaneous squamous cell carcinoma: a systematic review. Dermatol Surg. 2017;43(1):40–9.
125. Stevenson ML, Wang CQ, Abikhair M, Roudiani N, Felsen D, Krueger JG, et al. Expression of programmed cell death ligand in cutaneous squamous cell carcinoma and treatment of locally advanced disease with pembrolizumab. JAMA Dermatol. 2017;153(4):299–303.
126. Deinlein T, Lax SF, Schwarz T, Giuffrida R, Schmid-Zalaudek K, Zalaudek I. Rapid response of metastatic cutaneous squamous cell carcinoma to pembrolizumab in a patient with xeroderma pigmentosum: case report and review of the literature. Eur J Cancer. 2017;83:99–102.
127. Degache E, Crochet J, Simon N, Tardieu M, Trabelsi S, Moncourier M, et al. Major response to pembrolizumab in two patients with locally advanced cutaneous squamous cell carcinoma. J Eur Acad Dermatol Venereol. 2017 May 30. doi: 10.1111/jdv.14371. [Epub ahead of print].
128. Chen J, Ruczinski I, Jorgensen TJ, Yenokyan G, Yao Y, Alani R, et al. Nonmelanoma skin cancer and risk for subsequent malignancy. J Natl Cancer Inst. 2008;100(17):1215–22.
129. Wu S, Cho E, Li WQ, Qureshi AA. History of keratinocyte carcinoma and risk of melanoma: a prospective cohort study. J Natl Cancer Inst. 2017 Apr 1;109(4):1–8.

Chapter 5
Melanoma In Situ

Charles Thomas Darragh and Anna S. Clayton

Abstract Melanoma in situ (MIS) is defined as a malignant melanocytic tumor restricted to the epidermis. According to recent database statistics, it is the fastest-growing cancer in the United States with a 9.5% annual incidence increase. Melanoma in situ is not a dangerous tumor and is classified as stage 0. Patients diagnosed with MIS have the same life expectancy as the general population. It is important to remember the ABCDEs of melanoma when evaluating for lesions suspicious of melanoma in situ. There are several clinical subtypes, most notably lentigo maligna, which is found on sun-damaged sites. Diagnosis of MIS is made with histopathology, often with accompanying immunohistochemical stains including SOX 10 and Melan-A. It can be very difficult to determine severely sun-damaged skin versus MIS lesions under the microscope, and this remains a challenge for dermatopathologists. Once a diagnosis of MIS is made, it can be treated with several surgical options. These options include wide local excision, Mohs micrographic surgery, and staged excision or "slow Mohs." In certain circumstances, imiquimod or radiation could be considered for adjuvant therapy. After diagnosis of MIS, patients should be followed closely with every 3- to 6-month skin checks.

Keywords Melanoma in situ · ABCDEs · Lentigo maligna · Mohs micrographic surgery · Wide local excision · Staged excision · Imiquimod · Dermoscopy · Sox 10 · Dermatopathology

Overview and Incidence

Melanoma in situ (MIS) is defined as melanoma restricted to the epidermis without deeper invasion [1] (Fig. 5.1). Fortunately, MIS is not associated with a significant mortality risk. The life expectancy of patients affected is similar to that of the

C. T. Darragh (✉) · A. S. Clayton
Dermatology, Vanderbilt University of Medicine, Nashville, TN, USA
e-mail: Charles.t.darragh@vanderbilt.edu; Anna.clayton@vanderbilt.edu

© Springer International Publishing AG, part of Springer Nature 2018   97
A. Hanlon (ed.), *A Practical Guide to Skin Cancer*,
https://doi.org/10.1007/978-3-319-74903-7_5

Fig. 5.1 Melanoma in situ
marked prior to biopsy
(Photo courtesy of Dr.
Darrel Ellis)

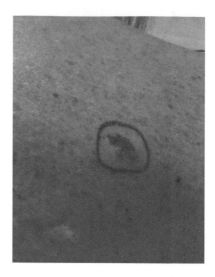

normal population [2]. Recent studies have looked at the Surveillance, Epidemiology, and End Results (SEER) database and have concluded that the incidence of MIS has increased 9.5% yearly [2]. This equates to the fastest-growing malignancy in terms of incidence in the SEER database [2, 3]. It far outpaces the annual increase in incidence of invasive melanoma, 3.6%, over the same time frame [2]. Similar increases in incidence have been documented worldwide [3–5]. Though beyond this textbook's scope, it is important to note that there is controversy as to whether MIS is truly increasing at this impressive rate. Some believe the increase in incidence is due to increases in biopsy rate as well as increased diagnostic scrutiny [6]. However, there is data to suggest there are elements of a true increase in MIS incidence [5, 7].

Epidemiology

MIS shows a greater predilection for the head and neck when compared to invasive melanoma [2, 3, 8] (Table 5.1). MIS is mostly a disease of Caucasian patients with 93.1% of cases seen in this population [2]. Males are affected more often than females, except in lentigo maligna subtype where there is a female predominance [2, 9–11]. More recent data recapitulates MIS most commonly presenting on the face overall, but women have a higher percentage of MIS on the trunk versus the face [12].

Risk Factors

- Risk factors for the development of melanoma in situ (Table 5.2) [13, 14]

Table 5.1 Distribution of MIS versus melanoma

Site	Melanoma in situ rates, % [2]	Invasive melanoma rates, % [8]
Head and neck	37.6%	18.2%
Trunk	24.9%	34.0%
Upper extremities	22.8%	23.4%
Lower extremities	14.0%	20.3%
Unknown/not specified	0.7%	4.2%

Table 5.2 Risk factors for development of melanoma in situ

Advanced patient age (>60)
Male sex
History of previous melanoma
Number of benign melanocytic nevi (>100 with highest risk)
Number of clinically atypical nevi (>5 with highest risk)
Fair skin, red or blond hair, blue eyes (Fitzpatrick skin type I)
High total lifetime sun exposure
Multiple blistering sunburns
Intermittent, intense sun exposure
Tanning bed use
Evidence of actinic damage especially history of actinic keratosis or nonmelanoma skin cancer
History of childhood cancer
Immunosuppression
First-degree relative with diagnosis of melanoma
Residence in sunnier climate/latitude near the equator

Clinical Features

When discussing any type of melanoma, including MIS, it is prudent to remember the ABCDEs that help aid in diagnosis of suspicious melanocytic lesions [15] (Fig. 5.2).

- A: asymmetry
- B: border
- C: color
- D: diameter
- E: evolving

A	Asymmetrical Lesion
B	Border irregularity
C	Color Variation
D	Diameter >6mm
E	Evolving

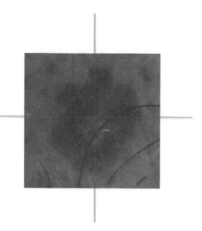

Fig. 5.2 ABCDEs of melanoma, many of which are exhibited in the example shown

Fig. 5.3 Melanoma in situ, with several ABCDE criteria (Photo courtesy of Dr. Wilfred Lumbang)

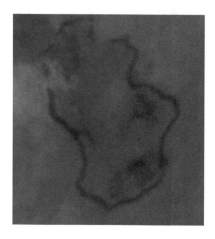

Data suggests the above criteria are clinically relevant in the recognition of MIS cases. A formal study of MIS clinical characteristics showed the following: 87% were asymmetric, 88% had an irregular border, 98% had nonuniform pigment, and 77% were larger than 6 millimeters (mm) [16] (Figs. 5.3 and 5.4). The size of the lesion appears to be the least sensitive of the criteria. In comparing clinical characteristics of MIS with invasive melanoma, a higher percentage of invasive melanoma is greater than 6 mm [17]. Diameter may be more relevant for invasive melanoma diagnosis, but one should remain suspicious of any pigmented lesion that displays many of the listed features, regardless of size.

Fig. 5.4 Melanoma in situ
(Photo courtesy of Dr.
Matthew Livingood)

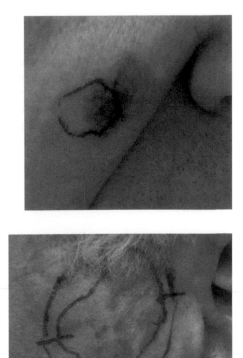

Fig. 5.5 Lentigo maligna
on sun-damaged skin

Lentigo Maligna

Lentigo maligna (LM) is a subcategory of MIS found exclusively on sun-damaged skin [3, 9, 11, 18] (Fig. 5.5). LM can be difficult to diagnose clinically because it is often found in the background of solar elastosis and dyspigmentation [9]. It tends to be fairly indolent and slow growing, progressing through a radial growth phase before it begins vertical growth or invasion [3, 11, 18]. Once a lentigo maligna becomes invasive, it is termed a lentigo maligna melanoma. Microscopically, LM can be very challenging to distinguish from severely sun-damaged skin because of pathologic similarities. Lentigo maligna is overwhelmingly found on the face with over 90% being found on the head and scalp in a series of 201 lesions [9]. Over half of these cases of lentigo maligna were found on the cheek [9]. LM was found to be larger when present among a background of freckles and other dyspigmentation [9], resulting in more difficult treatment choices.

Amelanotic MIS

Rarely, lesions of melanoma can be devoid of pigment. This is termed amelanotic and remains one of the most challenging lesions to recognize. Fortunately, amelanotic melanomas are thought to compromise only 1.8–8.1% of melanomas [19]. Diagnosis of amelanotic MIS is rare due to the delay that is often seen before identifying the lesion. Tumors are generally deeper at the time of the original diagnosis [18, 19].

Acral Lentiginous MIS

Like invasive melanoma, MIS can also be found on acral surfaces. In a recent cohort of 149 patients all with acral lentiginous melanoma, 20 (13%) were noted to be stage 0 consistent with acral MIS [20]. This subtype is noted to be more hyperplastic on histology with occasional prominent dendrites [21]. Of note, acral melanoma is the most common melanoma seen in patients of Asian and African descent. Similar to the amelanotic subtype, acral melanomas are often diagnosed at a more advanced stage [22].

Differential Diagnosis

- Melanoma in situ (Table 5.3) [9, 11, 15]

Table 5.3 Differential diagnosis for melanoma in situ

Solar lentigo
Pigmented actinic keratosis
Pigmented basal cell carcinoma
Seborrheic keratosis
Benign melanocytic nevus
Atypical (dysplastic) nevus
Ephelis
Benign lichen planus-like keratosis
Blue nevus
Recurrent nevus
Halo nevus
Extramammary Paget's disease
Bowen's disease
Ink spot lentigo (reticulated lentigo)

Diagnosis

The most up-to-date NCCN guidelines recommend excisional biopsy with 1–3 mm of clear margins if possible to make the diagnosis of melanoma. This can be performed by elliptical incision, punch biopsy, or deep shave (saucerization) biopsy [14]. However, they do recognize that there are situations when this is not always feasible (certain anatomic areas and larger-sized lesions) or necessary (low clinical suspicion) [14]. A 2012 article by Silverstein and Mariwalla provides an excellent summary of appropriate situations for each type of biopsy as well and pros and cons of each technique [23]. The gold standard should always be elliptical excision when possible. Nevertheless, there are advantages to a deep shave (saucerization) biopsy. This procedure is quick, low-cost, easy to execute, and safe and does not require a patient return visit for suture removal [23, 24]. The dogma exists that deep shave biopsy has a tendency to transect the base of a pigmented lesion, therefore making it impossible to determine the precise depth of the lesion. However, recent research suggests that deep shave biopsy consistently provides a negative deep margin, especially when the intent of the biopsy is for complete removal [24]. In general punch biopsy has a much lower rate of clear margins, and the possibility exists that an accurate representation of the sample might not be obtained [23, 24]. Some pigmented lesions are too large for complete removal with biopsy, especially large lentigo maligna lesions on the face. In this situation, one option is the use of scouting punch biopsies to evaluate more of the worrisome pigmented lesion. When using this technique, select several areas to perform a punch biopsy [25]. All of these are evaluated for histopathology (Fig. 5.6). This allows the clinician to evaluate a larger percentage of the lesion without entire removal.

Fig. 5.6 Large pigmented lesion being evaluated using scouting biopsy technique

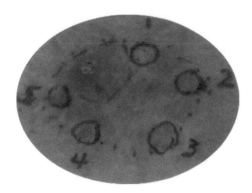

Prognosis

Several large studies have examined the prognosis of MIS and invasive melanoma and have found that 10-year mortality increases as thickness of the tumor increases [2, 26]. In over 93,000 cases of MIS diagnosed from 1973 to 2011, the overall melanoma-specific mortality was 0.6% with a mean follow-up of over 5 years [2]. Notably, this cohort of patients had the same life expectancy as the general population [2].

Pathology

Melanoma in situ is a diagnosis based solely on histopathologic interpretation. It is defined as a proliferation of atypical melanocytes confined to the epidermis without any evidence of dermal invasion [21] (Fig. 5.7a, b). This can only be determined with evaluation under the microscope. Criteria for histolopathologic diagnosis have been defined and can be found in Table 5.4 [21]. Differentiating lentigo maligna from surrounding chronically sun-damaged skin with background pigmentation is a diagnostic challenge. In this situation, it can be very challenging to differentiate lentigo maligna versus atypical melanocytic proliferation (AMP) [21]. Ackerman attempted to define 12 criteria to aid in the distinction of MIS/LM versus AMP (Table 5.5) [27]. A review of the criteria revealed that the most helpful criteria to distinguish the two entities were the presence of nesting and irregular distance between melanocytes and upward pagetoid scatter [28]. Imunnohistochemistry (IHC) can be helpful when making a diagnosis of MIS. Historically, Melan-A and melanoma antigen recognized by T-cells 1 (MART-1) have been used to aid in the diagnosis of MIS [29]. Both of these IHC stains recognize cytoplasmic proteins and have been discovered to overestimate the number of melanocytes. This is thought to be due to concomitant staining of pigmented keratinocytes as well as the dendrites of melanocytes [29, 30]. One study looking at the staining of actinic keratosis with Melan-A revealed diffuse staining throughout the actinic keratosis. Interestingly, Melan-A was also found to stain severely sun-damaged skin adjacent to the actinic keratosis [30]. One can imagine how this could lead to overdiagnosis of MIS especially given the issues detailed above. SOX10 and microphthalmia transcription factor 1 (MITF-1) are both nuclear stains that are increasing in popularity for the diagnosis of MIS [21]. Bonaccorsi and colleagues evaluated the usefulness of SOX10 and MITF-1 in evaluation of MIS versus actinic keratosis. They demonstrated reliable staining of MIS with both IHC stains, with MITF-1 being slightly more specific [29] (Fig. 5.8a–c). They also tested both stains on histologically proven actinic keratosis and found no adjacent staining of pigmented keratinocytes [29]. This allows a distinction between melanocytes of MIS and keratinocytes found in sun-damaged skin often found in the background of MIS and LM. Still, it is important to note that even with established criteria, IHC stains, and specialty

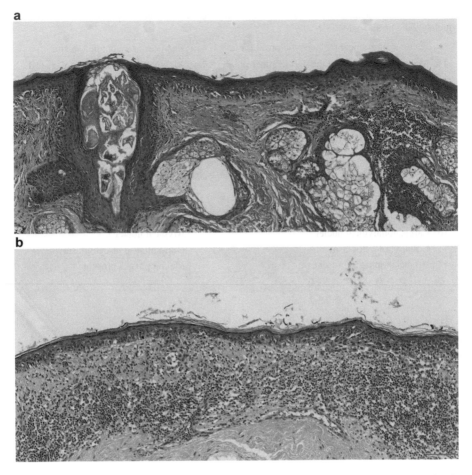

Fig. 5.7 (**a**, **b**) Representative dermatopathology images of melanoma in situ stained with classic hematoxylin and eosin stain (H/E stain) (Photo courtesy of Dr. Jeffrey Zwerner)

Table 5.4 Histopathologic criteria for diagnosis of melanoma in situ

Poor circumscription
Asymmetry

Predominance of individual melanocytes compared to nests with:
     Confluence along the dermoepidermal junction (DEJ)
     Effacement of rete ridges
     Pagetoid upward scatter

Nests of atypical melanocytes with
     Confluence
     Variability in size and shape
     Consumption of the epidermis

Haphazard distribution
Involvement of adnexa

Table 5.5 Histopathologic features to help distinguish melanoma in situ versus atypical melanocytic proliferation

	Features of atypical melanocytic proliferation	Features of melanoma in situ
1	Melanocytes mostly at the dermoepidermal junction (DEJ)	Melanocytes with pagetoid spread
2	Equidistant melanocytes	Asymmetric distance between melanocyte
3	Superficial descent down adnexa	Deep descent down adnexa
4	Non-confluence along DEJ	Confluence of melanocytes along DEJ
5	No nesting	Early nests of melanocytes
6	Uniform pigmentation	Nonuniform pigmentation
7	Preserved rete ridges	Flattened rete ridges
8	Uniform nuclei	Pleomorphic nuclei
9	Rare dendritic melanocytes	Dendritic melanocytes
10	Large, nonatypical nuclei	Atypical nuclei
11	Collapse of cytoplasm	Non-collapse of cytoplasm
12	No melanophages present	Melanophages present

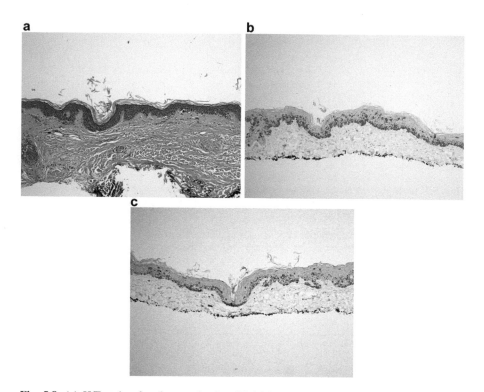

Fig. 5.8 (a) H/E stain of melanoma in situ. (b) Melanoma in situ stained with MART-1. (c) Melanoma in situ stained with SOX10 (Photos courtesy of Dr. Jeffrey Zwerner)

dermatopathology training, this remains one of the most challenging diagnostic dilemmas faced by our dermatopathology colleagues.

Treatment

The most recent NCCN guidelines on melanoma from January 2017 recommend wide excision of MIS with 0.5 centimeter (cm) to 1.0 cm margins if possible [14]. A sidenote explains, for large MIS or LM, margins of greater than 0.5 cm might be required and that it is reasonable to consider techniques that allow for complete examination of the margins [14]. There is inconsistency in the margins taken for MIS among dermatologists, reflected in a recent survey of over 550 providers [31]. There are numerous treatment options including surgery, topical therapy, and radiation (Fig. 5.9). These options include [21]:

- Wide local excision
- Staged excision (also known as "slow Mohs")

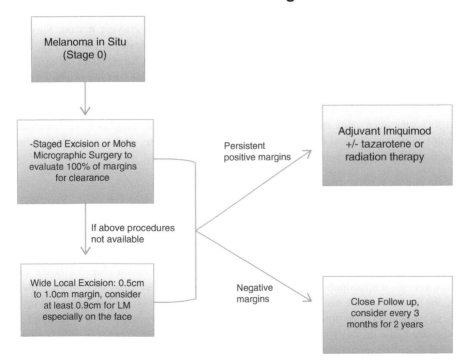

Fig. 5.9 Treatment algorithm for melanoma in situ

- Mohs micrographic surgery (MMS)
- Imiquimod
- Radiation therapy

Regardless of the surgical method used to remove MIS, it is essential to send the excision specimen or central debulking specimen (a component of a staged excision) for permanent vertical sectioning and histopathologic evaluation. A percentage of tumors originally thought to be MIS are upstaged to invasive melanoma upon examination of the entire specimen. A recent study examining 624 cases of MIS found 24 (4%) specimens that were upstaged after removal [32]. A recent review article cites rates ranging from 5% to 29%, with an average of 19% of lesions being upstaged after removal [21]. It is important to note that shave biopsy for diagnosis appears to lead to a higher rate of upstaging [33].

Wide Local Excision

Historically, wide local excision with appropriate margins has been the treatment of choice for MIS. The NCCN guidelines currently recommend 0.5–1.0 cm margins for removal [14]. Recent data suggests that 0.5 cm may be inadequate and more appropriate margins approach 0.8–0.9 cm [34]. Recurrence rates with 0.5 cm margins are reported to range from 6% to 20% [35]. A large 2012 study examined margin needed for clearance of 1120 MIS treated over a 26-year period. Surgical margins of 0.9 cm were required to clear 98.9% of MIS lesions. Conversely, only 86% of tumors were cleared with 0.6 cm margins [34]. A large series of head and neck MIS required surgical margins of 15 mm to clear 97% of tumors [36]. These larger margins may be attributed to subclinical spread often seen with LM. On the other hand, a study that evaluated only MIS on non-sun-exposed sites revealed 100% clearance rates in 155 tumors excised with 5 mm margins [37]. Clearance rates vary widely, and one should consider the size, site, and type of MIS when considering simple excision as a treatment for MIS [21].

Staged Excision ("Slow Mohs")

Staged excision describes a technique where the central tumor is outlined, followed by an outer rim of a few millimeters encircling the entire tumor (Fig. 5.10a–d). The central tumor specimen is sent for permanent bread loaf vertical sectioning. This is done to ensure there are no areas of invasion that would result in upstaging to invasive melanoma. The outer rim of tissue is then cut into several pieces depending on the size of the tumor. The pieces are laid en face and the entire outer margin is evaluated under the microscope. This technique is similar to MMS given the fact that the entire outer margin is examined. Most clinicians send these specimens for

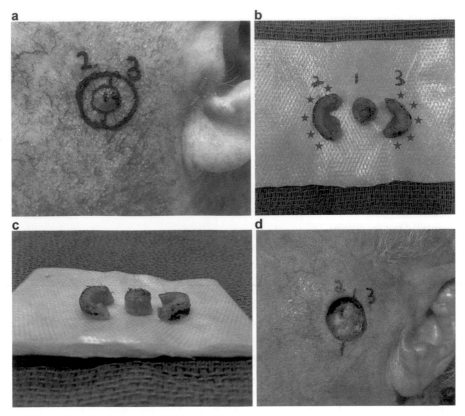

Fig. 5.10 (**a**) Preoperative markings for planned staged excision: section 1 will be sent for vertical frozen sections to ensure there is no invasive component; sections 2 and 3 will be prepared and sectioned so the entire outer margin is evaluated. (**b**) Sections 2 and 3 will be cut parallel to the outer edge (blue stars) to evaluate 100% of the outer margins (also known as en face processing). (**c**) Another view of the previous photo, to reiterate the tissue will be cut parallel to the outer edge which is inked black in this photo. (**d**) Postoperative defect, which will be left unrepaired until pathology is evaluated and margins are clear; if margins are still involved, another margin will be taken but only in the positive section (Photos courtesy of Dr. William Stebbins)

permanent sections, and the patient's wound is not repaired until a report is generated verifying clear margins, hence the term "slow Mohs." Recurrence rates are lower for staged excision compared to wide local excision, likely due to complete examination of the outer margin [38]. A larger cohort with 239 tumors treated had a recurrence rate of 1.7% with 32 months of follow-up [38]. The percentage of disease-free patients after treatment with staged excision ranges from 95.2% to 100% with variable follow-up [38]. There are other variations of staged excision most notably the square technique or spaghetti technique [39, 40] (Fig. 5.11). With this technique only the outer 2–3 mm edge is excised and sent for en face histopathologic evaluation. Once the margins are deemed clear, the central portion is excised and submitted, and the defect is repaired [39, 40].

Fig. 5.11 Staged excision, "spaghetti technique" – the central tumor is circled with a 1 cm margin; outside that margin is a 3 mm rim of tissue, which will be excised and separated into 12 separate pieces; they will be processed en face and evaluated by a dermatopathologist (by cutting the outer rim into 12 sections, it allows for more exact localization of positive margins if needed). Once the margins are clear, then the central tumor with the 1 cm margin will be excised (Photo courtesy of Dr. Wilfred Lumbang)

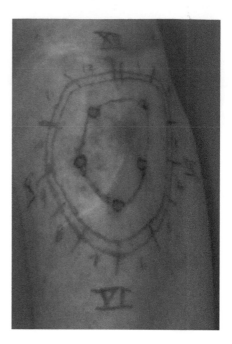

Mohs Micrographic Surgery (MMS)

Over the last several years, the use of MMS for MIS has increased dramatically [41]. Historically, recurrence rates for MMS have ranged from 0% to 10% [21]. When using MMS for the treatment of MIS, several factors need to be considered. It is integral for the Mohs surgeon and the histotechnician to have experience due to the difficulty of processing and reading melanocytes under frozen section [21, 42]. To help better delineate melanocytes on frozen sections, many Mohs labs utilize IHC stains such as MART-1. A large study using MART-1 and MMS reported on 863 primary MIS lesions for which there were only 3 recurrences (0.35%) with an average follow-up of over 3.5 years. This group also treated 119 recurrent MIS lesions and only had 1 recurrence (0.41%) [43]. The margins required for clearance from this large cohort of patients is significant. For MIS on the head and neck, 0.9 cm was required for clearance of 97% of tumors. Margins of 1.2 cm and 1.5 cm were required to clear 97% of lesions on the hands/feet and head/neck, respectively [43]. Another study recently published also looked at recurrence rates following MMS utilizing MART-1. Out of 436 MIS lesions treated with MMS, there were 2 recurrences (0.45%) [44]. Both of these larger studies showed recurrence rates significantly lower than wide local excision [43, 44].

Imiquimod

Imiquimod is an immunomodulator activating toll-like receptor 7 to induce a local immune reaction targeting MIS [15]. It is FDA approved for the treatment of genital warts, actinic keratosis, and superficial basal cell carcinoma [15]. Although it is considered off-label, imiquimod is used in the treatment of LM. Treatment regimens vary widely in frequency of application as well as duration of treatment [21]. Success of treatment differs with clearance rates ranging from 0% to 100% [21, 45]. A recent systematic review evaluated all lesions of LM in the literature that were treated with imiquimod as monotherapy. A total of 347 LM were included. Histologic and clinical clearance rates were reported as 76.2% and 78.3%, respectively, with the incidence of clinical recurrence found to be 2.3% at a mean of 34 months. The analysis found that LM lesions treated for more than 60 applications (8 times higher likelihood) or greater than 5 times a week (6 times higher likelihood) were statistically more likely to result in histologic clearance [45]. Along with monotherapy, imiquimod cream is used in conjunction with other treatment modalities, especially surgical excision and tazarotene [21]. In surgical excision it is often being used as adjuvant therapy following surgery with persistent positive margins [46]. In a cohort of 21 patients with residual LM following surgery, patients were first treated with imiquimod. However, if there was no significant clinical inflammation, topical retinoid tazarotene was then added with a goal of 12 weeks of an inflammatory response. Out of 21 LM tumors treated with this regimen, 20 exhibited no recurrence at a mean of 24 months [46]. Tazarotene can be added to help penetration of imiquimod, thereby increasing inflammation and theoretically improving clearance rates [47]. A randomized controlled trial comparing application of imiquimod alone versus imiquimod and tazarotene found that the combination was associated with a higher percentage of grade 2 inflammation, which coincided with a higher rate of histologically cleared LM tumors [47]. When thinking about imiquimod therapy, note that its use is off-label, and monotherapy results in much lower clearance rates than the previously mentioned surgical techniques [21, 47]. Imiquimod can be prescribed to treat MIS in cosmetically sensitive areas or in patients with contraindications to surgery.

Radiation Therapy

Historically, radiation therapy has been used sparingly in the treatment of MIS. Published rates of recurrence range anywhere from 0% to 20% depending on the size of the study [21]. A recent study out of the Melanoma Institute in Australia reviewed studies from 1941 to 2009 and identified 349 patients treated with primary radiotherapy for lentigo maligna that met inclusion criteria. Out of the 349 cases, there were 18 reported cases of recurrence (5%) along with 5 cases that progressed to lentigo maligna melanoma [48]. They also published treatment recommendations based on literature review and their own clinical experience. These recommendations include [48]:

• Treatment field to extend 1 cm beyond visible lesion.
• Treat to a depth of 5 mm.
• Need at least 35 gray (Gy), 50 Gy given for adjuvant therapy, and 54 Gy for primary treatment; do not exceed 60 Gy due to risk of side effects.

  – Given in 2–4 Gy intervals

Side effects are notable and include hypopigmentation, telangiectasias, alopecia, decreased skin elasticity, radiation dermatitis, and an increased future risk for other nonmelanoma skin cancers [21, 48]. Radiation therapy should be considered a second-line therapy to be used in situations where primary surgery is not feasible or as adjuvant therapy when it is not possible to obtain clear margins.

Follow-Up

Patients with invasive melanoma should be followed every 3 months for the first 2–3 years and then every 6 months thereafter [14, 49]. Such close follow-up has been shown to lead to thinner, less invasive subsequent melanomas [50]. Thinner melanomas correspond to a lower stage classification; therefore, close follow-up also leads to improved prognosis [50]. However, screening guidelines for MIS are not as well established, mostly due to the excellent prognosis of patients diagnosed with MIS. Patients with a history of MIS are at an increased risk of development of invasive melanoma when compared to the general population [2, 51]. A recent study examined the risk of developing a subsequent melanoma after an original diagnosis of melanoma versus MIS [52]. The authors reviewed the SEER database from 1973 to 2011 and found roughly 56,000 cases of MIS and 113,000 cases of invasive melanoma [52]. Furthermore, 6.5% or roughly 11,000 patients developed a second melanoma [52]. Interestingly, the study found a higher risk of all types of subsequent melanoma in the MIS group over the invasive melanoma group. They also found the risk of developing a second invasive melanoma to be roughly the same in the melanoma in situ group [52]. Although MIS is a disease with excellent prognosis, the argument can be made that these patients should be followed just as closely as invasive melanoma patients, given this equivalent risk of a second melanoma. Close follow-up leads to earlier diagnosis of subsequent melanomas and a better prognosis. Patients with a diagnosis of MIS are at a higher risk of invasive melanoma than the general population and have virtually the same risk of developing a subsequent melanoma as a patient diagnosed with a previous invasive melanoma. Practitioners should consider following MIS patients every 3 months for the first 2 years and then every 6 months thereafter just as they would an invasive melanoma patient.

References

1. Rapini RP. Practical dermatopathology. 2nd ed. Edinburgh: Elsevier/Saunders; 2012. p. 450.
2. Mocellin S, Nitti D. Cutaneous melanoma in situ: translational evidence from a large population-based study. Oncologist. 2011;16(6):896–903.
3. Higgins HW 2nd, Lee KC, Galan A, Leffell DJ. Melanoma in situ: part I. Epidemiology, screening, and clinical features. J Am Acad Dermatol. 2015;73(2):181–90. quiz 91-2.
4. Coory M, Baade P, Aitken J, Smithers M, McLeod GR, Ring I. Trends for in situ and invasive melanoma in Queensland, Australia, 1982–2002. Cancer Causes Control. 2006;17(1):21–7.
5. Helvind NM, Holmich LR, Smith S, Glud M, Andersen KK, Dalton SO, et al. Incidence of in situ and invasive melanoma in Denmark from 1985 through 2012: a National Database Study of 24,059 melanoma cases. JAMA Dermatol. 2015;151(10):1087–95.
6. Welch HG, Woloshin S, Schwartz LM. Skin biopsy rates and incidence of melanoma: population based ecological study. BMJ. 2005;331(7515):481.
7. Linos E, Swetter SM, Cockburn MG, Colditz GA, Clarke CA. Increasing burden of melanoma in the United States. J Invest Dermatol. 2009;129(7):1666–74.
8. Bradford PT, Freedman DM, Goldstein AM, Tucker MA. Increased risk of second primary cancers after a diagnosis of melanoma. Arch Dermatol. 2010;146(3):265–72.
9. Wei EX, Qureshi AA, Han J, Li TY, Cho E, Lin JY, et al. Trends in the diagnosis and clinical features of melanoma in situ (MIS) in US men and women: a prospective, observational study. J Am Acad Dermatol. 2016;75(4):698–705.
10. Tiodorovic-Zivkovic D, Argenziano G, Lallas A, Thomas L, Ignjatovic A, Rabinovitz H, et al. Age, gender, and topography influence the clinical and dermoscopic appearance of lentigo maligna. J Am Acad Dermatol. 2015;72(5):801–8.
11. Lesage C, Barbe C, Le Clainche A, Lesage FX, Bernard P, Grange F. Sex-related location of head and neck melanoma strongly argues for a major role of sun exposure in cars and photoprotection by hair. J Invest Dermatol. 2013;133(5):1205.
12. Cohen LM. Lentigo maligna and lentigo maligna melanoma. J Am Acad Dermatol. 1995;33(6):923–36. quiz 37-40.
13. Australian Cancer Network Melanoma Guidelines Revision Working Party. Clinical practice guidelines for the managment of melanoma in Australia and New Zealand. Cancer Council Australia and Australian Cancer Network, Sydney and New Zealand Guidelines Group, Wellington; 2008.
14. NCCN Clinical Practice Guidelines in Oncology (NCCN Guidelines) Melanoma Version 1.2017 [web page]. 2017. www.nccn.orgJanuary. [updated January 2017].
15. Bolognia J, Jorizzo JL, Schaffer JV. Dermatology. Available from: https://www.clinicalkey.com/dura/browse/bookChapter/3-s2.0-C20101670885
16. Bartoli C, Bono A, Clemente C, Del Prato ID, Zurrida S, Cascinelli N. Clinical diagnosis and therapy of cutaneous melanoma in situ. Cancer. 1996;77(5):888–92.
17. Rosina P, Tessari G, Giordano MV, Girolomoni G. Clinical and diagnostic features of in situ melanoma and superficial spreading melanoma: a hospital based study. J Eur Acad Dermatol Venereol. 2012;26(2):153–8.
18. Ara M, Maillo C, Martin R, Grasa MP, Carapeto FJ. Recurrent lentigo maligna as amelanotic lentigo maligna melanoma. J Eur Acad Dermatol Venereol. 2002;16(5):506–10.
19. Koch SE, Lange JR. Amelanotic melanoma: the great masquerader. J Am Acad Dermatol. 2000;42(5 Pt 1):731–4.
20. Jung HJ, Kweon SS, Lee JB, Lee SC, Yun SJ. A clinicopathologic analysis of 177 acral melanomas in Koreans: relevance of spreading pattern and physical stress. JAMA Dermatol. 2013;149(11):1281–8.
21. Higgins HW 2nd, Lee KC, Galan A, Leffell DJ. Melanoma in situ: Part II. Histopathology, treatment, and clinical management. J Am Acad Dermatol. 2015;73(2):193–203; quiz −4.
22. Goydos JS, Shoen SL. Acral Lentiginous Melanoma. Cancer Treat Res. 2016;167:321–9.
23. Silverstein D, Mariwalla K. Biopsy of the pigmented lesions. Dermatol Clin. 2012;30(3):435–43.

24. Mendese G, Maloney M, Bordeaux J. To scoop or not to scoop: the diagnostic and therapeutic utility of the scoop-shave biopsy for pigmented lesions. Dermatol Surg. 2014;40(10):1077–83.
25. Appert DL, Otley CC, Phillips PK, Roenigk RK. Role of multiple scouting biopsies before Mohs micrographic surgery for extramammary Paget's disease. Dermatol Surg. 2005;31(11 Pt 1):1417–22.
26. Balch CM, Soong SJ, Gershenwald JE, Thompson JF, Reintgen DS, Cascinelli N, et al. Prognostic factors analysis of 17,600 melanoma patients: validation of the American Joint Committee on Cancer melanoma staging system. J Clin Oncol. 2001;19(16):3622–34.
27. Ackerman AB, Briggs PL, Bravo F. Differential diagnosis in dermatopathology III. Philadelphia: Lea & Febiger; 1993. pp. xii, 202.
28. Weyers W, Bonczkowitz M, Weyers I, Bittinger A, Schill WB. Melanoma in situ versus melanocytic hyperplasia in sun-damaged skin. Assessment of the significance of histopathologic criteria for differential diagnosis. Am J Dermatopathol. 1996;18(6):560–6.
29. Buonaccorsi JN, Prieto VG, Torres-Cabala C, Suster S, Plaza JA. Diagnostic utility and comparative immunohistochemical analysis of MITF-1 and SOX10 to distinguish melanoma in situ and actinic keratosis: a clinicopathological and immunohistochemical study of 70 cases. Am J Dermatopathol. 2014;36(2):124–30.
30. El Shabrawi-Caelen L, Kerl H, Cerroni L. Melan-A: not a helpful marker in distinction between melanoma in situ on sun-damaged skin and pigmented actinic keratosis. Am J Dermatopathol. 2004;26(5):364–6.
31. Charles CA, Yee VS, Dusza SW, Marghoob AA, Oliveria SA, Kopf A, et al. Variation in the diagnosis, treatment, and management of melanoma in situ: a survey of US dermatologists. Arch Dermatol. 2005;141(6):723–9.
32. Gardner KH, Hill DE, Wright AC, Brewer JD, Arpey CJ, Otley CC, et al. Upstaging from melanoma in situ to invasive melanoma on the head and neck after complete surgical resection. Dermatol Surg. 2015;41(10):1122–5.
33. Egnatios GL, Dueck AC, Macdonald JB, Laman SD, Warschaw KE, DiCaudo DJ, et al. The impact of biopsy technique on upstaging, residual disease, and outcome in cutaneous melanoma. Am J Surg. 2011;202(6):771–7; discussion 7–8.
34. Kunishige JH, Brodland DG, Zitelli JA. Surgical margins for melanoma in situ. J Am Acad Dermatol. 2012;66(3):438–44.
35. de Vries K, Greveling K, Prens LM, Munte K, Koljenovic S, van Doorn MB, et al. Recurrence rate of lentigo maligna after micrographically controlled staged surgical excision. Br J Dermatol. 2016;174(3):588–93.
36. Felton S, Taylor RS, Srivastava D. Excision margins for melanoma in situ on the head and neck. Dermatol Surg. 2016;42(3):327–34.
37. Welch A, Reid T, Knox J, Wilson ML. Excision of melanoma in situ on nonchronically sun-exposed skin using 5-mm surgical margins. J Am Acad Dermatol. 2014;71(4):834–5.
38. Abdelmalek M, Loosemore MP, Hurt MA, Hruza G. Geometric staged excision for the treatment of lentigo maligna and lentigo maligna melanoma: a long-term experience with literature review. Arch Dermatol. 2012;148(5):599–604.
39. Johnson TM, Headington JT, Baker SR, Lowe L. Usefulness of the staged excision for lentigo maligna and lentigo maligna melanoma: the "square" procedure. J Am Acad Dermatol. 1997;37(5 Pt 1):758–64.
40. Gaudy-Marqueste C, Perchenet AS, Tasei AM, Madjlessi N, Magalon G, Richard MA, et al. The "spaghetti technique": an alternative to Mohs surgery or staged surgery for problematic lentiginous melanoma (lentigo maligna and acral lentiginous melanoma). J Am Acad Dermatol. 2011;64(1):113–8.
41. Viola KV, Rezzadeh KS, Gonsalves L, Patel P, Gross CP, Yoo J, et al. National utilization patterns of Mohs micrographic surgery for invasive melanoma and melanoma in situ. J Am Acad Dermatol. 2015;72(6):1060–5.
42. Zitelli JA, Moy RL, Abell E. The reliability of frozen sections in the evaluation of surgical margins for melanoma. J Am Acad Dermatol. 1991;24(1):102–6.

43. Valentin-Nogueras SM, Brodland DG, Zitelli JA, Gonzalez-Sepulveda L, Nazario CM. Mohs micrographic surgery using MART-1 immunostain in the treatment of invasive melanoma and melanoma in situ. Dermatol Surg. 2016;42(6):733–44.
44. Etzkorn JR, Sobanko JF, Elenitsas R, Newman JG, Goldbach H, Shin TM, et al. Low recurrence rates for in situ and invasive melanomas using Mohs micrographic surgery with melanoma antigen recognized by T cells 1 (MART-1) immunostaining: tissue processing methodology to optimize pathologic staging and margin assessment. J Am Acad Dermatol. 2015;72(5):840–50.
45. Mora AN, Karia PS, Nguyen BM. A quantitative systematic review of the efficacy of imiquimod monotherapy for lentigo maligna and an analysis of factors that affect tumor clearance. J Am Acad Dermatol. 2015;73(2):205–12.
46. Pandit AS, Geiger EJ, Ariyan S, Narayan D, Choi JN. Using topical imiquimod for the management of positive in situ margins after melanoma resection. Cancer Med. 2015;4(4):507–12.
47. Hyde MA, Hadley ML, Tristani-Firouzi P, Goldgar D, Bowen GM. A randomized trial of the off-label use of imiquimod, 5%, cream with vs without tazarotene, 0.1%, gel for the treatment of lentigo maligna, followed by conservative staged excisions. Arch Dermatol. 2012;148(5):592–6.
48. Fogarty GB, Hong A, Scolyer RA, Lin E, Haydu L, Guitera P, et al. Radiotherapy for lentigo maligna: a literature review and recommendations for treatment. Br J Dermatol. 2014;170(1):52–8.
49. Marsden JR, Newton-Bishop JA, Burrows L, Cook M, Corrie PG, Cox NH, et al. Revised U.K. guidelines for the management of cutaneous melanoma 2010. Br J Dermatol. 2010;163(2):238–56.
50. DiFronzo LA, Wanek LA, Morton DL. Earlier diagnosis of second primary melanoma confirms the benefits of patient education and routine postoperative follow-up. Cancer. 2001;91(8):1520–4.
51. Balamurugan A, Rees JR, Kosary C, Rim SH, Li J, Stewart SL. Subsequent primary cancers among men and women with in situ and invasive melanoma of the skin. J Am Acad Dermatol. 2011;65(5 Suppl 1):S69–77.
52. Pomerantz H, Huang D, Weinstock MA. Risk of subsequent melanoma after melanoma in situ and invasive melanoma: a population-based study from 1973 to 2011. J Am Acad Dermatol. 2015;72(5):794–800.

Chapter 6
Melanoma

Jennifer Divine and Anna S. Clayton

Abstract Melanoma most commonly presents as a new or changing pigmented lesion on sun exposed skin. The skin cancer can be categorized into varying subtypes based on its clinical appearance and anatomical location. The prognosis is similar amongst the subtypes with tumor thickness as the most important factor for survival. Melanoma staging depends upon the patient's symptoms, clinical exam and clinician's index of suspicion. Surgery is the first line treatment for localized melanoma. Advances in tumor genetics and immunology have led to the development of targeted therapies for metastatic disease.

Keywords Invasive · Melanoma · Nevi · Genetic mutations · *BRAF* · *MAPK* · *MEK* · *NRAS* · *Kit CDKN2A* · Risk factors · UV radiation · Dysplastic nevi · ABCD · Dermoscopy · Melanoma in situ · Nodular melanoma · Metastatic melanoma · Histology · Immunohistochemistry · Breslow depth · Staging · TNM · Prognosis · Survival · Sentinel lymph node · Wide local excision · Margins · Radiation therapy · Chemotherapy · Adjuvant therapy · Immunotherapy · Cytokines · Cancer vaccine · Oncolytic viral therapy · Targeted therapy

Introduction

Melanoma is the most lethal skin cancer. Melanoma most commonly presents on the skin but can arise in any location where melanocytes are present, including mucosa, uvea, and leptomeninges. Melanoma can present as a new or changing nevus. The prognosis depends upon how deeply the tumor invades the underlying dermis and subcutaneous structures. Invasive lesions carry the risk of metastasis and increased morbidity and mortality.

J. Divine (✉)
Divine Dermatology and Surgical Institute, Fort Collins, CO, USA

A. S. Clayton
Dermatology, Vanderbilt University of Medicine, Nashville, TN, USA

© Springer International Publishing AG, part of Springer Nature 2018   117
A. Hanlon (ed.), *A Practical Guide to Skin Cancer*,
https://doi.org/10.1007/978-3-319-74903-7_6

Epidemiology

Global incidence rates of melanoma are rising. In the United States, non-Hispanic whites account for over 95% of disease occurrences, but minority groups are more likely to present with advanced-stage disease [1]. Melanoma is more common in men than women. In patients less than 40 years old, women have a greater melanoma incidence than men likely due to differences in UV exposure and hormonal factors [1, 2]. Melanoma is one of the most common cancers in young adults and has an average age of onset nearly a decade before most solid organ malignancies [3]. With improved screening, incidence rates of thin melanomas <1 mm are increasing faster than thick lesions. Despite earlier detection, death rates from melanoma are increasing for white men, those aged >65 years, and for thin lesions. Death rates have stabilized for younger age groups and thick lesions [4].

Pathogenesis

Melanoma pathogenesis is traced to changes in copies of DNA and several distinct genomic aberrations based upon body location and variations in intensity and duration of UV exposure [5]. The mitogen-activated protein kinase (*MAPK*) pathway plays a key role in normal melanocyte function and melanoma transformation. The most common genetic alteration, present in 40–60% of all melanomas, is a single-codon substitution: V600E of the *BRAF* gene. This results in subsequent dysregulation of *MAPK* signaling pathway leading to cellular proliferation, growth, and migration [6]. *NRAS* lies just upstream of *BRAF* in the *MAPK* pathway and is the second most common mutation. *NRAS* and *BRAF* are predominant mutations in intermittently sun-exposed skin [5]. *CDKN2A* gene encodes downstream p16 tumor suppressor protein which plays an inhibitory role in the *MAPK* pathway. Mutation in the *CDKN2A* gene is the cause of rare cases of inherited familial melanoma but may also be acquired [7]. *KIT* gene encodes tyrosine kinase receptors which is the first step in *MAPK* and *P13K* signaling and plays a critical role in melanoma of chronically sun-exposed skin, mucosa, and uvea [8]. Other key mutations identified lie in the *GNAQ* and *ERBB4* gene [9]. These discoveries led to the development of molecular targeted therapies such as the BRAF kinase inhibitors dabrafenib and vemurafenib.

Risk Factors

Risk factors for melanoma are environmental and genetic. UV radiation is a known carcinogen responsible for over 85% of melanomas. Having more than five sunburns at any period in life doubles the risk of melanoma, while daily use of SPF 15 or above decreases the risk of invasive melanoma by 73% [10–12]. Intermittent intense UV exposure, often associated with shirtless recreational activities, increases the risk of melanoma on the trunk. Chronic lower level and continuous occupational UV exposure increases risk on the head and neck [1]. The risk of melanoma increases with the number of indoor tanning sessions and younger age when indoor tanning behavior starts [13].

The tendency to burn, light skin, light eyes, and light hair (especially red hair) are all phenotypic traits that increase susceptibility to UV radiation and therefore increase the risk of melanoma. Freckling and a large number of nevi indicate past UV exposure. Personal history of melanoma is a strong predictor for subsequent melanoma. Family history of melanoma has a twofold effect correlating with similar skin phenotype as well as an inborn genetic tendency for melanoma. Patients with dysplastic nevus syndrome (aka familial atypical multiple mole-melanoma syndrome) exemplify the strong impact of genetics. Inheritance may be autosomal dominant or sporadic. Two melanoma susceptibility genes are identified in melanoma-prone families: *CDKN2A* and more rarely *CDK4*. There are numerous remaining melanoma families without either of these mutations, so more research is needed [14, 15]. Melanoma in children, people with darker skin tones, and the existence of non-cutaneous melanomas (in the eye, mouth, nasal cavity, vagina, and anogenital locations) point to further unidentified genetic and possible environmental causes that require more research.

The immune system plays an important role in melanoma development and treatment. Immunosuppressed patients have an increased risk of developing melanoma, especially iatrogenically immunosuppressed solid organ transplant recipients and leukemia patients. Appropriately activated $CD8^+$ cytotoxic T cells recognize melanoma antigens and kill tumor cells resulting in complete or incomplete tumor regression. $CD4^+$ helper cells and antibodies also play key roles in host immunity to melanoma. Exploiting these host immune responses is the basis for immunotherapy [16, 17].

Clinical Presentation

Melanoma has a broad clinical presentation. Most commonly, melanoma presents on sun-exposed skin as a changing nevus or a new, changing pigmented lesion. First introduced in 1985, the ABCD acronym represented clinical features for melanoma diagnosis. Asymmetry (A), border irregularity (B), color variability (C), and diameter greater than 6 mm (D) are associated with worrisome clinical features for melanoma [18]. Diameter is a controversial parameter as melanomas can be smaller than 6 mm. Later, E was added to the acronym for evolution as a changing lesion is concerning [19]. The ABCDE of melanoma helped remind the public of melanoma's features but is not inclusive of all pigmented tumors. The acronym was expanded further to include elevated, firm (F), and growing(G) to encompass clinical features for nodular and amelanotic melanomas. Grob et al. observed that an

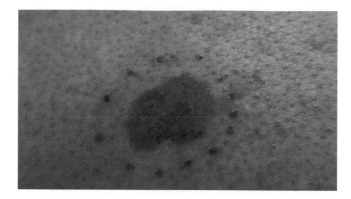

Fig. 6.1 Superficial spreading melanoma (Photo courtesy of Anna Dewan, MD)

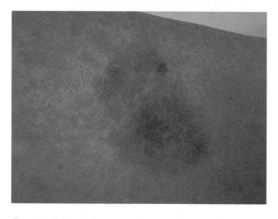

Fig. 6.2 Lentigo maligna melanoma (Photo courtesy of Darrel Ellis, MD)

individual's nevi resemble one another, and the clinically different or "ugly duckling" nevus is worrisome for melanoma [20]. For instance, a small, dark nevus is an outlier among a field of large, light brown nevi, the patient's signature nevi. The "ugly duckling" sign is especially helpful in evaluating patients with multiple nevi including familial melanoma syndrome.

The four most common types of invasive melanoma include superficial spreading (Fig. 6.1), nodular (Fig. 6.2), lentigo maligna (Fig. 6.3), and acral lentiginous melanoma (Fig. 6.4). Most invasive melanomas arise from melanoma in situ, a tumor with malignant melanocytes localized to the epidermis and/or hair follicle epithelium (Chapter 5). After a prolonged horizontal growth phase, melanoma in situ can transform into a vertical growth phase leading to invasive lentigo maligna, superficial spreading, or acral lentiginous subtypes. Clinical indications of invasion include areas of induration or a firm papule within the lesion.

Nodular melanoma grows quickly in a vertical manner and often appears as a dome-shaped, blue, black, or red firm papule most commonly on the trunk, head, or neck. Nodular melanoma accounts for 10–15% of melanomas but is responsible for over 40% of melanoma deaths. Median Breslow depth at the time of diagnosis is

Fig. 6.3 Nodular
melanoma (Photo courtesy
of Zachary Jones, MD)

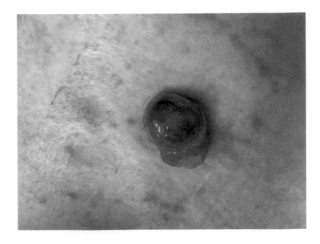

Fig. 6.4 Acral lentiginous
melanoma (Source:
Bristow IR, Acland
K. Acral lentiginous
melanoma of the foot and
ankle: A case series and
review of the literature.
Journal of Foot and Ankle
Research. 2008;1:11,
Fig. 1, Open Access under
the Creative Commons
Attribution License 2.0)

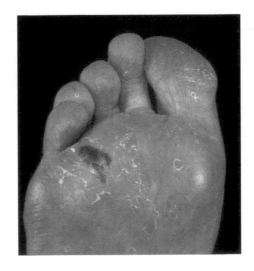

significantly greater (2.6 mm) than superficial spreading melanoma (0.6 mm) [21].
Breslow depth and ulceration at the time of diagnosis are the most critical factors
affecting prognosis of localized melanoma [22]. Nodular melanoma forming within
giant congenital nevi usually begins as a deep dermal process resulting in poor
survival [23].

Less common melanoma types include amelanotic melanoma (Fig. 6.5), mucosal melanoma, desmoplastic and neurotropic melanoma, and nail matrix melanoma
(Fig. 6.6). Amelanotic melanoma lacks pigment and presents as a pink to erythematous macule or patch. Mucosal melanoma can present in the mouth, nasopharynx,
and vagina. Desmoplastic and neurotropic melanoma can present as a flesh colored

Fig. 6.5 Amelanotic
melanoma (Clinical photo
of amelanotic melanoma
with adjacent seborrheic
keratosis)

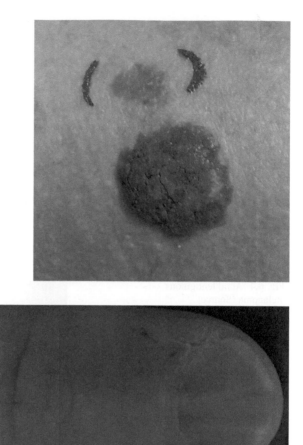

Fig. 6.6 Nail matrix
melanoma

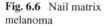

or pink to pigmented firm nodule. Desmoplastic and neurotropic melanoma can
have an overlying lentigo maligna. Nail matrix melanoma presents as new or evolving melanonychia. Involvement of the nail cuticle is a worrisome feature for
melanoma.

Diagnostic Techniques

Dermoscopy is an emerging field and has aided dermatologist in separating benign
from malignant lesions. Regular use of dermoscopy helps reveal malignant features
that are not visible to the naked eye leading to earlier melanoma diagnosis while
simultaneously decreasing excision of benign lesions if reassuring features are seen

[24]. Features suggesting invasion are asymmetry along two axes, two or more colors, and pseudopods [25]. Nodular melanomas are more likely to have symmetric shape and pigment network as seen clinically but may have large vessels, predominant peripheral vessels, homogenous blue pigmentation, blue-white veil, black color, pink color, and milky red-pink areas [26].

When malignancy is suspected, various biopsy techniques are employed. The American Academy of Dermatology guidelines state that the preferred biopsy technique is narrow excisional biopsy that encompasses the entire breadth of the lesion with clinically negative margins to the depth sufficient to ensure the lesion is not transected. This may be accomplished by elliptical or punch excision with sutures or shave removal to depth below the anticipated plane of lesion. While no one option is more correct, the outcome should always be to provide the pathologist with the entirety of the lesion (usually extending 1–3 mm past clinically evident pigment) to obtain the most correct and complete diagnosis to best guide patient care. Guidelines further state that partial sampling (incision biopsy) is acceptable in select clinical circumstances: facial or acral location, low clinical suspicion or uncertainty of diagnosis, or very large lesions [27].

Histology

Histologic examination of suspected melanoma is required to differentiate from clinical mimickers (solar lentigo, seborrheic keratosis, thrombosed hemangioma, dermatofibroma, pigmented actinic keratosis, pigmented squamous cell carcinoma, and pigmented basal cell carcinoma). Melanoma is defined by an increased number of atypical, pleomorphic, single or nested melanocytes. The changes range from extremely subtle to profound. Differentiation from dysplastic nevus, which also has atypical melanocytes, and from benign junctional melanocytic hyperplasia of sun-damaged skin, which has an increased number of single-cell but relatively normal-appearing melanocytes, remains a challenge and results in significant variability in pathologist interpretation [28–30]. When invasive lesions are arising from melanoma in situ, an asymmetric, poorly circumscribed proliferation of melanocytes of varying size and shape, often larger than their benign counterpart with abundant eosinophilic and finely granular cytoplasm, is seen in the overlying epidermis often extending far beyond the dermal component. Less often the cells are small or spindle-shaped. The melanocytes grow in linear arrays of single cells with occasional irregular and confluent nesting and uneven distribution along the dermal-epidermal junction (Fig. 6.7). Upward extension in the epidermis, referred to as pagetoid spread, and downward migration into adnexal structures are other indicators of malignancy (Fig. 6.8).

Compared to the wide lateral extension of epidermal tumor present in invasive melanoma arising from melanoma in situ, nodular melanomas have a well-defined overlying epidermal involvement that does not extend past the dermal component. This correlates with the clinical exam. Ulceration may be encountered. A complete

Fig. 6.7 Invasive
superficial spreading
melanoma (Photo courtesy
of Jeffrey Zwerner, MD,
PhD)

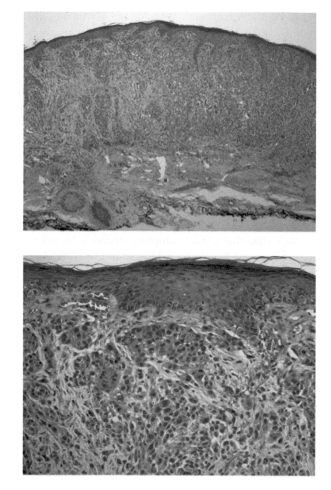

Fig. 6.8 Invasive
superficial spreading
melanoma (Photo courtesy
of Jeffrey Zwerner, MD,
PhD)

lack of epidermal involvement raises concerns for a metastatic lesion. Otherwise, the invasive components are indistinguishable. Nests of melanocytes that do not mature with increasing depth characterize dermal invasion. In benign compound and intradermal nevi, the size of the nests and size of the nuclei taper with depth down to lymphocyte-sized single cells at the base. In contrast, melanocytes at the base of an invasive melanoma remain in large nests and sheets with the same large nuclei and abundant cytoplasm seen in the more superficial portion. The Breslow depth is measured in millimeters from the granular layer of the epidermis (or the surface of ulceration) to the deepest area of tumor invasion [31]. Mitotic activity varies widely and necrotic melanocytes can be present. An asymmetrical lymphocytic inflammatory infiltrate supports the diagnosis of melanoma. It can be brisk, mild, or even absent. Areas of regression might be identified. Pleomorphic spindle-shaped cells, epithelioid cells, and balloon cells can all be seen in a single lesion [32]. Structured pathology reporting protocols aim to improve clinical management,

Table 6.1 College of
American Pathologists
melanoma reporting protocol

Procedure
Specimen laterality
Tumor site
Tumor size
Macroscopic satellite nodules
[a]Macroscopic pigmentation
Histologic type
Maximum tumor thickness
[a]Anatomic level
Ulceration
Margins
Mitotic rate
Microsatellitosis
Lymph-vascular invasion
[a]Perineural invasion
[a]Tumor-infiltrating lymphocytes
[a]Tumor regression
[a]Growth phase
Lymph nodes (only if present in specimen)
TNM staging

[a]Data elements are not required. However, these elements may be clinically important but are not yet validated or regularly used in patient management

data collection, and research worldwide. In the United States, the College of American Pathologists encourages all pathologists to include details shown in Table 6.1 in every melanoma report.

A wide spectrum of histologic morphology of melanoma promotes the use and development of immunohistochemistry to distinguish it from the many mimickers and aid in differentiating benign from malignant melanocytic proliferations. Histologic differential diagnosis of melanoma includes numerous malignant entities including carcinomas like neuroendocrine tumors, sarcomas, lymphomas, and germ cell tumors, as well as a variety of benign tumors. S100 is a widely used marker with excellent sensitivity for melanoma but poor specificity, staining nerve sheath, myoepithelial, adipocyte, and Langerhans cell tumors. It is the most sensitive marker for desmoplastic melanoma [33]. HMB-45, a monoclonal antibody to melanoma, is less sensitive but more specific than S100 and can be used to distinguish benign from malignant melanocytic lesions [34]. MelanA/MART1 is highly sensitive and specific for melanocytes but stains benign and malignant cells alike. Ki-67, a stain for active cellular proliferation, remains the most useful stain in distinguishing benign from malignant melanocytes [35]. Some studies suggest that the density of

Ki-67 immunoreactivity may serve as a prognostic indicator for metastasis [36]. Other less commonly used markers include tyrosinase, MITF, NKI/C3, and vimentin.

Staging and Prognosis

The American Joint Committee on Cancer (AJCC) published the eighth edition of the melanoma staging system in 2017 [37]. The updated staging system incorporates the seventh edition with new evidence-based recommendations. The staging system includes primary tumor (T) characteristics, regional lymph node (N), and distant metastatic sites (M) to determine the patient's prognosis. Primary tumor thickness and histopathologic evidence of ulceration determine the tumor (T) classification (Table 6.2). Tx and T0 were added to the primary tumor staging in the eighth addition. Tx designates when the primary tumor thickness cannot be assessed and T0 when there is no evidence of a primary tumor. The tumor mitotic rate is an important prognostic factor in all tumor categories but is no longer included in the staging system. T1 tumors were subdivided in the eighth edition to incorporate differences in melanoma-specific survival in patients with thin melanomas [38]. Regional lymph node involvement is classified as not clinically present but found microscopically or clinically detected and confirmed histologically (Table 6.3). The specific size of metastasis is no longer associated with lymph node staging.

Table 6.2 American Joint Committee on Cancer eighth edition melanoma staging guidelines

Primary tumor (T)		
T classification	Thickness (mm)	Ulceration status
TX	Not applicable	Not applicable
T0	Not applicable	Not applicable
Tis	Not applicable	Not applicable
T1	≤1.0 mm	Unknown
T1a	<0.8 mm	Without ulceration
T1b	<0.8 mm	With ulceration
	0.8 to 1 mm	With or without ulceration
T2	>1 to 2 mm	Unknown
T2a	>1 to 2 mm	Without ulceration
T2b	>1 to 2 mm	With ulceration
T3	>2 to 4 mm	Unknown
T3a	>2 to 4 mm	Without ulceration
T3b	>2 to 4 mm	With ulceration
T4	>4 mm	Unknown
T4a	>4 mm	Without ulceration
T4b	>4 mm	With ulceration

Used with permission of the American Joint Committee on Cancer (AJCC), Chicago, Illinois. The original and primary source for this information is the AJCC Cancer Staging Manual, Eighth Edition (2017) published by Springer International Publishing

Table 6.3 American Joint Committee on Cancer eighth edition melanoma staging guidelines

Regional lymph node (N)

N category	Number of tumor-involved regional lymph nodes	Presence of in-transit, satellite and/or microsatellite metastases
NX	Regional nodes not assessed	No
N0	No regional metastases detected	No
N1	One tumor-involved node or in-transit, satellite, or microsatellite metastases with no tumor-involved nodes	
N1a	One clinically occult node detected by SLN	No
N1b	One clinically detected	No
N1c	No regional node disease	Yes
N2	Two to three tumor-involved nodes or in-transit, satellite, or microsatellite metastases with one tumor-involved node	
N2a	Two to three clinically occult nodes detected by SLN biopsy	No
N2b	Two or three, at least one of which was clinically detected	No
N2c	One clinically occult or clinically detected node	Yes
N3	Four or more tumor-involved nodes or in-transit, satellite, or microsatellite metastases with two or tumor-involved nodes, or any number of matted nodes without or with in-transit, satellite, and/or microsatellite metastases	
N3a	Four or more clinically occult nodes detected by SLN	No
N3b	Four or more, at least one of which was clinically detected, or presence of any number matted nodes	No
N3c	Two or more clinically occult or clinically detected and /or presence of any number of matted nodes	Yes

Used with permission of the American Joint Committee on Cancer (AJCC), Chicago, Illinois. The original and primary source for this information is the AJCC Cancer Staging Manual, Eighth Edition (2017) published by Springer International Publishing

Microsatellite, satellite, and in-transit and/or subcutaneous metastases are types of melanoma metastases between the primary tumor and the draining lymph node basin. These localized metastases are stratified according to the number of tumor-involved lymph nodes. Distant metastases are categorized by anatomical location. In the eighth edition, the metastases staging includes serum lactate dehydrogenase (LDH), an important independent factor for patients with metastatic melanoma. Melanoma metastasis is divided into M1a, metastases to distant skin, subcutaneous or lymph node; M1b, lung metastases; M1c, metastases to other visceral sites, excluding the central nervous system; and M1d, metastases to the central nervous system, with or without involvement of other sites (Table 6.4). The M1d is a new category and is associated with a poor prognosis. LDH serum levels subcategorize the metastasis groups into either 0 for a non-elevated LDH or 1 for an elevated LDH.

The TNM classification is then translated into clinical staging when clinical and radiologic data is the only evaluation of lymph nodes and pathological staging when

Table 6.4 American Joint Committee on Cancer Eighth Edition Melanoma Staging Guidelines

Distant metastasis (M)		
M category	Anatomic site	Lactate dehydrogenase level
M0	None	Not applicable
M1	Evidence of distant metastasis	See below
M1a	Distant metastasis to the skin, soft tissue including muscle, and/or nonregional lymph node	Not recorded or unspecified
M1a(0)	Distant metastasis to the skin, soft tissue including muscle, and/or nonregional lymph node	Not elevated
M1a(1)	Distant metastasis to the skin, soft tissue including muscle, and/or nonregional lymph node	Elevated
M1b	Distant metastasis to the lung with or without M1a sites of disease	Not recorded or unspecified
M1b(0)	Distant metastasis to the skin, soft tissue including muscle, and/or nonregional lymph node	Not elevated
M1b(1)	Distant metastasis to the skin, soft tissue including muscle, and/or nonregional lymph node	Elevated
M1c	Distant metastasis to non-CNS visceral sites with or without M1a or M1b sites of disease	Not recorded or unspecified
M1c(0)	Distant metastasis to non-CNS visceral sites with or without M1a or M1b sites of disease	Not elevated
M1c(1)	Distant metastasis to non-CNS visceral sites with or without M1a or M1b sites of disease	Elevated
M1d	Distant metastasis to CNS with or without M1a, M1b, or M1c sites of disease	Not recorded or unspecified
M1d(0)	Distant metastasis to non-CNS visceral sites with or without M1a or M1b sites of disease	Not elevated
M1d(1)	Distant metastasis to non-CNS visceral sites with or without M1a or M1b sites of disease	Elevated

Used with permission of the American Joint Committee on Cancer (AJCC), Chicago, Illinois. The original and primary source for this information is the AJCC Cancer Staging Manual, Eighth Edition (2017) published by Springer International Publishing

pathologic information about regional lymph nodes is available (Table 6.5). The clinical and pathologic stage can then be used to provide the clinician and patient with a survival prognosis (Table 6.5). Melanoma in situ is stage 0. Stage I patients have ≤1 mm of invasion with or without ulceration or 1–2 mm of invasion without ulceration and are considered low risk. Stage II patients have increased risk of mortality with increasing Breslow depth and presence of ulceration. Stage III patients have regional metastasis and the most variable survival range. Stage IV patients have distant metastatic disease.

Independent and confounding risk factors that impact survival include tumor thickness, ulceration, anatomical location of the primary tumor, age at diagnosis, and gender. For localized disease (stages I and II), Breslow depth is the most powerful prognostic indicator for survival in patients with lesions ≤1 mm, while ulceration, age, and site are the most significant predictive factor for lesions 2–4 mm

Table 6.5 Clinical and pathological staging of melanoma with 5- and 10-year survival [27, 42]

Stage	5-year survival (%)	10-year Survival (%)	Clinical staging			Pathologic staging		
0			Tis	N0	M0	Tis	N0	M0
IA	97	95	T1a	N0	M0	T1a	N0	M0
1B	92	86	T1b T2a	N0	M0	T1b T2a	N0	M0
IIA	81	67	T2b T3a	N0	M0	T2b T3a	N0	M0
IIB	70	57	T3b T4a	N0	M0	T3b T4a	N0	M0
IIC	53	40	T4b	N0	M0	T4b	N0	M0
III			Any T	N1–3	M0			
IIIA	78	68				T1-4a T1-4a	N1a N2a	M0
IIIB	59	43				T1-4b T1-4b T1-4a T1-4a T1-4a	N1a N2a N1b N2b N2c	M0
IIIC	40	24				T1-4b T1-4b T1-4b Any T	N1b N2b N2c N3	M0
IV	15–20	10–15	Any T	Any N	Any M1	Any T	Any N	Any M1

Used with permission of the American Joint Committee on Cancer (AJCC), Chicago, Illinois. The original and primary source for this information is the *AJCC Cancer Staging Manual*, Eighth Edition (2017) published by Springer International Publishing

[27]. Older patients are more likely to present with thicker and ulcerated melanomas and are more likely to carry comorbidities that affect survival. Older patients are also more likely to be male and have a poor prognosis. Women tend to develop melanoma at a younger age, seek care at earlier stages, and have better outcomes. Tumors on the head, neck, and trunk are higher risk and occur more frequently in people older than 65 and in men. Those on the extremities occur more frequently in younger patients and females. Stage I disease has excellent 5-year survival at 92–97%. Stage II 5-year survival drops significantly with increasing thickness and ulceration from 81% for stage IIA down to 53% for stage IIC [39].

For patients with regional metastasis (stage III) which includes regional lymph node, satellite, and/or in-transit metastasis, three factors are most important for survival and listed in descending significance: (1) the number of metastatic nodes, (2) the tumor burden of the affected nodes, and (3) the ulceration of the primary tumor. Survival is best predicted with delineation of 1, 2, 3, and 4+ nodes. Ulceration is the only primary tumor characteristic that is an independent risk factor for survival of stage III patients. This heterozygous group of patients has a wide range of 5-year survival rates from 78% for stage IIIA down to 59% and 40% for stages IIIB and

IIIC, respectively. Stage IIIA patient survival is more closely linked to primary tumor characteristics such as thickness and ulceration, like stage II patients, and more closely matches stage II survival rates than those of stages IIIB and IIIC [31].

Stage IV disease is defined as distant metastasis. It has very poor 5-year survival rates at 15–20%. Metastasis to non-visceral sites (distant skin, subcutaneous tissue, and lymph nodes) has improved survival over metastasis to visceral sites. Metastasis to the lung has a slight 1-year survival advantage with rates more similar to non-visceral sites but drops to match that of other visceral sites by 2 years. Recently, elevated serum LDH is an independent and highly predictive indicator for poor survival [31].

Routine blood tests and imaging screening of asymptomatic patient with melanoma of any thickness are generally not recommended. Serum LDH is insensitive and nonspecific at detecting metastatic disease and only provides additional prognostic value when distant metastasis is already known. Routine chest radiograph is nonspecific, does not correlate with sentinel lymph node results, is cost ineffective, exposes patients to unnecessary radiation, and may result in unnecessary follow-up imaging or procedures. Workup should be driven based upon physical exam finding, review of system complaints, and index of suspicion [40].

Sentinel Lymph Node

Sentinel lymph node (SLN) biopsy for melanoma is controversial. It was developed as a conservative alternative to lymph node dissection, a practice that started in 1892 and carries 37% complication rate including lymphedema and infection. Sentinel lymph node biopsy is currently offered as an elective procedure for patients with primary tumor thickness ≥1 mm, or <1 mm with ulceration, and clinically negative lymph node exam. It provides prognostic information and predicts the status of the other regional lymph nodes. SLN biopsy is not offered when regional lymph node involvement is blatant or when distant spread is already known. SLN biopsy is not therapeutic and does not improve survival outcomes. If SLN biopsy is positive, a complete lymph node dissection is recommended, and the patient can be stratified into the correct stage III substage, allowing for survival information and clinical trial enrollment for emerging adjuvant therapy. SLN is not risk-free, however. It carries a 10% complication rate including delayed wound healing, infection, false negative results if the cancer has already metastasized to other lymph nodes in the basin or distant organs, false positives due to the normal and relatively common presence of benign nevi in the lymph nodes, and anaphylaxis to the blue dye [41–43].

Advocates for SLN biopsy claim benefits including more accurate staging. This provides patients, their family, and providers with information which may impact treatment of the melanoma as well as other comorbidities. SLN status is often used to identify patient who may benefit from additional therapies and allows for clinical trial enrollment. Positive SLN allows the opportunity for early complete lymph node dissection. Some studies show early complete lymph node dissection improves morbidity and mortality over waiting until clinically evident lymphadenopathy is present in some patient subsets. Although no improved short-term or long-term survival exists with SLN biopsy, some have also found an increased disease-free survival time and an arguably improved quality of life during that period, making SLN biopsy preferred over observation alone [41, 44]. Other studies have not found improved survival with early complete lymph node dissection or improved disease-free survival with SLN biopsy [45, 46]. A recent prospective trial examining observation versus complete lymph node dissection after a positive SLN showed that immediate complete lymph node dissection increased the rate of regional disease control but did not increase melanoma-specific survival in sentinel lymph node positive patients [47].

Those opposed to SLN biopsy argue that Breslow thickness and ulceration provide adequate stratification information. Only 17% of patients who undergo SLN biopsy have positive results, and the vast majority of patients have N1a or N2a disease that matches their clinically stage I and II counterparts well enough. SLN biopsy has several potential complications. It is expensive, especially if general anesthesia is used. A positive SLN may lead to an unnecessary complete lymph node dissection which can cause greater adverse events. The premise behind the SLN biopsy was to have a procedure that would improve survival. But with evidence showing no survival benefit, less invasive and less expensive testing on primary and circulating tumor cells that could provide similar prognostic information would be preferred but is still under development [48, 49].

Treatment

Surgical

Surgical excision is the treatment of choice for primary localized melanoma. Wide local excision (WLE) is recommended as tumor cells often spread several millimeters, and at times even centimeters, past the clinically apparent melanoma. The goal is to achieve complete removal and reduce local recurrence of disease. Current guidelines recommend a 1 cm margin for lesions of ≤1 mm thickness, 1–2 cm margin for lesions 1.01–2.0 mm thickness, and 2 cm margins for tumors of >2 mm thickness. Greater than 2 cm margins is of no advantage. Surgical excision should extend to the depth of the muscular fascia whenever reasonable or at least to the level of the deep adipose tissue if abundant adipose tissue is present. Histologic examination should be thorough, and Mohs micrographic surgery or request for tissue specimen be cut "en face" by surgical pathology can be considered. Both techniques allow for 100% of the deep and lateral margin to be examined, rather than the <1% that is routinely examined with standard bread-loafing technique [27].

Radiation Therapy

Radiation therapy is used with notable success for unresectable local disease and as palliative care for distant metastasis. Whole brain radiotherapy, surgical resection, and more recently stereotactic radiosurgery are mainstay treatments for cerebral metastasis [50, 51]. Other indications include bone metastasis and spinal cord compression. Radiation therapy is not recommended as adjuvant therapy after lymph node dissection [52].

Chemotherapy

For patients with metastatic melanoma (stages III and IV), traditional cytotoxic chemotherapy agents have limited efficacy and use. Dacarbazine is the only FDA-approved chemotherapy agent for melanoma to be tried in advanced disease for palliative measures to slow tumor growth or temporarily decrease tumor burden, but a survival advantage has not been proven. Dacarbazine along with temozolomide, nab-paclitaxel, paclitaxel, cisplatin, carboplatin, and vinblastine may also be used alone or in combination with each other or added to newer therapies known as bio-chemotherapy or chemoimmunotherapy. Melphalan and actinomycin-D are used for isolated-limb-perfusion chemotherapy which can increase efficacy and reduce systemic toxicities for extremity-localized advanced disease [53, 54].

Immunotherapy

Due to poor response to cytotoxic chemotherapy and the recognized importance of host immunity in melanoma, particular attention has been paid to immunotherapy (modalities that boost patients own tumor-fighting capabilities). In addition to the medications already on the market described below, numerous other therapies are currently in clinical trial.

Cytokines

Cytokines interleukin-2 (IL-2) and interferon-alpha (IFN-alpha) were the first FDA-approved immune-stimulating drugs. Interleukin-2 enhances CD8+ T cells and NK cells and produces a 15–20% objective response rate and ~5% long-term, durable complete response. IL-2 must be given intravenously at high doses with substantial side effects limiting its use including fever, chills, malaise, flushing, hypotension, and capillary leak syndrome [55, 56]. Interferon-alpha has been more extensively studied but with conflicting results leading to a sudden rise and then fall in popularity. Dosing schedules for high-dose, intermediate-dose, low-dose, and pegylated formulations have been suggested. Some evidence of a dose-response relationship exists with a significant recurrence-free survival with increased doses. It remains unclear if a worthwhile overall survival benefit is present [57]. Mechanism of action includes direct antiproliferative effect on tumor cells, enhanced NK activity, increased T helper lymphocytes and tumor-specific CD8+ T cells, and increased tumor-infiltrating T lymphocytes [58]. Side effects of interferon-alpha include fever, chills, malaise, nausea and vomiting, hepatitis, neutropenia, depression, and suicide. Further research is needed to determine optimal dose, duration, and appropriate patient profile for optimized response to this toxic medication [59].

Checkpoint Inhibitors

Immune checkpoint inhibitors are among the fastest-growing categories of immunotherapy. T-cell activation requires stimulation by antigen-presenting cells. In addition to co-stimulatory molecules, inhibitory molecules are also present on T cells and antigen-presenting cells to control the level of immune response and avoid autoimmunity. Similar inhibitory molecules are present on tumor cells and can prevent killing of tumor cells by T cells. Blocking these inhibitory signals acts to remove the brakes of this antitumor arm of the immune systems. Checkpoint inhibitors come with a slow response time and may take several months to begin shrinking tumors. It is not uncommon for tumors to swell within those first months and thus appear larger on scans, a concept known as pseudo-progression.

Ipilimumab, an anti-CTLA-4 monoclonal antibody, is the first checkpoint inhibitor FDA approved for the treatment of metastatic or unresectable melanoma. Ipilimumab binds to CTLA-4 on the surface of activated T cells to prevent antigen-presenting cell inhibition of T-cell activation through the CTLA-4/CD80/CD86 interaction. Early trials showed improved overall survival from 6.4 months in the control group to 10.1 months in the treatment arm. Long-term data is increasing with patients surviving 2, 5, and even 10 years showing a durable response [60, 61]. Objective response rates range from 7% to 15% as a single agent and increase to 20.8% when combined with dacarbazine and up to 57.6% when combined with nivolumab [60, 62, 63].

Nivolumab and pembrolizumab followed as the next generation of checkpoint inhibitors to be FDA approved in 2014. Programmed cell death protein 1 (PD-1) is a T-cell surface molecule that functions to recognize self and suppress autoimmunity. Programmed death-ligand 1 (PDL-1) present on melanoma cells binds to PD-1 on activated antigen-specific T cells and prevents tumor cell-mediated immune responses. Nivolumab and pembrolizumab are humanized monoclonal antibodies which bind to PD-1 and prevent its binding with PDL-1. In the absence of PDL-1 and PD-1 ligation, T cells remain in an active state and cytotoxic to the tumor. Pembrolizumab has demonstrated an overall objective response rate of 33%

including those who failed ipilimumab and upward of 45% for treatment-naïve patients [64]. In addition to a greater response rate over ipilimumab, pembrolizumab also has significantly longer progression-free survival [65]. Nivolumab has equal response rates of pembrolizumab at 33% irrespective of prior therapy and BRAF status [66]. As mentioned previously, combination therapy of ipilimumab with nivolumab produces an additive effect with nearly 60% response rate and is quickly becoming the gold standard of therapy when available [63].

Blocking T-cell checkpoints comes with the risk of immune-mediated side effects. Autoimmune-mediated dermatitis, mucositis, colitis, hepatitis, pneumonitis, and endocrinopathies have been observed as the overactive immune system attacks other body organs besides the intended cancer cells. Less commonly nephritis, pancreatitis, meningitis, myelitis, cardiomyositis, as well as a variety of bone marrow suppression and ophthalmic inflammation can occur. Immune-mediated adverse events are typically transient but can be severe or fatal. For moderate (grade 2) reactions, checkpoint inhibitors should be withheld until symptoms decrease or resolve. Corticosteroids should be started if the reaction has not improved in 1 week. For patients with severe or life-threatening (grade 3 or 4) reaction, checkpoint inhibitors should be permanently discontinued, and high-dose corticosteroids should be started immediately. If corticosteroids fail to promptly improve symptoms within a few days, infliximab should be considered [64]. In the largest set of reported data, ipilimumab immune-mediated adverse events were reported in 85% of patients, with 35% requiring corticosteroids and 10% requiring infliximab. Pembrolizumab has shown significantly fewer grade 3–5 adverse reactions than ipilimumab (10–13.3% compared to 19.9%) [65]. Nivolumab grade 3 and 4 adverse events occurred in 2.8–11.7% of patients [66, 67].

Oncolytic Virus Therapy and Therapeutic Vaccines

Oncolytic virus therapy is another promising new approach for cancer treatment. The concept emerged in the 1970s when the bacille Calmette-Guérin (BCG) vaccine was injected intralesionally with anecdotal but nonstatistically significant reproducible results. The research persisted, and talimogene laherparepvec, a genetically engineered herpesvirus (HSV-1), became the first and currently only FDA-approved oncolytic virus therapy for metastatic melanoma, approved in 2015 [68]. The virus is modified to remove two genes, one responsible for immune system evasion and another for the ability to replicate within healthy cells. The gene for human granulocyte-macrophage colony-stimulating factor (GM-CSF) is added as well with hopes of boosting immune recognition. The virus is injected directly into the tumor where it preferentially replicates within cancer cells until the cancer cells rupture. The effect is twofold with both direct cancer cell death and increased tumor antigen presentation after tumor cell particles are released. Phase III trial shows an overall response rate of 26.4% and a durable response rate at 16.3%. There was no statistically significant difference in the overall survival between the treatment arm and control arm. Adverse events include fever, chills, and fatigue but are mostly mild to moderate. Grade 3 and 4 adverse events only occurred in 2% with no deaths [67, 68].

Therapeutic cancer vaccines aim to boost the immune system's capability to recognize and destroy tumor through cytotoxic T cells or antibody-mediated cell death. Therapeutic vaccination is far less effective than preventative cancer vaccines, such as those for HPV and hepatitis B, at stimulating an immune response. For those patients with proven immune response by enzyme-linked immunospot assays, overall survival was increased from 10.8 to 21.3 months [69].

Other Avenues of Immunotherapy: Adoptive Cell Therapy, Monoclonal Antibodies, and Adjuvant Immunotherapy

Advancements in immunotherapy are ongoing. In adoptive cell therapy, T cells are removed from the patients, genetically modified with melanoma receptors or otherwise enhanced in activity or number, and then reintroduced back into the patient. Monoclonal antibodies directed to tumor antigens to promote immune response are under development as well. Other adjuvant immunotherapies in clinical trial include the use of innate immunity Toll-like receptors 3, 8, and 9.

Targeted Molecular Therapy

Understanding of the molecular pathways involved in the pathogenesis of melanoma has led to the development of *MAPK* pathway inhibitors with targets including *BRAF*, *MEK*, *NRAS*, and *KIT*. *BRAF* mutations are present in up to 66% of all melanomas. Vemurafenib and dabrafenib are FDA-approved monoclonal antibodies that target mutated *BRAF* molecules. When compared to treatment with dacarbazine, *BRAF* inhibitors have a remarkable higher response rate and significantly greater median overall survival [70, 71]. Despite their impressive initial responses, when given as monotherapy, inhibition is eventually overcome, and resistance develops. Common adverse events include cutaneous squamous cell carcinoma, keratoacanthoma type, rash, photosensitivity, arthralgia, diarrhea, and fatigue. Severe adverse events are rare.

Trametinib and cobimetinib are inhibitors of *MEK*, an enzyme downstream of *BRAF* in the *MAPK* pathway. Trametinib shows modest activity when used as monotherapy for patients with *BRAF* mutations but is subpar to *BRAF* inhibitors. Cobimetinib has not been studied as monotherapy. *MEK* inhibitors are generally well tolerated, and adverse events include rash, diarrhea, fatigue, edema, cardiac dysfunction, and interstitial lung disease. Similar to *BRAF* inhibitors, resistance develops.

To overcome high rates of resistance, improve response rates, and decrease toxicity, clinical trials with dual therapy with *BRAF + MEK* inhibitors were conducted. Combination therapies with dabrafenib plus trametinib and vemurafenib plus cobimetinib have objective response rates of 79% and 68%, respectively. Both combinations have improved progression-free survival and overall survival compared to *BRAF* monotherapy. Resistance remains nearly inevitable and an unresolved hurdle. Side effects are reduced when dabrafenib is combined with trametinib but unchanged when vemurafenib is combined with cobimetinib [72, 73]. Head-to-head comparison of the two combinations has not been performed, but indirect comparison suggests vemurafenib plus cobimetinib is of equal efficacy but associated with increased adverse events [74].

Existing *KIT* inhibitors such as imatinib and nilotinib appear to have a narrow but significant role in melanomas harboring such mutations [75]. *NRAS* inhibitors are currently in trial. In addition, inhibition of *mTOR* and *AKT* also shows promise [76, 77]. Combination therapy with targeted molecular inhibitors and immunotherapy are being studied.

References

1. Erdei E, Torres SM. A new understanding in the epidemiology of melanoma. Expert Rev Anticancer Ther. 2010;10(11):1811–23. https://doi.org/10.1586/era.10.170.
2. Bradford PT, Anderson WF, Purdue MP, Goldstein AM, Tucker MA. Rising melanoma incidence rates of the trunk among younger women in the United States. Cancer Epidemiol Biomark Prev Publ Am Assoc Cancer Res Cosponsored Am Soc Prev Oncol. 2010;19(9):2401–6. https://doi.org/10.1158/1055-9965.epi-10-0503.
3. Siegel RL, Miller KD, Jemal A. Cancer statistics, 2016. CA Cancer J Clin. 2016;66(1):7–30. https://doi.org/10.3322/caac.21332.
4. Jemal A, Saraiya M, Patel P, Cherala SS, Barnholtz-Sloan J, Kim J, Wiggins CL, Wingo PA. Recent trends in cutaneous melanoma incidence and death rates in the United States, 1992-2006. J Am Acad Dermatol. 2011;65(5 Suppl 1):S17-25.e11–3. https://doi.org/10.1016/j.jaad.2011.04.032.
5. Curtin JA, Fridlyand J, Kageshita T, Patel HN, Busam KJ, Kutzner H, Cho KH, Aiba S, Brocker EB, LeBoit PE, Pinkel D, Bastian BC. Distinct sets of genetic alterations in melanoma. N Engl J Med. 2005;353(20):2135–47. https://doi.org/10.1056/NEJMoa050092.
6. Millington GW. Mutations of the BRAF gene in human cancer, by Davies et al. (Nature 2002; 417: 949-54). Clin Exp Dermatol. 2013;38(2):222–3. https://doi.org/10.1111/ced.12015.
7. Goldstein AM, Chan M, Harland M, Gillanders EM, Hayward NK, Avril MF, Azizi E, Bianchi-Scarra G, Bishop DT, Bressac-de Paillerets B, Bruno W, Calista D, Cannon Albright LA, Demenais F, Elder DE, Ghiorzo P, Gruis NA, Hansson J, Hogg D, Holland EA, Kanetsky PA, Kefford RF, Landi MT, Lang J, Leachman SA, Mackie RM, Magnusson V, Mann GJ, Niendorf K, Newton Bishop J, Palmer JM, Puig S, Puig-Butille JA, de Snoo FA, Stark M, Tsao H, Tucker MA, Whitaker L, Yakobson E. High-risk melanoma susceptibility genes and pancreatic cancer, neural system tumors, and uveal melanoma across GenoMEL. Cancer Res. 2006;66(20):9818–28. https://doi.org/10.1158/0008-5472.can-06-0494.
8. Curtin JA, Busam K, Pinkel D, Bastian BC. Somatic activation of KIT in distinct subtypes of melanoma. J Clin Oncol. 2006;24(26):4340–6. https://doi.org/10.1200/JCO.2006.06.2984.
9. Bello DM, Ariyan CE, Carvajal RD. Melanoma mutagenesis and aberrant cell signaling. Cancer Control. 2013;20(4):261–81.

10. Parkin DM, Mesher D, Sasieni P. 13. Cancers attributable to solar (ultraviolet) radiation exposure in the UK in 2010. Br J Cancer. 2011;105(Suppl 2):S66–9. https://doi.org/10.1038/bjc.2011.486.
11. Pfahlberg A, Kolmel KF, Gefeller O, Febim Study G. Timing of excessive ultraviolet radiation and melanoma: epidemiology does not support the existence of a critical period of high susceptibility to solar ultraviolet radiation- induced melanoma. Br J Dermatol. 2001;144(3):471–5.
12. Green AC, Williams GM, Logan V, Strutton GM. Reduced melanoma after regular sunscreen use: randomized trial follow-up. J Clin Oncol. 2011;29(3):257–63. https://doi.org/10.1200/JCO.2010.28.7078.
13. Ghivasand R, Ruegg CS, Welderpass E, Green AC, Lund E, Velerod MB. Indoor tanning and melanoma risk: long-term evidence from a Prospective Population Based Cohort Study. Am J Epidemol. 2017;185(3):147–56.
14. Friedman RJ, Farber MJ, Warycha MA, Papathasis N, Miller MK, Heilman ER. The "dysplastic" nevus. Clin Dermatol. 2009;27(1):103–15. https://doi.org/10.1016/j.clindermatol.2008.09.008.
15. Silva JH, Sa BC, Avila AL, Landman G, Duprat Neto JP. Atypical mole syndrome and dysplastic nevi: identification of populations at risk for developing melanoma – review article. Clinics (Sao Paulo). 2011;66(3):493–9.
16. Nestle FO, Burg G, Dummer R. New perspectives on immunobiology and immunotherapy of melanoma. Immunol Today. 1999;20(1):5–7.
17. Zhang M, Graor H, Yan L, Kim J. Identification of melanoma-reactive CD4+ T-cell subsets from human melanoma draining lymph nodes. J Immunother. 2016;39(1):15–26. https://doi.org/10.1097/CJI.0000000000000103.
18. Friedman RJ, Rigel DS, Kopf AW. Early detection of malignant melanoma: the role of physician examination and self-examination of the skin. CA Cancer J Clin. 1985;35:130–51.
19. Abbasi NR, Shaw HM, Rigel DS, Friedman RJ, McCarthy WH, Osman I, Kopf AW, Polsky D. Early diagnosis of cutaneous melanoma: revisiting the ABCD criteria. JAMA. 2004;29(22):2771–6.
20. Grob JJ, Bonerandi JJ. The 'ugly duckling' sign: identification of the common characteristics of nevi in an individual as a basis for melanoma screening. Arch Dermatol. 1998;134(1):103–4.
21. Mar V, Roberts H, Wolfe R, English DR, Kelly JW. Nodular melanoma: a distinct clinical entity and the largest contributor to melanoma deaths in Victoria, Australia. J Am Acad Dermatol. 2013;68(4):568–75. https://doi.org/10.1016/j.jaad.2012.09.047.
22. Thompson JF, Soong SJ, Balch CM, Gershenwald JE, Ding S, Coit DG, Flaherty KT, Gimotty PA, Johnson T, Johnson MM, Leong SP, Ross MI, Byrd DR, Cascinelli N, Cochran AJ, Eggermont AM, McMasters KM, Mihm MC Jr, Morton DL, Sondak VK. Prognostic significance of mitotic rate in localized primary cutaneous melanoma: an analysis of patients in the multi-institutional American joint committee on cancer melanoma staging database. J Clin Oncol. 2011;29(16):2199–205. https://doi.org/10.1200/JCO.2010.31.5812.
23. Jen M, Murphy M, Grant-Kels JM. Childhood melanoma. Clin Dermatol. 2009;27(6):529–36. https://doi.org/10.1016/j.clindermatol.2008.09.011.
24. Vestergaard ME, Macaskill P, Holt PE, Menzies SW. Dermoscopy compared with naked eye examination for the diagnosis of primary melanoma: a meta-analysis of studies performed in a clinical setting. Br J Dermatol. 2008;159(3):669–76. https://doi.org/10.1111/j.1365-2133.2008.08713.x.
25. Gallegos-Hernandez JF, Ortiz-Maldonado AL, Minauro-Munoz GG, Arias-Ceballos H, Hernandez-Sanjuan M. Dermoscopy in cutaneous melanoma. Cir Cir. 2015;83(2):107–11. https://doi.org/10.1016/j.circir.2015.04.004.
26. Menzies SW, Moloney FJ, Byth K, Avramidis M, Argenziano G, Zalaudek I, Braun RP, Malvehy J, Puig S, Rabinovitz HS, Oliviero M, Cabo H, Bono R, Pizzichetta MA, Claeson M, Gaffney DC, Soyer HP, Stanganelli I, Scolyer RA, Guitera P, Kelly J, McCurdy O, Llambrich A, Marghoob AA, Zaballos P, Kirchesch HM, Piccolo D, Bowling J, Thomas L, Terstappen K, Tanaka M, Pellacani G, Pagnanelli G, Ghigliotti G, Ortega BC, Crafter G, Ortiz AM, Tromme I, Karaarslan IK, Ozdemir F, Tam A, Landi C, Norton P, Kacar N, Rudnicka

L, Slowinska M, Simionescu O, Di Stefani A, Coates E, Kreusch J. Dermoscopic evalua-tion of nodular melanoma. JAMA Dermatol. 2013;149(6):699–709. https://doi.org/10.1001/jamadermatol.2013.2466.

27. Bichakjian CK, Halpern AC, Johnson TM, Foote Hood A, Grichnik JM, Swetter SM, Tsao H, Barbosa VH, Chuang TY, Duvic M, Ho VC, Sober AJ, Beutner KR, Bhushan R, Smith Begolka W, American Academy of Dermatology. Guidelines of care for the management of primary cutaneous melanoma. American Academy of Dermatology. J Am Acad Dermatol. 2011;65(5):1032–47. https://doi.org/10.1016/j.jaad.2011.04.031.

28. Hendi A, Brodland DG, Zitelli JA. Melanocytes in long-standing sun-exposed skin: quantita-tive analysis using the MART-1 immunostain. Arch Dermatol. 2006;142(7):871–6. https://doi.org/10.1001/archderm.142.7.871.

29. Duffy K, Grossman D. The dysplastic nevus: from historical perspective to management in the modern era: part I. Historical, histologic, and clinical aspects. J Am Acad Dermatol. 2012;67(1):1.e1–16. quiz 17–8. https://doi.org/10.1016/j.jaad.2012.02.047.

30. Patrawala S, Maley A, Greskovich C, Stuart L, Parker D, Swerlick R, Stoff B. Discordance of histopathologic parameters in cutaneous melanoma: clinical implications. J Am Acad Dermatol. 2016;74(1):75–80. https://doi.org/10.1016/j.jaad.2015.09.008.

31. Balch CM, Soong SJ, Gershenwald JE, Thompson JF, Reintgen DS, Cascinelli N, Urist M, McMasters KM, Ross MI, Kirkwood JM, Atkins MB, Thompson JA, Coit DG, Byrd D, Desmond R, Zhang Y, Liu PY, Lyman GH, Morabito A. Prognostic factors analysis of 17,600 melanoma patients: validation of the American Joint Committee on Cancer melanoma staging system. J Clin Oncol. 2001;19(16):3622–34. https://doi.org/10.1200/JCO.2001.19.16.3622.

32. Smoller BR. Histologic criteria for diagnosing primary cutaneous malignant melanoma. Mod Pathol. 2006;19(Suppl 2):S34–40. https://doi.org/10.1038/modpathol.3800508.

33. Schmitt FC, Bacchi CE. S-100 protein: is it useful as a tumour marker in diagnostic immuno-cytochemistry? Histopathology. 1989;15(3):281–8.

34. Gown AM, Vogel AM, Hoak D, Gough F, McNutt MA. Monoclonal antibodies spe-cific for melanocytic tumors distinguish subpopulations of melanocytes. Am J Pathol. 1986;123(2):195–203.

35. Ohsie SJ, Sarantopoulos GP, Cochran AJ, Binder SW. Immunohistochemical characteristics of melanoma. J Cutan Pathol. 2008;35(5):433–44. https://doi.org/10.1111/j.1600-0560.2007.00891.x.

36. Moretti S, Spallanzani A, Chiarugi A, Fabiani M, Pinzi C. Correlation of Ki-67 expression in cutaneous primary melanoma with prognosis in a prospective study: different correlation according to thickness. J Am Acad Dermatol. 2001;44(2):188–92. https://doi.org/10.1067/mjd.2001.110067.

37. Gershenwald JE, Scolyr RA, Hess KR, et al. Melanoma of the skin. In: Amin MD, editor. AJCC cancer staging manual. 8th ed. Chicago: American Joint Committee on Cancer; 2017. p. 563.

38. Maurichi A, Miceli R, Camerini T, et al. Prediction of survival in patients with thin melanoma: results from a multi-institution study. J Clin Oncol. 2014;32:2479.

39. Schuchter L, Schultz DJ, Synnestvedt M, Trock BJ, Guerry D, Elder DE, Elenitsas R, Clark WH, Halpern AC. A prognostic model for predicting 10-year survival in patients with primary melanoma. The Pigmented Lesion Group. Ann Intern Med. 1996;125(5):369–75.

40. Wang TS, Johnson TM, Cascade PN, Redman BG, Sondak VK, Schwartz JL. Evaluation of staging chest radiographs and serum lactate dehydrogenase for localized melanoma. J Am Acad Dermatol. 2004;51(3):399–405. https://doi.org/10.1016/j.jaad.2004.02.017.

41. Morton DL, Thompson JF, Cochran AJ, Mozzillo N, Nieweg OE, Roses DF, Hoekstra HJ, Karakousis CP, Puleo CA, Coventry BJ, Kashani-Sabet M, Smithers BM, Paul E, Kraybill WG, McKinnon JG, Wang HJ, Elashoff R, Faries MB, MSLT Group. Final trial report of sentinel-node biopsy versus nodal observation in melanoma. N Engl J Med. 2014; 370(7):599–609. https://doi.org/10.1056/NEJMoa1310460.

42. Biddle DA, Evans HL, Kemp BL, El-Naggar AK, Harvell JD, White WL, Iskandar SS, Prieto VG. Intraparenchymal nevus cell aggregates in lymph nodes: a possible diagnostic pitfall with malignant melanoma and carcinoma. Am J Surg Pathol. 2003;27(5):673–81.

43. Carson KF, Wen DR, Li PX, Lana AM, Bailly C, Morton DL, Cochran AJ. Nodal nevi and cutaneous melanomas. Am J Surg Pathol. 1996;20(7):834–40.

44. Morton DL, Thompson JF, Cochran AJ, Mozzillo N, Elashoff R, Essner R, Nieweg OE, Roses DF, Hoekstra HJ, Karakousis CP, Reintgen DS, Coventry BJ, Glass EC, Wang HJ, MSLT Group. Sentinel-node biopsy or nodal observation in melanoma. N Engl J Med. 2006;355(13):1307–1317. https://doi.org/10.1056/NEJMoa060992.

45. Wong SL, Morton DL, Thompson JF, Gershenwald JE, Leong SP, Reintgen DS, Gutman H, Sabel MS, Carlson GW, McMasters KM, Tyler DS, Goydos JS, Eggermont AM, Nieweg OE, Cosimi AB, Riker AI, GC D. Melanoma patients with positive sentinel nodes who did not undergo completion lymphadenectomy: a multi-institutional study. Ann Surg Oncol. 2006;13(6):809–16. https://doi.org/10.1245/ASO.2006.03.058.

46. Kingham TP, Panageas KS, Ariyan CE, Busam KJ, Brady MS, Coit DG. Outcome of patients with a positive sentinel lymph node who do not undergo completion lymphadenectomy. Ann Surg Oncol. 2010;17(2):514–20. https://doi.org/10.1245/s10434-009-0836-3.

47. Faries MB, Thompson JF, Andtbacka RH, Mozzillo N, et al. Complete dissection or observation for sentinel-node metastasis in melanoma. N Engl J Med. 2017;376(23):2211–22.

48. Torjesen I. Sentinel node biopsy for melanoma: unnecessary treatment? BMJ. 2013;346:e8645. https://doi.org/10.1136/bmj.e8645.

49. Balch CM, Gershenwald JE, Soong SJ, Thompson JF, Atkins MB, Byrd DR, Buzaid AC, Cochran AJ, Coit DG, Ding S, Eggermont AM, Flaherty KT, Gimotty PA, Kirkwood JM, McMasters KM, Mihm MC Jr, Morton DL, Ross MI, Sober AJ, Sondak VK. Final version of 2009 AJCC melanoma staging and classification. J Clin Oncol. 2009;27(36):6199–206. https://doi.org/10.1200/JCO.2009.23.4799.

50. Schild SE. Role of radiation therapy in the treatment of melanoma. Expert Rev Anticancer Ther. 2009;9(5):583–6. https://doi.org/10.1586/era.09.21.

51. Samlowski WE, Watson GA, Wang M, Rao G, Klimo P Jr, Boucher K, Shrieve DC, Jensen RL. Multimodality treatment of melanoma brain metastases incorporating stereotactic radiosurgery (SRS). Cancer. 2007;109(9):1855–62. https://doi.org/10.1002/cncr.22605.

52. Fuhrmann D, Lippold A, Borrosch F, Ellwanger U, Garbe C, Suter L. Should adjuvant radiotherapy be recommended following resection of regional lymph node metastases of malignant melanomas? Br J Dermatol. 2001;144(1):66–70.

53. Yang AS, Chapman PB. The history and future of chemotherapy for melanoma. Hematol Oncol Clin North Am. 2009;23(3):583–597, x. https://doi.org/10.1016/j.hoc.2009.03.006.

54. Kroon HM. Treatment of locally advanced melanoma by isolated limb infusion with cytotoxic drugs. J Skin Cancer. 2011;2011:106573. https://doi.org/10.1155/2011/106573.

55. Zloza A, Dharmadhikari ND, Huelsmann EJ, Broucek JR, Hughes T, Kohlhapp FJ, Kaufman HL. Low-dose interleukin-2 impairs host anti-tumor immunity and inhibits therapeutic responses in a mouse model of melanoma. Cancer Immunol Immunother. 2017;66(1):9–16. https://doi.org/10.1007/s00262-016-1916-4.

56. Schwartz RN, Stover L, Dutcher J. Managing toxicities of high-dose interleukin-2. Oncology (Williston Park). 2002;16(11 Suppl 13):11–20.

57. Wheatley K, Ives N, Hancock B, Gore M, Eggermont A, Suciu S. Does adjuvant interferon-alpha for high-risk melanoma provide a worthwhile benefit? A meta-analysis of the randomised trials. Cancer Treat Rev. 2003;29(4):241–52.

58. Ferrantini M, Capone I, Belardelli F. Interferon-alpha and cancer: mechanisms of action and new perspectives of clinical use. Biochimie. 2007;89(6–7):884–93. https://doi.org/10.1016/j.biochi.2007.04.006.

59. Sabel MS, Sondak VK. Pros and cons of adjuvant interferon in the treatment of melanoma. Oncologist. 2003;8(5):451–8.

60. Hodi FS, O'Day SJ, McDermott DF, Weber RW, Sosman JA, Haanen JB, Gonzalez R, Robert C, Schadendorf D, Hassel JC, Akerley W, van den Eertwegh AJ, Lutzky J, Lorigan P, Vaubel

JM, Linette GP, Hogg D, Ottensmeier CH, Lebbe C, Peschel C, Quirt I, Clark JI, Wolchok JD, Weber JS, Tian J, Yellin MJ, Nichol GM, Hoos A, Urba WJ. Improved survival with ipilimumab in patients with metastatic melanoma. N Engl J Med. 2010;363(8):711–23. https://doi.org/10.1056/NEJMoa1003466.

61. Schadendorf D, Hodi FS, Robert C, Weber JS, Margolin K, Hamid O, Patt D, Chen TT, Berman DM, Wolchok JD. Pooled analysis of long-term survival data from phase II and phase III trials of Ipilimumab in Unresectable or metastatic melanoma. J Clin Oncol. 2015;33(17):1889–94. https://doi.org/10.1200/JCO.2014.56.2736.

62. Robert C, Thomas L, Bondarenko I, O'Day S, Weber J, Garbe C, Lebbe C, Baurain JF, Testori A, Grob JJ, Davidson N, Richards J, Maio M, Hauschild A, Miller WH Jr, Gascon P, Lotem M, Harmankaya K, Ibrahim R, Francis S, Chen TT, Humphrey R, Hoos A, Wolchok JD. Ipilimumab plus dacarbazine for previously untreated metastatic melanoma. N Engl J Med. 2011;364(26):2517–26. https://doi.org/10.1056/NEJMoa1104621.

63. Larkin J, Chiarion-Sileni V, Gonzalez R, Grob JJ, Cowey CL, Lao CD, Schadendorf D, Dummer R, Smylie M, Rutkowski P, Ferrucci PF, Hill A, Wagstaff J, Carlino MS, Haanen JB, Maio M, Marquez-Rodas I, McArthur GA, Ascierto PA, Long GV, Callahan MK, Postow MA, Grossmann K, Sznol M, Dreno B, Bastholt L, Yang A, Rollin LM, Horak C, Hodi FS, Wolchok JD. Combined nivolumab and Ipilimumab or monotherapy in untreated melanoma. N Engl J Med. 2015;373(1):23–34. https://doi.org/10.1056/NEJMoa1504030.

64. Ribas A, Hamid O, Daud A, Hodi FS, Wolchok JD, Kefford R, Joshua AM, Patnaik A, Hwu WJ, Weber JS, Gangadhar TC, Hersey P, Dronca R, Joseph RW, Zarour H, Chmielowski B, Lawrence DP, Algazi A, Rizvi NA, Hoffner B, Mateus C, Gergich K, Lindia JA, Giannotti M, Li XN, Ebbinghaus S, Kang SP, Robert C. Association of pembrolizumab with tumor response and survival among patients with advanced melanoma. JAMA. 2016;315(15):1600–9. https://doi.org/10.1001/jama.2016.4059.

65. Robert C, Schachter J, Long GV, Arance A, Grob JJ, Mortier L, Daud A, Carlino MS, McNeil C, Lotem M, Larkin J, Lorigan P, Neyns B, Blank CU, Hamid O, Mateus C, Shapira-Frommer R, Kosh M, Zhou H, Ibrahim N, Ebbinghaus S, Ribas A, KEYNOTE-006 Investigators. Pembrolizumab versus Ipilimumab in Advanced Melanoma. N Engl J Med. 2015;372(26):2521–32. https://doi.org/10.1056/NEJMoa1503093.

66. Larkin J, Lao CD, Urba WJ, McDermott DF, Horak C, Jiang J, Wolchok JD. Efficacy and safety of nivolumab in patients with BRAF V600 mutant and BRAF wild-type advanced melanoma: a pooled analysis of 4 clinical trials. JAMA Oncol. 2015;1(4):433–40. https://doi.org/10.1001/jamaoncol.2015.1184.

67. Linardou H, Gogas H. Toxicity management of immunotherapy for patients with metastatic melanoma. Ann Transl Med. 2016;4(14):272. https://doi.org/10.21037/atm.2016.07.10.

68. Andtbacka RH, Kaufman HL, Collichio F, Amatruda T, Senzer N, Chesney J, Delman KA, Spitler LE, Puzanov I, Agarwala SS, Milhem M, Cranmer L, Curti B, Lewis K, Ross M, Guthrie T, Linette GP, Daniels GA, Harrington K, Middleton MR, Miller WH Jr, Zager JS, Ye Y, Yao B, Li A, Doleman S, VanderWalde A, Gansert J, Coffin RS. Talimogene laherparepvec improves durable response rate in patients with advanced melanoma. J Clin Oncol. 2015;33(25):2780–8. https://doi.org/10.1200/JCO.2014.58.3377.

69. Kirkwood JM, Lee S, Moschos SJ, Albertini MR, Michalak JC, Sander C, Whiteside T, Butterfield LH, Weiner L. Immunogenicity and antitumor effects of vaccination with peptide vaccine+/−granulocyte-monocyte colony-stimulating factor and/or IFN-alpha2b in advanced metastatic melanoma: Eastern Cooperative Oncology Group Phase II Trial E1696. Clin Cancer Res. 2009;15(4):1443–51. https://doi.org/10.1158/1078-0432.CCR-08-1231.

70. Chapman PB, Hauschild A, Robert C, Haanen JB, Ascierto P, Larkin J, Dummer R, Garbe C, Testori A, Maio M, Hogg D, Lorigan P, Lebbe C, Jouary T, Schadendorf D, Ribas A, O'Day SJ, Sosman JA, Kirkwood JM, Eggermont AM, Dreno B, Nolop K, Li J, Nelson B, Hou J, Lee RJ, Flaherty KT, McArthur GA, BRIM-3 Study Group. Improved survival with vemurafenib in melanoma with BRAF V600E mutation. N Engl J Med. 2011;364(26):2507–16. https://doi.org/10.1056/NEJMoa1103782.

71. Hauschild A, Grob JJ, Demidov LV, Jouary T, Gutzmer R, Millward M, Rutkowski P, Blank CU, Miller WH Jr, Kaempgen E, Martin-Algarra S, Karaszewska B, Mauch C, Chiarion-Sileni V, Martin AM, Swann S, Haney P, Mirakhur B, Guckert ME, Goodman V, Chapman PB. Dabrafenib in BRAF-mutated metastatic melanoma: a multicentre, open-label, phase 3 randomised controlled trial. Lancet. 2012;380(9839):358–65. https://doi.org/10.1016/S0140-6736(12)60868-X.

72. Long GV, Stroyakovskiy D, Gogas H, Levchenko E, de Braud F, Larkin J, Garbe C, Jouary T, Hauschild A, Grob JJ, Chiarion-Sileni V, Lebbe C, Mandala M, Millward M, Arance A, Bondarenko I, Haanen JB, Hansson J, Utikal J, Ferraresi V, Kovalenko N, Mohr P, Probachai V, Schadendorf D, Nathan P, Robert C, Ribas A, DeMarini DJ, Irani JG, Swann S, Legos JJ, Jin F, Mookerjee B, Flaherty K. Dabrafenib and trametinib versus dabrafenib and placebo for Val600 BRAF-mutant melanoma: a multicentre, double-blind, phase 3 randomised controlled trial. Lancet. 2015;386(9992):444–51. https://doi.org/10.1016/S0140-6736(15)60898-4.

73. Larkin J, Ascierto PA, Dreno B, Atkinson V, Liszkay G, Maio M, Mandala M, Demidov L, Stroyakovskiy D, Thomas L, de la Cruz-Merino L, Dutriaux C, Garbe C, Sovak MA, Chang I, Choong N, Hack SP, McArthur GA, Ribas A. Combined vemurafenib and cobimetinib in BRAF-mutated melanoma. N Engl J Med. 2014;371(20):1867–76. https://doi.org/10.1056/NEJMoa1408868.

74. Daud A, Gill J, Kamra S, Chen L, Ahuja A. Indirect treatment comparison of dabrafenib plus trametinib versus vemurafenib plus cobimetinib in previously untreated metastatic melanoma patients. J Hematol Oncol. 2017;10(1):3. https://doi.org/10.1186/s13045-016-0369-8.

75. Carvajal RD, Antonescu CR, Wolchok JD, Chapman PB, Roman RA, Teitcher J, Panageas KS, Busam KJ, Chmielowski B, Lutzky J, Pavlick AC, Fusco A, Cane L, Takebe N, Vemula S, Bouvier N, Bastian BC, Schwartz GK. KIT as a therapeutic target in metastatic melanoma. JAMA. 2011;305(22):2327–34. https://doi.org/10.1001/jama.2011.746.

76. Meier F, Busch S, Lasithiotakis K, Kulms D, Garbe C, Maczey E, Herlyn M, Schittek B. Combined targeting of MAPK and AKT signalling pathways is a promising strategy for melanoma treatment. Br J Dermatol. 2007;156(6):1204–13. https://doi.org/10.1111/j.1365-2133.2007.07821.x.

77. Lasithiotakis KG, Sinnberg TW, Schittek B, Flaherty KT, Kulms D, Maczey E, Garbe C, Meier FE. Combined inhibition of MAPK and mTOR signaling inhibits growth, induces cell death, and abrogates invasive growth of melanoma cells. J Invest Dermatol. 2008;128(8):2013–23. https://doi.org/10.1038/jid.2008.44.

Chapter 7
Merkel Cell Carcinoma

Sheena Tsai and Jeremy S. Bordeaux

Abstract Merkel cell carcinoma (MCC) is a rare, aggressive skin cancer. The incidence has increased over the past 20 years, and this may be attributed to increased ultraviolet (UV) light exposure. MCC is more common among Caucasians, males, and individuals older than 69 years of age. Immunosuppressed patients are at a higher risk for MCC. MCC may present clinically as a dome-shaped red or blue nodule. The mnemonic "AEIOU" describes common clinical features: asymptomatic, expanding rapidly, immunosuppression, older than 50 years, and ultraviolet-exposed/fair skin. MCC most commonly presents on the head and neck, followed by the extremities and trunk. Diagnosis is made via biopsy, and the first-line treatment is surgical removal of the primary tumor. Sentinel lymph node biopsy (SLNB) is recommended for all patients: patients with negative sentinel lymph nodes (SLNs) may undergo wide local excision (WLE), Mohs micrographic surgery (MMS), or radiation to the primary tumor site. Patients with positive SLNs may undergo WLE or MMS, followed by complete lymph node dissection (CLND) and/or radiation to the nodal basin. Patients with metastatic disease may undergo chemotherapy or immunotherapy. Prognosis for MCC patients depends on the stage of disease: survival rates decrease as the stage advances. Due to the high recurrence rate of MCC, patients are encouraged to see their dermatologists frequently.

Keywords Merkel cell carcinoma · Skin cancer · Epidemiology · Clinical features · Diagnosis · Histopathology · Staging · Treatment · Prognosis

Introduction

Merkel cell carcinoma (MCC) is a rare, aggressive skin cancer most commonly presenting on sun-exposed skin. MCC has multiple synonyms: primary cutaneous neuroendocrine carcinoma, small cell primary cutaneous carcinoma, and cutaneous

S. Tsai · J. S. Bordeaux (✉)
University Hospitals Cleveland Medical Center and Case Western Reserve University School of Medicine, Cleveland, OH, USA
e-mail: jeremy.bordeaux@uhhospitals.org

© Springer International Publishing AG, part of Springer Nature 2018
A. Hanlon (ed.), *A Practical Guide to Skin Cancer*,
https://doi.org/10.1007/978-3-319-74903-7_7

trabecular carcinoma. MCC occurs when Merkel cells have unregulated growth. Merkel cells are localized to the basal layer of the epidermis, at the skin's dermo-epidermal junction [1–4]. They are receptors for light touch sensation and are innervated by heavily myelinated Aβ sensory nerves [5].

Epidemiology

Merkel cell carcinoma incidence has tripled over the past two decades in the United States to 1500 cases per year [6]. The increased incidence is attributed to greater UV exposure, increasing numbers of immunocompromised persons, and more specific diagnostic techniques. Excessive UV radiation is attributed to sun exposure, tanning beds, and light-based therapies such as psoralens with UV light (PUVA). Infection with Merkel cell polyomavirus (MCPyV) is an important risk factor, as up to 80% of patients are found to be MCPyV positive [7]. MCC occurs most commonly in elderly individuals, with a mean age at diagnosis of 69 years [8]. For men younger than 65 years old, it is found mostly on the trunk and limbs, whereas it is found most commonly on the head and neck in males 65 years of age and older [9]. MCC affects males more often than females (2:1 ratio in Caucasians and African Americans; 1.5:1 in all other ethnic groups) [10]. Fair skin is a risk factor, with more than nine out of ten cases being found in Caucasians [11].

Immunosuppression is a risk factor for MCC: patients with HIV have a 13-fold increase in relative risk of MCC, and solid organ transplant recipients have a 10-fold increase. Patients with chronic lymphocytic leukemia (CLL) also have an increased risk of developing MCC [12].

Clinical Features

MCC usually presents as a rapidly growing, asymptomatic, dome-shaped red or blue nodule on chronically sun-damaged skin (Fig. 7.1) [13]. The differential diagnosis includes basal cell carcinoma (BCC), melanoma, epidermoid cyst, small cell lung carcinoma, cutaneous lymphoma, neuroblastoma, and sarcoma [14].

MCC presents most frequently in the head and neck (41%–50%) (Fig. 7.1), followed by the extremities (32%–38%) (Fig. 7.2) and trunk (12%–14%) [13]. The primary tumor's size varies greatly: in one study, 21.3% of patients had a primary tumor with a diameter of less than 1 cm; 43.3% of patients had tumors with a diameter between 1 and 2 cm; 35.3% of patients had tumors measuring greater than 2 cm [15]. If MCC is suspected, a thorough lymph node exam is performed to evaluate for clinical lymph node metastasis.

Fig. 7.1 Merkel cell
carcinoma by the eyelid

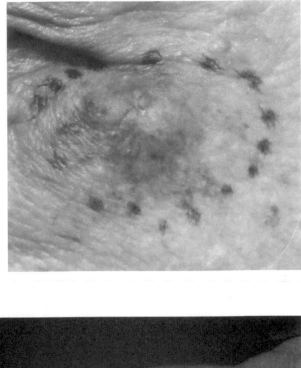

Fig. 7.2 Merkel cell
carcinoma on lower
extremity

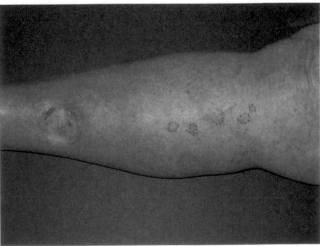

Histopathology

Merkel cells are clear oval cells localized to the dermo-epidermal junction where
they associate with dermal nerves to function as mechanoreceptors of light touch
(Figs. 7.3 and 7.4). Merkel cells are found throughout the skin but have increased
density in glabrous skin and hair follicles [15a]. Merkel cells within the hair follicles and oral mucosa are not associated with nerves. On light microscopy, Merkel

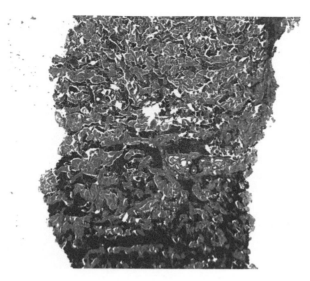

Fig. 7.3 H&E of Merkel cell carcinoma, 4× magnification

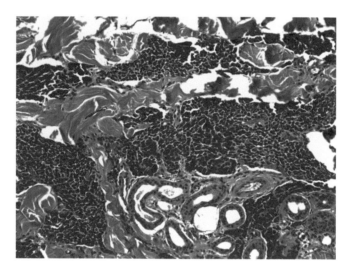

Fig. 7.4 H&E of Merkel cell carcinoma, 20× magnification

cells are virtually undetectable by the naked eye. However, on electron microscopy, Merkel cells are characterized by lobulated nuclei, a cytoskeleton consisting of intermediate filaments, microvilli that extend into nearby keratinocytes to allow increased sensitivity for mechanical stimuli, and membrane-bound cytoplasmic granules [16]. On immunohistochemistry, Merkel cells' intermediate filaments stain for cytokeratins (CK) 8, 18, 19, and 20 [17]. In normal Merkel cells, CK 20 staining is observed in a diffuse pattern, whereas it is observed in a perinuclear pattern in MCC. Additionally, the cytoplasmic granules stain positively for synaptophysin, chromogranin A, and neuron-specific enolase; they stain negatively for desmin and S100.

Diagnosis and Staging

Shave, incisional, or excisional biopsy is recommended for evaluation of skin lesions clinically suspicious for MCC. MCC is diagnosed histologically with dermal clusters of round or ovoid cells with hyperchromatic nuclei—a typical finding in neuroendocrine neoplasms. However, due to variable histopathologic features, cytokeratin immunohistochemistry staining is used to differentiate MCC from other neuroendocrine tumors.

Sentinel lymph node biopsy (SLNB) is recommended in the evaluation and treatment of MCC whether clinical lymphadenopathy is noted. MCC often metastasizes to the draining lymph node basin. Lymph node involvement is an important factor for survival and is a necessary component for MCC staging [18]. Positive SLNs are found in up to 33% of patients on initial presentation [19]. Chest X-rays and computerized tomography (CT)/positron emission tomography (PET) scans may be performed for patients with primary tumors greater than 2 cm to survey for MCC metastases or to evaluate for small cell lung carcinoma, a neuroendocrine tumor that can metastasize to the skin.

The TNM (tumor thickness, nodal involvement, metastasis) staging system for MCC is outlined in Table 7.1. Staging is based on clinical size of the primary tumor, presence or absence of SLNB, presence or absence of tumor metastasis in the SLN, presence or absence of lymph node involvement, and presence or absence of distant metastases.

Primary Tumor (T)

The T category defines the dimensions of the primary tumor and/or how far the tumor has invaded into other tissues, specifically bone, muscle, fascia, or cartilage. Tumors with dimensions of <2 cm (T1) have a better prognosis than those with dimensions of >2 cm (T2–T3). T2 tumors measure greater than 2 cm but less than 5 cm. T3 tumors are over 5 cm in dimension. Lastly, T4 tumors invade underlying bone, muscle, fascia, or cartilage [20].

Table 7.1 Staging of Merkel cell carcinoma, AJCC 8th edition

Stage	Primary tumor thickness	Nodal involvement	Metastasis
0	In situ	No regional lymph node metastasis	No distant metastasis
I Clinical[a]	≤ 2 cm maximum tumor dimension	Nodes negative by clinical exam only	No distant metastasis
I Pathologic[b]	≤ 2 cm maximum tumor dimension	Nodes negative by pathologic exam	No distant metastasis
IIA Clinical	> 2 cm tumor dimension	Nodes negative by clinical exam only	No distant metastasis
IIA Pathologic	> 2 cm tumor dimension	Nodes negative by pathologic exam	No distant metastasis
IIB Clinical	Primary tumor invades bone, muscle, fascia, or cartilage	Nodes negative by clinical exam only	No distant metastasis
IIB Pathologic	Primary tumor invades bone, muscle, fascia, or cartilage	Nodes negative by pathologic exam	No distant metastasis
III Clinical	Any size/depth	Nodes positive by clinical exam only	No distant metastasis
IIIA Pathologic	Any size/depth	Nodes positive by pathologic exam only (nodes not apparently positive on clinical exam)	No distant metastasis
	Not detected ("unknown primary")	Nodes positive by clinical exam and confirmed via pathologic exam	No distant metastasis
IIIB Pathologic	Any size/depth	Nodes positive by clinical exam and confirmed via pathologic exam or in-transit metastasis[c]	No distant metastasis
IV Clinical	Any	+/− regional nodal involvement	Distant metastasis detected via clinical exam
IV Pathologic	Any	+/− regional nodal involvement	Distant metastasis confirmed via pathologic exam

Used with permission of the American Joint Committee on Cancer (AJCC), Chicago, Illinois. The original and primary source for this information is the AJCC Cancer Staging Manual, Eighth Edition (2017), published by Springer International Publishing

[a]Detected via inspection, palpation, and/or imaging

[b]Detected via sentinel lymph node biopsy, lymphadenectomy, or fine needle biopsy; pathologic confirmation of metastatic disease may be via biopsy of the suspected metastasis

[c]In-transit metastasis: a tumor distinct from the primary lesion and located either between the primary lesion and the draining regional lymph nodes or distal to the primary lesion

Nodal Involvement (N)

The N category is characterized by regional lymph node involvement detected either by clinical or pathologic exam; the 8th Edition AJCC Staging System has this defined in the stage itself (Table 7.2) [20]. N0 designates no lymph node involvement, while cN0 designates negative clinical lymph node exam, and pN0 designates negative pathologic lymph node exam. This distinction is critical, as patients with clinically positive nodes have worse outcomes than those with positive pathologic or microscopic nodes.

Lymph node metastasis, whether detected clinically or histologically, is denoted as N1. Pathologic lymph node staging is further divided into N1a if there are micrometastases (isolated tumor cells in a lymph node) without clinical lymphadenopathy or N1b if there are macrometastases with clinical lymphadenopathy and histologic confirmation. Patients with N1b staging have a worse prognosis than those with N1a. In-transit metastases are denoted as N2.

Metastasis (M)

The M category is characterized by distant metastases most often to the brain, liver, lung, and bone. This category distinguishes stage IV from all the other stages. Metastases beyond the regional lymph nodes denote M1; to the skin, subcutaneous tissues, or distant lymph nodes, M1a; to the lungs, M1b; and to visceral sites, M1c [20].

Table 7.2 Staging for nodal involvement (N) category

Clinical staging	Pathologic staging	Nodal involvement (N)
NX	NX	Regional lymph nodes not able to be assessed
N0	N0	No regional lymph node metastasis
	cN0	Lymph nodes negative by clinical exam[a]
	pN0	Lymph nodes negative by pathologic exam
N1	N1	Metastasis in regional lymph nodes
	N1a	Micrometastasis[b]
	N1b	Macrometastasis[c]
N2	N2	In-transit metastasis[d]
N3	N3	In-transit metastasis with lymph node metastasis

Used with permission of the American Joint Committee on Cancer (AJCC), Chicago, Illinois. The original and primary source for this information is the AJCC Cancer Staging Manual, Eighth Edition (2017) published by Springer International Publishing
[a]Clinical exam performed via palpation, inspection, or imaging
[b]Micrometastasis defined as isolated tumor cells in a lymph node
[c]Macrometastasis defined as clinical detectable nodes, confirmed by lymphadenectomy or needle biopsy
[d]In-transit metastasis defined as tumor distinct from primary lesion and located either between the primary lesion and regional lymph nodes or distal to the primary lesion

Staging

Tables 7.3 and 7.4 show the final staging based on the TNM system. Staging is specific for either clinical or pathologic exam. Stage I is for tumors less than or equal to 2 cm. Stage II is for tumors greater than 2 cm. Stage IIC denotes tumors that have invaded the bone, muscle, fascia, or cartilage but have no lymph node involvement or distant metastases. Stage III is any tumor size with regional lymph node involvement. Stage III is subdivided into either micrometastases or macrometastases. Stage IV is characterized by metastasis beyond the draining lymph node basin, irrespective of primary tumor size and draining lymph node involvement [20].

Treatment

Surgery is the first-line treatment for MCC [15]. Intraoperative SLNB is recommended for all MCC carcinoma patients due to the procedure's low morbidity and mortality and the high rate of lymph node metastasis associated with MCC.

Table 7.3 Final staging based on TNM system, for clinical exam

Final stage	Tumor thickness (T)	Nodal involvement (N)	Metastasis (M)
0	Tis	N0	M0
I	T1	N0	M0
IIA	T2/T3	N0	M0
IIB	T4	N0	M0
III	Any T	N1–N3	M0
IV	Any T	Any N	M1

Used with permission of the American Joint Committee on Cancer (AJCC), Chicago, Illinois. The original and primary source for this information is the AJCC Cancer Staging Manual, Eighth Edition (2017), published by Springer International Publishing

Table 7.4 Final staging based on TNM system, for pathologic exam

Final stage	Tumor thickness (T)	Nodal involvement (N)	Metastasis (M)
0	Tis	N0	M0
I	T1	N0	M0
IIA	T2/T3	N0	M0
IIB	T4	N0	M0
IIIA	Any T	N1a	M0
IIIA	T0	N1b	M0
IIIB	Any T	N1b, N2, N3	M0
IV	Any T	Any N	M1

Used with permission of the American Joint Committee on Cancer (AJCC), Chicago, Illinois. The original and primary source for this information is the AJCC Cancer Staging Manual, Eighth Edition (2017) published by Springer International Publishing

Patients with negative SLNs can undergo either wide local excision (WLE) or Mohs micrographic surgery (MMS) for surgical treatment of T1 tumors. WLE with 1–2 cm margins is recommended. If the tumor is in a cosmetically sensitive area, MMS is a surgical option. In MMS, the clinical tumor is removed with a 2–4 mm margin of normal skin. The tissue is processed to study the entire margin. The MMS technique ensures complete removal of the tumor while sparing normal adjacent tissue [21].

For patients with a positive SLN, there are three treatment options: complete lymph node dissection (CLND), CLND and radiation of the nodal basin, or radiation of the nodal basin.

Radiation is typically prescribed in conjunction with surgery or as the sole treatment if the patient is a nonsurgical candidate. Factors to consider in deciding upon radiation treatment include the patient's level of immunosuppression, the primary tumor's size, SLN status, tumor depth, and technicalities of therapy (location of tumor, lack of SLNB) [15]. Radiation is not recommended in patients with a low risk of recurrence (e.g., negative SLNB, clear surgical margins, or primary tumor <1 cm). However, radiation is highly recommended for primary tumor sites or SLNs in patients with a high risk of recurrence (macroscopic nodal disease, multiple node involvement, positive margins at resection, primary tumor>2 cm). Surgery with radiation to the regional lymph nodes can decrease the rate of recurrence 3.7-fold [22, 23]. For primary lesions on the head and neck, radiation is recommended even with negative SLNs, as SLNBs performed in this area may not be reliable. For primary lesions on the trunk or extremities, radiation may not be necessary if the SLNs are negative, as tracking the draining lymph node is more reliable.

Chemotherapy is not often used as the primary or adjuvant treatment of MCC as there is no randomized controlled studies to guide care [24]. If chemotherapy is used, it is for palliative care rather than a primary or adjuvant therapy. Patients treated with cytotoxic chemotherapy have a median progression-free survival of only 3 months [25]. There are no Food and Drug Administration (FDA)-approved chemotherapies for advanced MCC, but current standard therapy is platinum with etoposide [25].

Immunotherapy is a promising, new treatment for MCC. Programmed death ligand 1 (PDL-1) is overexpressed in many MCC tumors [26]. PDL-1 binds to programmed death-1 (PD-1) to inhibit lymphocyte tumor responses. Checkpoint inhibitor immunotherapy with PD-1 receptors nivolumab and pembrolizumab showed a recurrence-free period of 8 months and 9.7 months in MCC patients, respectively [27, 28]. Avelumab, a monoclonal antibody that binds PDL-1, is the only FDA-approved drug for the treatment of MCC. In 88 MCC patients previously treated with chemotherapy, 20 patients had a partial tumor response; 8 had a complete tumor response with avelumab. Importantly, the responses were durable with 40% having a progression-free survival and 60% an overall survival at 6 months [29]. Immunotherapy is reserved for metastatic disease and not as an adjuvant therapy following surgery.

Outcomes/Prognosis

The 5-year survival rates for MCC are stage-dependent. For stage IA and IB, the 5-year survival rates are 80% and 60%, respectively. As disease progresses, the survival rate decreases to 50% in stage II and to 25% in stage IV [30]. MCC often recurs. Local recurrence or lymph node metastasis usually presents within the first year. Patients are recommended to have regular dermatology exams with clinical lymph node evaluation every 2–3 months for the first year and every 6 months following.

References

1. Smith KR. The ultrastructure of the human Haarscheibe and Merkel cell. J Invest Dermatol. 1970;54:150–9.
2. Hashimoto K. The ultrastructure of the skin of human embryos. X. Merkel tactile cells in the finger and nail. J Anat. 1972;111:99–120.
3. Kurosumi K, Kurosumi U, Suzuki H. Fine structures of Merkel cells and associated nerve fibers in the epidermis of certain mammalian species. Arch Histol Jpn. 1969;30:295–313.
4. Halata Z, Grim M, Bauman KI. Friedrich Sigmund Merkel and his "Merkel cell", morphology, development, and physiology: review and new results. Anat Rec. 2003;271:225–39.
5. Iggo A, Muir AR. The structure and function of a slowly adapting touch corpuscle in hairy skin. J Physiol. 1969;200:763–96.
6. Lemos B, Nghiem P. J Investig Dermatol. 2007;127:2100.
7. Feng H, Shuda M, Chang Y, Moore PS. Clonal integration of a polyomavirus in human Merkel cell carcinoma. Science. 2008;319(5866):1096–100.
8. Miller RW, Rabkin CS. Merkel cell carcinoma and melanoma: etiological similarities and differences. Cancer Epidemiol Biomark Prev. 1999;8:153–8.
9. Hussain SK, Sundquist J, Hemminki K. Incidence trends of squamous cell and rare skin cancers in the Swedish national cancer registry point to calendar year and age-dependent increases. J Invest Dermatol. 2010;130:1323–8.
10. Medina-Franco H, Urist MM, Fiveash J, Heslin MJ, et al. Multimodality treatment of Merkel cell carcinoma: case series and literature review of 1024 cases. Ann Surg Oncol. 2001;8:204–8.
11. Key statistics for Merkel cell carcinoma [Internet]. American Cancer Society. 2016 [cited 12 December 2016]. Available from: http://www.cancer.org/cancer/skincancer-merkelcell/detailedguide/skin-cancer-merkel-cell-carcinoma-key-statistics.
12. Tadmor T, Aviv A, Polliack A. Merkel cell carcinoma, chronic lymphocytic leukemia and other lymphoproliferative disorders: an old bond with possible new viral ties. Ann Oncol. 2011;22:250–6.
13. Duprat JP, Landman G, Salvajoli JV, Brechtbühl ER. A review of the epidemiology and treatment of Merkel cell carcinoma. Clinics (Sao Paulo). 2011;66(10):1817–23.
14. Wang TS, Byrne PJ, Jacobs LK, Taube JM. Merkel cell carcinoma: update and review. Semin Cutan Med Surg. 2011;30:48–56.
15. Heath M, Jaimes N, Lemos B, et al. Clinical characteristics of Merkel cell carcinoma at diagnosis in 195 patients: the AEIOU features. J Am Acad Dermatol. 2008;58:375–81.
16. Kim DK, Holbrook KA. The appearance, density and distribution of Merkel cells in human embryonic and fetal skin: their relation to sweat gland and hair follicle development. J Invest Dermatol. 1995;104(3):411–416.

17. Eispert AC, Fuchs F, Brandner JM, et al. Evidence for distinct populations of human Merkel cells. Histochem Cell Biol. 2009;132:83–93.
18. Moll R, Löwe A, Cytokeratin LJ. 20 in human carcinomas. A new histodiagnostic marker detected by monoclonal antibodies. Am J Pathol. 1992;140:427–47.
19. Hill AD, Brady MS, Coit DG. Intraoperative lymphatic mapping and sentinel lymph node biopsy for Merkel cell carcinoma. Br J Surg. 1999;86(4):518–21.
20. Messina JL, Reintgen DS, Cruse CW, et al. Selective lymphadenectomy in patients with Merkel cell (cutaneous neuroendocrine) carcinoma. Ann Surg Oncol. 1997;4(5):389–95.
21. Edge S, Greene FL, Byrd DR, Brookland RK, et al., editors. AJCC cancer staging manual. 8th ed. New York: Springer; 2017.
22. Overview of Mohs Micrographic Surgery: Mohs Surgery Patient Education [Internet]. Skincancermohssurgery.org. 2016 [cited 13 December 2016]. Available from: http://www.skincancermohssurgery.org/about-mohs-surgery/overview-of-mohs-micrographic-surgery.
23. Lewis KG, Weinstock MA, Weaver AL, et al. Adjuvant local irradiation for Merkel cell carcinoma. JAMA Dermatol. 2006;142:693–700.
24. Mojica P, Smith D, Ellenhorn JD. Adjuvant radiation therapy is associated with improved survival in Merkel cell carcinoma of the skin. J Clin Oncol. 2007;25:1043–7.
25. Voog E, Biron P, Martin JP, et al. Chemotherapy for patients with locally advanced or metastatic Merkel cell carcinoma. Cancer. 1999;85:2589–95.
26. Lipson EJ, Vincent JG, Loyo M, Kagohara LT, et al. PD-L1 expression in the Merkel cell microenvironment association with inflammation, Merkel cell polyomavirus and overall survival. Cancer Immunol Res. 2013;1:10.
27. Walocko FM, Scheier BY, Harms PW, et al. Metastatic Merkel cell carcinoma response to nivolumab. J Immunother Cancer. 2016;4:79.
28. Nghiem PT, Bhatia S, Lipson EJ, et al. PD-1 blockade with pembrolizumab in advanced Merkel-cell carcinoma. N Engl J Med. 2016;374:2542–52.
29. Kaufman HL, Russell J, Hamid O, Bhatia S, et al. Avelumab in patients with chemotherapy refractory metastatic Merkel cell carcinoma: a multicenter, single-group, open-label, phase 2 trial. Lancet Oncol. 2016;17(10):1374–85.
30. Survival rates for Merkel cell carcinoma, by stage [Internet]. American Cancer Society. 2016 [cited 12 December 2016]. Available from: http://www.cancer.org/cancer/skincancer-merkelcell/detailedguide/skin-cancer-merkel-cell-carcinoma-survival-rates.

Chapter 8
Cutaneous Lymphomas

Trisha Bhat, Jeffrey P. Zwerner, and Amy Musiek

Abstract Cutaneous B-cell and T-cell lymphomas are distinct subtypes of non-Hodgkin lymphoma (NHL). They are cancers of lymphocytes that primarily involve the skin, the most common single-organ location of extranodal NHL (Groves et al., J Natl Cancer Inst. 2000;92(15):1240–1251). Cutaneous lymphomas may remain limited to the skin for long periods of time but can spread to blood, lymph nodes, and viscera in cases of advanced disease. Cutaneous T-cell lymphomas (CTCL), involving malignant clonal T cells that present primarily in the skin, comprise more than 75% of all primary cutaneous lymphomas (Willemze et al., Blood. 2005;105(10):3768–3785). CTCL includes variants with indolent, aggressive, and variable clinical behavior, with mycosis fungoides (MF) and Sézary syndrome (SS) together comprising more than 50% of all CTCLs (Willemze et al., Blood. 2005;105(10):3768–3785). The second most common type of CTCL, CD30+ lymphoproliferative disorders, comprises 20% of all cutaneous lymphomas. Cutaneous B-cell lymphoma (CBCL) is less common and often presents as indolent disease.

Keywords Cutaneous T-cell lymphoma · Mycosis fungoides · Sézary syndrome · Folliculotropic mycosis fungoides · Pagetoid reticulosis (Woringer-Kolopp) · Granulomatous slack skin · Hypopigmented mycosis fungoides · Cutaneous B-cell lymphoma · Primary cutaneous follicular center lymphoma · Primary cutaneous marginal zone B-cell lymphoma · Primary cutaneous large B-cell lymphoma (PCLBCL) · Leg-type

T. Bhat
Washington University in St. Louis, School of Medicine, St. Louis, MO, USA

J. P. Zwerner
Department of Medicine, Division of Dermatology, Vanderbilt University, Nashville, TN, USA

A. Musiek (✉)
Dermatology, Washington University in St. Louis, School of Medicine, St. Louis, MO, USA
e-mail: amusiek@wustl.edu

© Springer International Publishing AG, part of Springer Nature 2018
A. Hanlon (ed.), *A Practical Guide to Skin Cancer*,
https://doi.org/10.1007/978-3-319-74903-7_8

Epidemiology

MF/SS make up 4% of NHL, with approximately 0.96 CTCL cases per 100,000 patients and 3000 new cases every year. The annual incidence of CTCL has continued to rise since the early 1970s, likely due to absolute increases in number of cases but also due to improved and increased physician detection and diagnosis; higher incidence has been shown to correspond to physician and medical specialist density [3, 4]. Annual overall incidence of CTCL increased from 6.4 in 1973–2002 to 7.7 persons per million in 2001–2005, with MF incidence alone accounting for 4.1 persons per million [1, 5]. Accounting for early-stage MF that is often not reported to tumor registries, Zic et al. estimate 3000 new cases of MF annually between 2000 and 2013 [6]. However, annual percent change in overall incidence of CTCL has stabilized since 1998, with similar incidence stabilization seen across race, sex, age, diagnosis, and registry lines. Five-year CTCL survival rates have also increased over time [7]. The median age at diagnosis is 55–65 years, and two-thirds of patients present with early-stage disease (IB-IIA). CTCL disproportionately affects African Americans, the elderly, and males, with a 2:1 male:female ratio [3, 5, 8]. The most significant clinical prognostic factors are TNMB classification and clinical stage, presence or lack of extracutaneous disease, and patient age [9].

Pathogenesis

In normal skin, T cells are recruited after an insult, such as an arthropod bite or exposure to a contact allergen, and their receptors recognize specific antigens and initiate an immune reaction. Downstream inflammatory responses lead to activation of naïve T cells in the lymph nodes to antigen-specific effector/memory cells which can then home to the skin. These skin effector/memory T cells are CD3+, CD4+, CD7−, CD26−, CLA+, CXCR3+, and CCR4+. Cutaneous lymphocyte antigen (CLA), an E-selectin ligand, interacts with E-selectin receptor (ELAM-1) on post-capillary venules in the dermis, allowing T lymphocytes to slow down and roll along endothelial venule walls [10, 11]. CXC chemokine receptor 3 (CXCR3) and CC-chemokine receptor 4 (CCR4) both bind to skin-manufactured chemokines, helping lymphocytes to chemotax and home to the skin [11–14].

Tropism of any malignant lymphoma to the skin is based on both the dysregulated skin-homing behavior of the lymphocytes involved and their ability to attain clonal dominance and proliferate within the skin. In MF, the defect is found in mature effector memory T cells that are present in and do not leave the skin; in SS, affected cells are central memory T cells that migrate between the skin, lymph nodes, and blood [15].

Malignant CLA$^+$ T lymphocytes express particularly high levels of CC-chemokine receptor 4 (CCR4) as well as CXCR3 [6, 11, 16–18] (Fig. 8.1) . Additionally, MF skin lesions often express high levels of the CCR4 ligands CCL17 (TARC) and CCL22 (MDC) [16, 19, 20]. Increased expression of CCR4 and CXCR3 on T

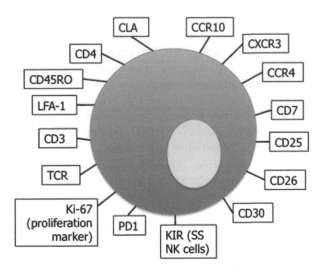

Fig. 8.1 Malignant T lymphocyte [6, 11]

lymphocytes and increased expression of their chemotactic ligands in the skin may help to explain the dysregulated skin-homing behavior and enhanced epidermotropism of MF T cells [21]. Notably, this epidermotropism is lost in late-stage CTCL; tumor-stage tissue exhibits decreased expression of CCR4 and CXCR3 but increased expression of CCR7, a receptor involved in lymphatic entry [18].

The mechanism behind constitutive activation and proliferation of malignant T lymphocytes in CTCL remains unclear, though the prevalence of Langerhans cells in the hallmark Pautrier's microabscesses seen on histopathology (detailed below) may suggest their involvement [11]. Langerhans cells, immature dendritic cells that reside in the skin, may provide persistent stimulation to T cells in the skin, allowing for constitutive activation and clonal expansion [22].

Malignant T cells in mycosis fungoides also exhibit Th2-type activity, expressing high levels of the Th2 cytokines IL-4, IL-5, and IL-10 that are important in mechanisms of allergy and responses against extracellular parasites. The Th2 response also decreases cytotoxicity, intracellular microbicidal activity, and cell-mediated immunity by downregulating Th1 differentiation and cytokine production [11, 23]. Additionally, Stat3 and Stat5, components of the JAK-STAT signaling pathway used to transmit cytokine signaling information, are dysregulated and show constitutive activation even in early CTCL. Meanwhile, Fas expression and signaling, important in cell-mediated cytotoxicity, are decreased, corresponding to decreased sensitivity to apoptotic stimuli; this may allow tumor cells to accumulate [24–27]. Malignant T lymphocytes are also resistant to the growth suppression effects of transforming growth factor (TGF)-β [11]. Malignant lymphocytes can also escape elimination by cell-mediated cytotoxicity by exploiting the immunosuppressive cell surface protein PD-1, which is involved in the functional impairment of immune cells that would normally be activated against MF/SS cells. PD-1 is found on the surface of malignant T lymphocytes in many forms of CTCL but is most notably seen in the majority of cases of early-stage MF.

No reliable genetic abnormality has been uniformly detected in early-stage CTCL. In later-stage MF/SS, various sites of common chromosomal structural aberration have been identified through comparative genomic hybridization analysis. Somatic copy number variants (SCNVs) appear to drive CTCL, comprising 92% of all driver mutations [28]. The most frequent losses are found in chromosomes 1p, 17p, 10q/10, and 19 as well as rare deletions in 1p31p36 and 10q26; 17p deletions involve deletion of tumor suppressor TP53 and allow for uncontrolled growth. The most frequent gains are found in chromosomes 4/4q, 18, and 17q/17 [29]. Many of these gains and losses involve specific, identifiable genes that can thus be implicated in CTCL pathogenesis. In a study of 40 leukemic CTCL patients, Choi et al. analyzed recurrent changes in single amino acids and recurrent protein-altering changes in specific genes to identify *CD28*, *RHOA*, *PLCG1*, *BRAF*, *STAT5B*, *TP53*, *DNMT3A*, *FAS*, *NFKB*, *ARID1A*, *ZEB1*, and *CDKN2A* as possible CTCL drivers [28].

Disease progression has been associated with widespread hypermethylation of tumor suppressor genes and their promoters. Hypermethylation of *BCL7a*, *PTPRG*, and *thrombospondin 4* genes, as well as promoter hypermethylation of tumor suppressor genes *p73*, *p16*, *CHFR p15*, and *TMS1*, leads to loss of function and inactivation of these genes, with consequences for DNA repair, the cell cycle, and apoptotic signaling pathways [30]. Amplification of oncogenes has also been observed, particularly amplification of 8q containing the *MYC* oncogene [28, 31].

Staging

Staging evaluation for CTCL entails a comprehensive physical exam, complete blood count, metabolic panel, and imaging [11]. Physical examination includes evaluating the size and type of skin lesions, palpating peripheral lymph nodes, and palpating for masses and organomegaly [32, 33]. The standard staging classification system for CTCL, including both mycosis fungoides and Sézary syndrome, is the tumor-node-metastasis-blood (TNMB) system, encompassing cutaneous, lymph node, visceral, and peripheral blood involvement [34].

T (Tumor)

The T classification comprises both the body surface area involved and lesional thickness (Table 8.1). Patients with only patches and plaques are classified as T1 (lesions covering less than 10% of skin surface) or T2 (lesions covering more than 10% skin surface), with the area of a single hand with the thumb removed equivalent to 1% of total body surface area. Patches are skin lesions of any size that lack induration or elevation above surrounding skin (Table 8.2, *Patch Stage A*), while plaques are indurated or elevated (Table 8.2, *Patch Stage B*). T1 can be divided into

Table 8.1 Tumor classification

T1a	Patches only <10% total BSA
T1b	Plaques ± patches only <10% total BSA
T2a	Patches only >10% total BSA
T2b	Plaques ± patches only >10% total BSA
T3	Tumor >1 cm in diameter
T4	Erythroderma >80% BSA

T1a (patch only) and T1b (plaque ± patch), and T2 can be divided into T2a (patch only) and T2b (plaque ± patch). Patients with at least one cutaneous tumor – a solid or nodular lesion greater than or equal to 1 cm in diameter with deep infiltration in the skin and/or vertical growth – are classified as T3 (Table 8.2, *Tumor Stage*) [35, 36]. The presence of erythroderma, defined as skin involvement of more than 80% of the total body surface area, defines T4.

N (Node)

Lymph node biopsies are rare in the routine diagnosis of CTCL and are typically only performed in patients for whom a diagnosis is in question [32]. The TNMB system classifies most patients as N0, with no clinically abnormal nodes, or NX, with clinically abnormal lymph nodes that have not been histologically confirmed by biopsy. NX patients may have enlarged nodes secondary to dermatopathic changes, lymphoma, or other reactive diseases. In patients with lymphadenopathy, defined as nodes 1.5 cm or larger in diameter or nodes that are firm or irregular, excisional node biopsies are used preferentially over fine needle aspirations because the presence and extent of lymph node involvement affects both staging and prognosis. N1 denotes enlarged lymph nodes that are histologically uninvolved (Dutch grade 1 or NCI LN_{0-2}). N2 denotes enlarged lymph nodes that are histologically involved but without changes in nodal architecture (Dutch grade 2 or NCI LN_3). N3 denotes enlarged lymph nodes that are histologically involved with effacement of nodal architecture (Dutch grade 3–4 or NCI LN_4) [33].

M (Metastasis)

The M classification denotes extracutaneous metastasis. M0 indicates that lymphoma cells have not spread outside the skin or lymph nodes, while M1 indicates visceral involvement. M1 classification requires documentation of the involvement of only one organ, typically liver or spleen, outside of the skin and nodes [36].

Table 8.2 Clinical manifestations of MF and SS

	Clinical presentation	Prognosis and management	Predominant T cell subset

Classic MF	Patches (Fig. 8.2)
	Plaques (Fig. 8.3)
	Tumors (Fig. 8.4)
	Erythroderma
	Pruritus
	Skin ulcers
		Indolent clinical behavior
		Worse prognosis at more advanced stages
		Antihistamines, topical therapies, and psychotropic drugs for pruritus
		Skin-directed therapies for early-stage MF
		  • Class I topical steroids
		  • PUVA
		  • nb-UVB
		  • Topical mechlorethamine
		Therapies for advanced stage MF:
		  • Bexarotene
		  • TSEBT
		  • Vorinostat or romidepsin
		  • Brentuximab
		  • IFN-α
		  • ECP
		  • Multimodal combination therapy
			CD4+

Folliculotropic MF (FMF) (Fig. 8.5)	Pilosebaceous areas: head, neck, upper torso [83]
	Slowly enlarging solitary patch, plaque, or tumor
	Cystic and comedonal lesions
	Alopecia
	Mucinorrhea
	Pruritus
		More aggressive than conventional MF with increased risk of disease progression
		Difficult to achieve full response with skin-directed therapies
		Antihistamines, topical therapies, and psychotropic drugs for pruritus
		Systemic therapies for early-stage FMF:
		  • PUVA with oral bexarotene or acitretin
		  • PUVA with IFN-α
		  • TSEBT ± retinoids or IFN
		Systemic therapies for advanced stage FMF:
		  • Irradiation
		  • Allogeneic stem cell transplantation
		  • Chemotherapy
			CD4+

Pagetoid reticulosis (Woringer-Kolopp disease)	Extremities; acral skin. Solitary psoriasis-like or hyperkeratotic patch or plaque	Indolent clinical behavior with favorable prognosis Skin-directed therapies appropriate • Topical steroids • Topical mechlorethamine • PUVA • nb-UVB • Directed radiation • Localized electron beam therapy for solitary/limited areas	CD4+ or CD8+
Granulomatous slack skin	Groin and underarm. Folds of lax skin in major skin folds	Indolent, slowly progressive with favorable prognosis See classic therapies: • PUVA • Radiation • Systemic steroids • IFN-α	CD4+ or CD8+
Hypopigmented MF	Irregular but clearly defined hypopigmented patches. Some pruritus. Largely asymptomatic	Indolent clinical course with favorable prognosis and repigmentation Therapy: • nb-UVB • PUVA • Topical chemotherapy	Primarily CD8+
Sézary syndrome (SS) (Fig. 8.6)	Aggressive clinical behavior. Erythroderma. Hyperkeratosis of palms and soles. Thinning of hair. Ectropion. Severe pruritus. Enlarged lymph nodes. Frequent *Staphylococcus aureus* infections [84]	Aggressive clinical course with poor prognosis Systemic therapies: • IFN-α • Bexarotene • Romidepsin • Combination therapies Refractory disease: • Brentuximab vedotin • Low-dose alemtuzumab • Allogeneic stem cell transplantation Skin-directed therapy often added	CD4+

PUVA Psoralen plus UV-A, *nb-UVB* Narrow-band UVB, *TSEBT* Total skin electron beam therapy; *IFN* interferon, *ECP* Extracorporeal photopheresis

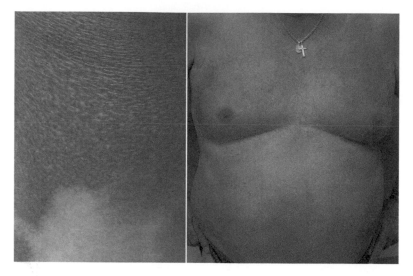

Fig. 8.2 Patch stage classic MF

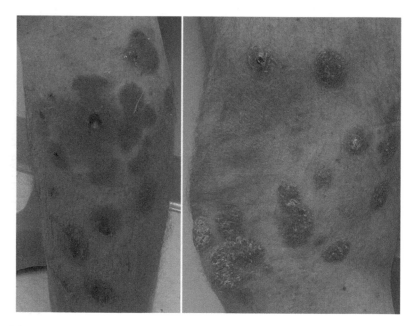

Fig. 8.3 Plaque stage classic MF

Fig. 8.4 Tumor stage classic MF

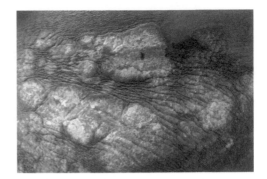

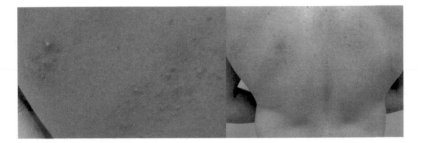

Fig. 8.5 Folliculotropic MF

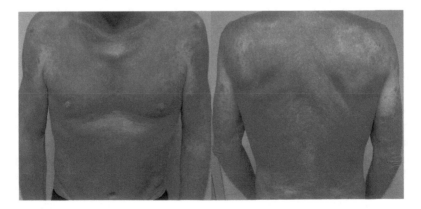

Fig. 8.6 Sézary syndrome

B (Blood)

Blood involvement is evaluated by complete blood count with analysis of Sézary cells by light microscopy and peripheral blood flow cytometry. Sézary cells appear as atypical cerebriform mononuclear T lymphocytes on light microscopy. They also exhibit altered expression of normal T-cell markers, including deletion of CD3, CD7, and/or CD26 on the surface of CD4+ cells [37–39]. However, neoplastic phenotypes are not uniform, and a single SS patient may present with more than one clone. Benign inflammatory conditions may also present with CD7− T lymphocytes in the blood, further confounding Sézary cell identification [40, 41]. Loss of CD26 may be a more specific marker to identify and quantify neoplastic lymphocytes [34, 37]. Though classification of lymphocytes as atypical is subjective, once significant blood involvement with more than 20% Sézary cells is determined, it is prognostically relevant independent of T and N classifications [9].

Modified ISCL/EORTC classifications define B_0 as 5% or fewer Sézary cells. B_1 is defined as more than 5% Sézary cells in combination with (1) the absence of clonal rearrangement of the T-cell receptor (TCR), (2) less than 1.0 K/μL absolute Sézary cells, or (3) both. B_2 is defined as clonal rearrangement of the TCR in the blood as well as either 1.0 K/μL absolute Sézary cells, increased CD4+ or CD3+ cells with a CD4/CD8 ratio of 10 or more, or increase in abnormal CD4+ cells [33, 42].

Histology and Immunohistochemistry

In MF, neoplastic lymphocytes typically present in a lichenoid or band-like pattern within the superficial dermis. Most are small- to intermediate-sized with hyperchromatic, cerebriform nuclei, though cytologic atypia may not be seen in the early stages of disease. Papillary dermal fibroplasia is a common finding. Neoplastic lymphocytes often align along the dermal-epidermal junction and extend into the epidermis [43]. The intraepidermal lymphocytes have surrounding haloes and may form small nests termed Pautrier's microabscesses (Fig. 8.7). A hallmark feature of mycosis fungoides is the relative lack of spongiosis relative to the number of intraepidermal lymphocytes. Notably, epidermotropism may not be present in tumor-stage disease [11]. Large cell transformation (LCT), a poor prognostic feature in MF, is characterized by lymphocytes at least four times the size of a typical lymphocyte exceeding 25% of the total lymphoid infiltrate or present in discrete clusters [44]. Classic MF T lymphocytes are CD3+, CD4+, CD45RO+, and CD8− and exhibit variable loss of CD7, a mature T-cell marker (Fig. 8.8). There is an increase in the CD4/CD8 T-cell ratio, though CD8 expression may be observed in rare variant forms of MF [32, 45, 46].

Folliculotropic mycosis fungoides (FMF) is morphologically similar to conventional MF, exhibiting CD4+ T lymphocytes with cerebriform nuclei, Th2 cytokines, epitheliotropism, and frequent Pautrier's abscesses. However, in FMF,

Fig. 8.7 Patch/plaque
mycosis fungoides.
Lymphocytes are tagging
along the dermal-
epidermal junction and
Pautrier's microabscesses
are seen

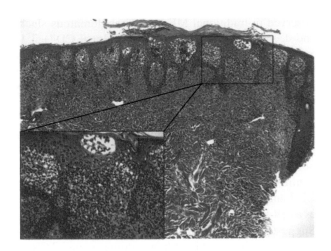

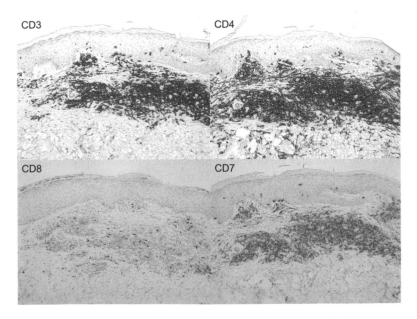

Fig. 8.8 Immunohistochemistry of a Sézary syndrome patient. Staining highlights an elevated
CD4/CD8 ratio and a loss of CD7

folliculotropism with or without follicular mucinosis is present. Additionally,
eosinophils and plasma cells are more conspicuous within the reactive infiltrate.
FMF may also contain abundant CD1a + Langerhans cells in the follicular epithelium [47, 48]. Pagetoid reticulosis, a variant of MF that typically involves the acral
sites, is characterized histologically by a level of epidermotropism that is rarely

observed in traditional MF [49]. Granulomatous slack skin exhibits a superficial and deep granulomatous infiltrate of clonal CD4+ T lymphocytes, macrophages, and multinucleate giant cells that often contain host lymphocytes or elastic fibers within their cytoplasm [50]. Hypopigmented MF exhibits similar histopathological features to classic patch and plaque MF; however, the atypical lymphocytic population is often CD8 positive [51].

SS is extremely difficult to diagnose by histology alone, as it lacks the characteristic features of MF, including epidermotropism and lack of spongiosis. It is not atypical for SS patients to require multiple biopsies before a definitive diagnosis is achieved. Immunohistochemical markers are often required to make or confirm a diagnosis, particularly a CD4/CD8 ratio of greater than 10 and a loss of CD7 and CD26 expression [34, 37]. KIR3DL2/CD158k has also been identified as a cell-specific marker for the evaluation of circulating tumoral burden in SS [52]. Suggestive pathology in combination with erythroderma, generalized lymphadenopathy, peripheral blood flow cytometry, and TCR gamma gene rearrangement is often necessary to make a final diagnosis [42, 53, 54].

Clinical

Significant clinical questions in CTCL diagnosis and treatment remain, even as therapeutics and outcomes improve. Differential diagnoses for the typical clinical and histological presentation of CTCL include various benign conditions, including atopic dermatitis, drug eruptions, and psoriasis, and thus defining tools to differentiate CTCL from its mimics are of vital importance. Clinical management must also be customized to the patient's prognostic factors as well as current available therapies [55].

The most useful factor in differentiating CTCL from its inflammatory mimics is correlation between clinical observations and pathology. Additionally, ancillary studies such as polymerase chain reaction (PCR) allow evaluation of the T-cell receptor (TCR) gene. However, PCR analysis of TCRγ chain rearrangement can be misleading, as several inflammatory dermatoses also contain clonal T-cell proliferations, and PCR may not detect clones in all patients. Diagnostic utility can be improved by using two sets of primers to detect and evaluate both TCRγ and TCRβ rearrangements and by detecting and demonstrating the existence of identical clones from two separate skin sites [56, 57]. Some investigators also suggest that high-throughput sequencing exhibits greater sensitivity and specificity in detecting T-cell clonality and may be preferable over PCR, particularly in skin biopsy samples in which the percentage of suspected neoplastic T cells is low [58]. Other exploratory diagnostic tests include fluorescence in situ hybridization (FISH) to distinguish between malignant and inflammatory cells, IHC for immunophenotypic markers, and miRNA expression profiles [55, 59].

Prognostic Considerations to Guide Clinical Management

Clinical Factors

Key clinical factors predicting disease progression in CTCL include demographic factors, clinical stage (using TNMB classification), disease variant, and transformation to aggressive clinical behavior. Demographic factors predisposing to development and progression of MF/SS include old age, male sex (2:1 male:female ratio), and black race [5, 8, 60, 61]. Patients at later stages of disease fare worse than patients with early-stage disease. Different clinical variants of disease also differ in terms of prognosis, with pagetoid reticulosis, granulomatous slack skin, and hypopigmented MF exhibiting indolent clinical behavior with a more favorable prognosis and folliculotropic mycosis fungoides (Table 8.2, *Folliculotropic MF*) and Sézary syndrome (Table 8.2, *Sézary syndrome*) exhibiting aggressive clinical behavior, with a correspondingly worse prognosis. Transformation to aggressive clinical behavior also predisposes to disease progression and poorer outcomes [9, 60, 62–64].

Histology and Laboratory

Histologically, large cell transformation is associated with decreased survival [65–67]. Folliculotropism also predisposes to more aggressive disease behavior and poorer outcomes [48]. Elevated lactate dehydrogenase (LDH), elevated β_2-microglobulin, and increased IgE (eosinophilia) also all correlate with poor outcomes in MF [65, 68]. For example, SS patients show elevated serum IgE and peripheral eosinophilia [69]. Increased soluble cytokine and cytokine receptor levels in the serum, particularly those of IL-6, also act as indicators of poor prognosis [70].

Increased levels of Ki-67, CD25, and/or CD30 are also predictive of poor prognosis. Ki-67 is a cellular marker for proliferation, with surface expression increased among rapidly proliferating malignant T lymphocytes; increased dermal Ki-67 is a negative prognostic indicator [71, 72]. CD25 is the alpha subunit of the receptor for the T cell growth factor IL-2, and surface expression is increased in advanced-stage MF; increased serum concentration of CD25 predicts increased tumor burden and poor prognosis [73–75]. CD30 is a tumor marker and member of the tumor necrosis factor (TNF) superfamily, with high levels of surface expression in transformed MF; elevated serum CD30 is a negative prognostic indicator [70, 76, 77]. CD30 expression is not limited to transformed MF; increased levels of dermal CD30 expression in nontransformed MF also predict adverse outcome [72].

Conversely, the presence of host tumor-infiltrating CD8+ cytotoxic T lymphocytes (TILs) and regulatory T cells (Tregs) correlate with improved prognosis and increased rate of survival in CTCL patients. When divided by T stage, patients with early-stage disease show higher proportions of host TILs on biopsy than those with advanced-stage disease. Higher proportions of TILs also correlate to better prognoses and survival rates within each T stage [78]. Higher levels of host Tregs in the tumor microenvironment are also correlated with increased survival rates for MF patients, a result that is not seen in other cancers with solid tumors [79].

Gene Expression Patterns

Gene expression patterns can also be used to distinguish indolent MF from aggressive MF tumors. Indolent MF exhibits increased expression of genes involved in epidermal differentiation as well as genes with tumor suppressor function, including negative cell cycle regulators and genes involved in apoptosis and DNA repair. Aggressive MF tumors show increased expression of genes regulating T-cell proliferation and survival. This includes genes involved in drug resistance; tumor necrosis factor (TNF) pathways, including CD40L and TNF-dependent apoptotic regulators; cytokine signaling molecules, including STAT4; and other oncogenes and inhibitors of apoptosis [80–82].

Management

Clinical symptoms and signs of disease as well as histological, laboratory, and molecular analysis lead to a diagnosis, which then allows for prognostication. Other helpful diagnostic tests include IHC panels and molecular analyses of skin biopsies for TCR rearrangements. Assessment of peripheral blood for Sézary cells using Sézary cell preparation, flow cytometry for abnormal immunophenotypes, and PCR for TCR gene rearrangement (an assessment of clonality) and biopsies of suspicious lymph nodes may be helpful in cases where skin alone is not diagnostic [11, 32]. CTCL clinical stage determines prognosis and entails different treatment approaches; management and treatment can therefore be selected once staging evaluation is completed (Table 8.2).

Overall goals in CTCL treatment are varied but may include the elimination of all patches, plaques, and tumors; the reduction of cancerous lymphocytes; the prevention of malignant T lymphocyte migration; the blockage of tumor cell growth; the restoration of immune balance and competence; and/or palliation of symptoms. Palliation of symptoms, particularly pain, pruritus, burning, and cosmetic disfigurement, becomes increasingly important in late-stage disease. Patients with asymptomatic, historically indolent, and limited patch disease may choose "watchful waiting," while patients with more extensive or advanced CTCL, including more extensive plaques, tumors, or erythroderma, may require faster and more multidisciplinary approaches. The cumulative and overlapping toxicities of different treatment modalities limit the duration and extent of treatment and therapy that can be provided.

Mycosis fungoides is managed using specific skin-directed and systemic treatments as well as symptomatic treatments, emollients, and antipruritics. Generally, skin-directed therapies are indicated for stage I patients, while systemic therapies or combination therapies (skin-directed with systemic or systemic with systemic) are indicated for patients with late-stage or refractory disease.

Reliable skin responses are observed in skin-directed therapies for CTCL up to stage IIA [85]. Patients with less than 3% body surface area affected can be treated with topical steroids. Appropriate skin-directed therapies for patients with more than 3% BSA affected include narrowband UVB (nb-UVB), psoralen and ultraviolet A (PUVA), and topical mechlorethamine (nitrogen mustard). nb-UVB is particularly effective and well-tolerated for patch and very limited plaque disease [86]. PUVA is effective in inducing long-term remission, with disease-free survivals of 74% and 50% at 5 and 10 years, respectively [87]. Topical mechlorethamine (nitrogen mustard) can also be used safely for patients with T1 or T2 disease [88]. Refractory disease can be managed with bexarotene gel, imiquimod, or local radiation therapy [32, 89].

Stage IB and IIA patients can also be treated with nb-UVB, PUVA, or nitrogen mustard. Refractory disease may require total skin electron beam therapy (TSEBT), HDAC inhibitor (romidepsin), brentuximab vedotin, bexarotene gel, or interferon (IFN). Topical bexarotene can be used alone or in combination with nb-UVB, PUVA, or nitrogen mustard [32].

For more extensive disease between stages IIB and IIIB, TSEBT or systemic therapy is appropriate; skin-directed therapy is often added. For patients with tumors, erythroderma, or high BSA affected, low-dose (≤ 30 Gy) TSEBT reduces disease burden with acceptable toxicity [90]. Other options include bexarotene, which can be used alone or in combination with nb-UVB, PUVA, or nitrogen mustard. Patients with blood involvement (B1 or B2) should be treated with extracorporeal photopheresis (ECP) in combination with other therapies, including interferons, retinoids, or both [32]. ECP is a leukapheresis procedure that isolates the patient's white blood cells and exposes them to a photosensitizer and UV radiation, resulting in apoptosis, particularly of activated and abnormal T lymphocytes. The apoptotic cells are then re-infused into the patient's blood and taken up and presented by antigen-presenting dendritic cells and macrophages, resulting in regulatory lymphocyte activation. ECP therefore both depletes the blood of abnormal T lymphocytes and activates antigen-specific regulatory lymphocytes, helping to restore immune balance. More extensive disease may also be treated with low-dose pralatrexate or brentuximab vedotin. Chemotherapy can be used for treatment of late-stage disease but should be restricted until other options are exhausted, as it must be administered more often and shows only modest increases in effectiveness compared to interferon and HDAC inhibitor therapies [91]. Enrollment in a clinical trial or allogeneic stem cell transplant may be considered in cases of refractory or progressive disease [32, 92, 93].

Stage IV patients should be started on ECP, alone or in combination with IFN-α, retinoids, or both. Refractory disease requires enrollment in a clinical trial or consideration of allogeneic transplant [32, 92, 93]. SS patients can also be progressed to low-dose alemtuzumab, which is effective in patients with blood involvement but ineffective in early-stage MF [94].

Supportive Therapy

CTCL causes associated symptoms that can compromise patients' quality of life, including pruritus, fatigue, skin sloughing, erythema, and increased risk of infection. Therapies used to pursue remission also carry associated toxicities and can induce dermatitis (bexarotene) or nausea (romidepsin); interrupt daily activities (phototherapy); require long-term, tedious full-body application (nitrogen mustard); cause alopecia (radiotherapy) or neuropathy (brentuximab vedotin); or pose high risks of mortality (transplant) [95]. Using combination therapies brings the additional complication of managing side effects from each therapy involved. Supportive therapy aims to mitigate symptoms that result from the disease itself as well as from the therapies being used to treat it.

CTCL also carries an increased risk of infection, which is a common cause of death in CTCL patients [96, 97]. To avoid methicillin-resistant *Staphylococcus aureus* (MRSA) and other forms of antibiotic resistance, prophylactic systemic antibiotics are not advised; rather, management involves repeated skin cultures in cases of suspicious skin erosions, with antibiotic use targeted to specific identified bacteria. Proper skincare, including appropriate use of emollients, use of sunscreen and minimization of sun exposure, and use of topical antibiotics, can help to fortify the skin barrier against colonization. Dilute bleach baths combined with topical antibiotics also minimize bacterial colonization and can be used to prevent infection [32].

Severe pruritus and xerosis are also common side effects of CTCL disease and therapy. Supportive measures include topical corticosteroids, emollients, oral antipruritics and antihistamines, and more simple remedies, including refrigeration of OTC topical ointments. Refractory pruritus also responds to narrowband UVB therapy and, anecdotally, to medications traditionally used as antidepressants (mirtazapine, dopexin), antiseizure medication (gabapentin), and anti-emetics (aprepitant) [98–100].

Other serious risks of CTCL treatment include nausea from HDAC inhibitors like romidepsin, neuropathy from brentuximab vedotin, and tumor lysis syndrome from monoclonal antibodies in patients with high tumor burden. Nausea and vomiting can be managed with 5-HT3 receptor antagonists alone or in combination with a benzodiazepine. In neuropathic patients, neuropathy should be monitored regularly to adjust brentuximab dosage, and pregabalin can be used along with selective serotonin-norepinephrine reuptake inhibitors to mitigate symptoms. Tumor lysis syndrome should be managed with rehydration therapy and management of electrolytes and uric acid.

Emerging Therapies

Malignant T lymphocytes express high levels of CC-chemokine receptor 4 (CCR4), which binds to skin-manufactured cytokines and may contribute to the enhanced epidermotropism of MF/SS T cells [16, 21, 101]. Anti-CCR4 monoclonal

Table 8.3 Adapted from Thornton 2016 and Rozati 2016 [110, 111]

1. Molecular targets
(a) Topical JAK and STAT signaling pathway inhibitors target cytokine signaling.
(b) IPH4102 is an antibody against KIR3DL2, a Sézary cell marker [112].
(c) MRG-106 is an inhibitor of miR-155, a microRNA that may be important in malignant T lymphocyte proliferation and development [113].
(d) Resimmune is an anti-CD3 immunotoxin [114].
2. Topical treatments
(a) Remetinostat is a topical HDAC inhibitor [115].
(b) SGX301 contains a synthetic hypericin, a photosensitizer activated by safe ranges of visible light. It is in phase II trials for clinical use [116].
(c) Topical resiquimod is a toll-like receptor agonist that enhances T-cell effector function [117].
3. Biologics
(a) E7777 (improved purity denileukin diftitox) is in phase III trials for clinical use [118].
4. Allogeneic hematopoietic stem cell transplantation [119]
5. Personalized medicine: After sequencing patient genome and isolating individual mutations and molecular targets

antibodies induce destruction of CCR4-expressing CTCL cells via antibody-dependent cellular toxicity and inhibition of CCL22-induced T lymphocyte epidermotropism. Mogamulizumab (KW-0761) is a humanized monoclonal antibody (mAb) against CCR4, supporting the use of mogamulizumab to combat CCR4-expressing malignant lymphocytes in CTCL [102, 103]. The effectiveness of mogamulizumab has been demonstrated in phase I and II randomized controlled trials [104, 105].

PD-1 (program death-1) is also found on the surface of malignant T lymphocytes in many forms of CTCL and may play a role in malignant T cells' ability to suppress host immune function. Increased levels of PD-1 are found in more advanced stages of disease, and PD-1 blockade has been found to enhance IFN-gamma production and cell-mediated immunity [106, 107]. Pembrolizumab, a humanized monoclonal antibody against PD-1, can therefore be used to enhance host immune function against MF/SS cancer cells. Phase II clinical trials for pembrolizumab use in patients with refractory or relapsed MF/SS are currently in progress; one ongoing phase II study with pembrolizumab in relapsed/refractory MF/SS shows response rates of 38% and high durability [108, 109].

Targeted molecular therapies are active areas of research for primary cutaneous T-cell lymphoma treatment (Table 8.3).

Prognosis

The prognosis of CTCL is heterogeneous and varies based on demographic factors, clinical stage (using TNMB classification), histology and laboratory values, and disease variant. Old age, male gender, and black race are negative prognostic factors [5, 8, 60, 61]. Decreased survival and increased risk of disease progression are also seen with advanced clinical stage, large cell transformation, and increased LDH [60]. Pagetoid reticulosis, granulomatous slack skin, and hypopigmented MF exhibit indolent clinical behavior with favorable prognoses, while FMF and SS exhibit aggressive clinical behavior and a correspondingly worse prognosis. Patients with SS show a 5-year overall survival rate of 10% [60].

Skin stage (T classification) is particularly predictive, with patients with patches only (T1a/T2a) showing statistically significant increases in survival and decreases in risk of disease progression compared to patients with patches and plaques (T1b/T2b) [60]. Patients with limited patch/plaque disease (stage IA), an indolent form of the disease, have life expectancies similar to control populations that are age-, sex-, and race-matched. Patients with more generalized patch/plaque disease without extracutaneous disease (stage IB or IIA) collectively have a median survival of approximately 12 years [120]. Though MF/SS is generally considered to be incurable, the estimated 65–85% of patients exhibiting early-stage (IA, IB, and IIA) disease do not progress to more advanced-stage disease [9, 66].

Median survival for patients with tumors or erythroderma (stage IIB, III, or IVA with grade LN3 lymph node histopathology) is only 2–3 years after diagnosis; median survival drops to less than 2 years for patients with extracutaneous disease involving the lymph nodes or viscera at time of diagnosis (stage IVA with grade LN4 lymph node histopathology or IVB) [120]. Thus, 5-year overall survival for MF varies widely from 18% to 94%. Differences in 5-year survival are most significant between stages IIIA and IIIB. Conversely, overall survival and disease-specific survival rates are similar for stages IIB/IIIA and IIIB/IVA, respectively [60].

Cutaneous B-Cell Lymphoma

Cutaneous B-cell lymphomas (CBCLs) are largely indolent and may appear as erythematous to violaceous rashes or nodules. Recurrence is common even after initial complete remission, but prognosis is generally favorable. Indolent forms of primary cutaneous B-cell lymphoma (PCBCL) include primary cutaneous follicular center lymphoma (PCFCL) and primary cutaneous marginal zone lymphoma (PCMZL) (Table 8.4). Leg-type primary cutaneous large B-cell lymphoma (PCLBCL), which is more aggressive and develops more quickly than PCFCL and PCMZL, also appears as red or violaceous nodules or tumors but can be classified based on immunohistochemistry and histology, regardless of anatomic location of the lesions involved. Other types of PCLBCL are extremely rare; non-leg PCLBCL includes intravascular large B-cell lymphoma, T-cell-rich large B-cell lymphoma, plasmablastic lymphoma, and anaplastic B-cell lymphoma (Table 8.4).

Table 8.4 Primary cutaneous B-cell lymphomas

	Entity	Clinical	Pathologic	Immunophenotype and genetic features	Diagnosis
Indolent	Primary cutaneous follicular center lymphoma (PCFCL) (Fig. 8.9)	• Firm, erythematous, painless, non-pruritic papules, plaques, or tumors • Typically single lesion <5 cm in diameter • Often head, neck, and trunk • Ulceration and extracutaneous involvement uncommon • Slow progression with long latency period [121–124]	• Dermal and subcutaneous infiltrate sparing epidermis • Medium- and large-sized centrocytes (large cleaved follicle center cells) • Variable number of centroblasts (large follicle center cells with prominent nucleoli) • Growth in follicular, follicular and diffuse, or diffuse pattern • If follicular: no mantle zone [125]	• Positive for: CD19, CD20, CD79a, BCL-6, HGAL • Negative for: Ig, CD5, BCL-2, MUM1/IRF4 • No uniform genetic abnormality • Some nodal FCLs may exhibit a t(14;18) translocation and/ or *bcl-2* gene rearrangement [125–129]	• Excisional biopsy or punch biopsy >4mm • Clinical, pathologic, and IHC correlation • Must be clonal (not reactive) infiltrate • Combination of BCL-6 with HGAL on IHC favors diagnosis of PCFCL over PCLBCL, leg type • Must be B-cell lineage, not T-cell or NK-cell – Confirmed if CD20+CD79a+CD3- • Must be limited to skin [125, 130]

	Primary cutaneous marginal zone B-cell lymphoma (PCMZL) (Fig. 8.10)	• Red, pink, or violaceous papules, plaques, or nodules
		• Often trunk or upper extremities
		• Multifocal skin lesions common
		• Cutaneous relapse common, even after remission
		• Ulceration uncommon
		• Extracutaneous involvement uncommon [129, 131]
			• Nodular to diffuse infiltrates throughout, except epidermis
			• Grenz zone without infiltration or significant involvement
			• Infiltrate: marginal zone B cells, small lymphocytes, lymphoplasmacytoid cells, and plasma cells
			  – Marginal zone B cells: abundant, pale cytoplasm, irregular nuclei, inconspicuous nucleoli
			• Many reactive T cells
			• Some centroblast- or immunoblast-like cells
			• Reactive germinal centers
			• PAS-positive, Ig-containing Dutcher bodies (intranuclear) or Russell bodies (intracytoplasmic) inclusions in cases with many lymphoplasmacytoid cells
			• Follicular structure colonization, lymphoepithelial lesions, large cell transformation (LCT) all uncommon [126, 132]
				• Post-germinal center B cells:
				  – Positive for: CD20, CD22, CD79a, BCL2
				  – Negative for: CD3, CD5, CD10, BCL6
				• Reactive germinal center B-cells:
				  – Positive for: BCL6, CD10
				  – Negative for: BCL2
				• No uniform genetic abnormality [126, 132]
					• Excisional biopsy or punch biopsy >4mm
					• Clinical, pathologic, and IHC correlation
					• Must be clonal (not reactive) infiltrate
					• Must be B-cell lineage, not T-cell or NK-cell
					  – Confirmed if CD20+CD79a+CD3-
					• Must be limited to skin [126]

(continued)

Table 8.4 (continued)

	Entity	Clinical	Pathologic	Immunophenotype and genetic features	Diagnosis
Intermediate/ aggressive	Primary cutaneous large B-cell lymphoma (PCLBCL), leg-type	• Red or blue nodules or tumors extending deep into body • Legs, usually lower legs • No evidence of extracutaneous involvement at time of diagnosis, but more likely to become open sores and disseminate outside of the skin • More aggressive: develops over weeks or months [133, 134]	• Diffuse, non-epidermotropic infiltrate – May extend subcutaneously • Monotonous population or large confluent sheets of centroblasts and immunoblasts with large nuclei (nuclear size equal to or exceeding normal macrophage nuclei) • Very few reactive T cells, only in perivascular areas [125, 133]	• Positive for: CD19, CD20, CD22, CD79a • May be positive for: BCL-2, Mum1, FOXP1, MYC, BCL-6 • May express cytoplasmic IgM and IgD and monotypic Ig light chains • No uniform genetic abnormality [121, 125, 135–140]	• Excisional biopsy or punch biopsy >4mm • Clinical, pathologic, and IHC correlation • "B" symptoms (fever, weight loss, night sweats), abnormal blood counts, or elevated LDH suggest systemic lymphoma rather than DLBCL • IHC testing should include BCL-2, Mum1, IgM, Ig light chains, FOXP1 if available – Positive IHC for BCL-2 and Mum1/ IRF4 favors diagnosis of PCLBCL, leg type over PCFCL • Characteristic dermatopathology indicates diagnosis of PCLBCL, leg type regardless of location on body [130, 134]

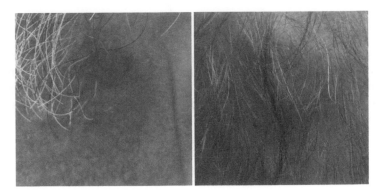

Fig. 8.9 Primary cutaneous follicular center lymphoma (PCFCL)

Fig. 8.10 Primary cutaneous
marginal zone B-cell lymphoma
(PCMZL)

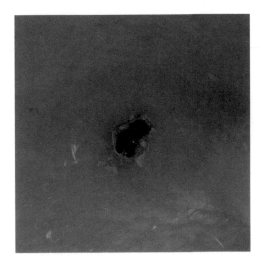

Treatment for Cutaneous B-Cell Lymphoma

Therapy considerations for B-cell lymphoma are based on the intent of therapy. Patients with solitary lesions often seek a curative option, which may include radiation therapy and/or excisional surgery. Patients with multiple lesions often seek a more palliative approach, including intralesional steroid injections, intralesional rituximab injections, and systemic single-agent rituximab. Chemotherapy with or without rituximab is the treatment of choice for aggressive cutaneous B-cell lymphomas [141].

PCFCL

Low-dose radiation is safe and effective for patients with solitary lesions. Complete excision alone with deferral of radiation until disease recurrence is also appropriate [123]. Intralesional corticosteroid injection and topical therapies may also be used. Patients with more extensive, symptomatic skin involvement can be treated effectively with single-agent rituximab [141].

PCMZL

PCMZL can be managed similarly, with radiation therapy for single lesions and single-agent rituximab for patients with more extensive, symptomatic skin involvement [141].

PCLBCL, LT

PCLBCL, leg-type, can be treated with first-line R-CHOP (rituximab, cyclophosphamide, doxorubicin, vincristine, and prednisone) with or without radiation therapy [123, 137, 141, 142]. Relapsed and refractory disease will require a second-line multi-agent chemotherapy regimen or a clinical study [143].

CD30+ Lymphoproliferative Disorders

CD30+ cutaneous lymphoproliferative disorders, accounting for approximately 30% of all CTCLs, include lymphomatoid papulosis (LyP) and primary cutaneous anaplastic large cell lymphoma (pcALCL) [2]. Both LyP and pcALCL are generally defined by T-cell expression of CD30 and a benign course with a favorable prognosis. Patients with CD30+ lymphoproliferative disorders show 5-year overall survival rates of 76–96% [144, 145]. Diagnosis can be challenging, as there is often no distinct histopathological distinction between LyP and pcALCL, and the malignant lymphocytes seen in LyP and pcALCL may be immunophenotypically similar to those seen in the cutaneous infiltrates of other CD30+ inflammatory and neoplastic diseases [146]. Therefore, clinical characteristics, clinicopathologic correlation, and clinical course over time must be used for definitive diagnosis and therapeutic selection [147].

Lymphomatoid Papulosis

Lymphomatoid papulosis (LyP) is a clinically benign condition with spontaneous regression. However, it is often recurrent and is associated with various other lymphomas, including MF, other systemic NHL, and Hodgkin's lymphoma (HL) [145]. The disease manifests as self-healing crops of erythematous papules (primary) and rare nodules (minor) that may or may not be grouped (Fig. 8.11). The lesions may become necrotic, ulcerative, and/or hemorrhagic. LyP patients do not present with associated fever, sweats, or weight loss, and such symptoms should raise concern for a systemic lymphoma [148, 149].

Many histologic subtypes, including LyP types A–F and LyP with 6p23.5 rearrangement, have been observed. Of note, several histologic patterns can be seen in the same patient. Type B is most similar to MF, exhibiting epidermotropism of small hyperchromatic cells and chronic dermal inflammation. Types A and C include large, atypical lymphocytes similar in appearance to Reed-Sternberg cells. Type A, the most common form of LyP, includes a mixed inflammatory infiltrate and is often confused histologically with an arthropod bite reaction. Type C includes sheets of large, atypical cells in a pattern indistinguishable from ALCL [150]. Type D exhibits and is characterized by an epidermotropic population of CD8+ cells [151]. Type E exhibits an angiocentric and angiodestructive infiltrate comprised of small- to medium-sized atypical lymphocytes. Of note, type E LyP presents with eschar-like lesions that appear similar to aggressive cytotoxic T-cell lymphoma. Correct identification is necessary in order to avoid overtreatment. Type F LyP has been proposed as a sixth category and exhibits folliculotropism [152]. LyP with 6p23.5 rearrangement

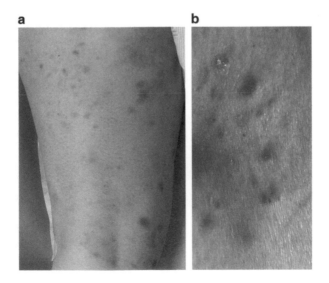

Fig. 8.11 Lymphomatoid papulosis

exhibits small- to medium-sized cerebriform lymphocytes and large pleomorphic dermal lymphocytes [153]. Most forms of LyP are CD30+ (some type B patients may be CD30−). Types A and C are CD3+, CD4+, CD8-, CD20-, and CD56-; type B is CD3+, CD4+, and CD8-; type D is CD8+; type E is often CD8+; and LyP with 6p23.5 rearrangement is CD4- and CD8- [152, 153].

The treatments for LyP include topical steroids, PUVA, low-dose methotrexate, bexarotene, and brentuximab vedotin [32].

pcALCL

In contrast to LyP, primary cutaneous anaplastic large cell lymphoma (pcALCL) exhibits less than 44% spontaneous regression [145]. pcALCL manifests in most patients as nodules and tumors that can manifest singly or in groups that grow rapidly and may ulcerate; rarely, patients may present with multifocal lesions (Fig. 8.12). Histologically, pcALCL is characterized by an epidermis-sparing reactive dermal infiltrate containing cohesive sheets of large CD30+ tumor cells; these cells contain large amounts of pale, eosinophilic cytoplasm and round, oval, or horseshoe-shaped nuclei with prominent nucleoli. A moderately dense reactive infiltrate composed of histiocytes, eosinophils, and small reactive lymphocytes appear in close vicinity to the large atypical cell infiltrate [145, 154]. Though pcALCL is of T-cell origin, many of the anaplastic cells exhibit an aberrant phenotype, with loss of both CD3 and CD45RO [155]. Most pcALCL cells are CD2+ and CD4+; though most are also CD8−, ALCL cells often express antigens typically associated with cytotoxic T cells, including TIA-1, granzyme B, and perforin [156, 157]. Therapies for pcALCL include radiation therapy, low-dose methotrexate, pralatrexate, bexarotene, and brentuximab vedotin for severe or refractory cases [32].

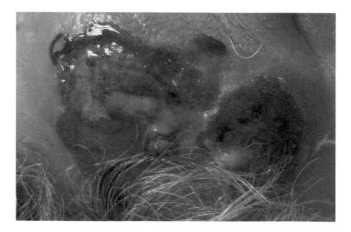

Fig. 8.12 Primary cutaneous anaplastic large cell lymphoma

References

1. Groves FD, Linet MS, Travis LB, Devesa SS. Cancer surveillance series: non-Hodgkin's lymphoma incidence by histologic subtype in the United States from 1978 through 1995. J Natl Cancer Inst. 2000;92(15):1240–51.
2. Willemze R, Jaffe ES, Burg G, Cerroni L, Berti E, Swerdlow SH, et al. WHO-EORTC classification for cutaneous lymphomas. Blood. 2005;105(10):3768–85.
3. Criscione VD, Weinstock MA. Incidence of cutaneous T-cell lymphoma in the United States, 1973-2002. Arch Dermatol. 2007;143(7):854–9.
4. National Center for Health Statistics. Health, United States. Health, United States, 2005: with chartbook on trends in the health of Americans. Hyattsville: National Center for Health Statistics (US); 2005.
5. Bradford PT, Devesa SS, Anderson WF, Toro JR. Cutaneous lymphoma incidence patterns in the United States: a population-based study of 3884 cases. Blood. 2009;113(21):5064–73.
6. Zic JA, Zwerner ZJ, McGirt LY, Mosse CA, Greer JP. Cutaneous T cell lymphoma: mycosis fungoides and sézary syndrome. In: Greer JP, Arber DA, Glader B, List AF, Means RT, Paraskevas F, Rodgers GM, editors. Wintrobe's clinical hematology. 13th ed. Philadelphia: Wolters Kluwer Health, Lippincott Williams & Wilkins; 2013.
7. Korgavkar K, Xiong M, Weinstock M. Changing incidence trends of cutaneous T-cell lymphoma. JAMA Dermatol. 2013;149(11):1295–9.
8. Sant M, Allemani C, Tereanu C, De Angelis R, Capocaccia R, Visser O, et al. Incidence of hematologic malignancies in Europe by morphologic subtype: results of the HAEMACARE project. Blood. 2010;116(19):3724–34.
9. Kim YH, Liu HL, Mraz-Gernhard S, Varghese A, Hoppe RT. Long-term outcome of 525 patients with mycosis fungoides and Sezary syndrome: clinical prognostic factors and risk for disease progression. Arch Dermatol. 2003;139(7):857–66.
10. Butcher EC, Picker LJ. Lymphocyte homing and homeostasis. Science (New York, NY). 1996;272(5258):60–6.
11. Kim EJ, Hess S, Richardson SK, Newton S, Showe LC, Benoit BM, et al. Immunopathogenesis and therapy of cutaneous T cell lymphoma. J Clin Invest. 2005;115(4):798–812.
12. Flier J, Boorsma DM, van Beek PJ, Nieboer C, Stoof TJ, Willemze R, et al. Differential expression of CXCR3 targeting chemokines CXCL10, CXCL9, and CXCL11 in different types of skin inflammation. J Pathol. 2001;194(4):398–405.
13. Groom JR, Luster AD. CXCR3 ligands: redundant, collaborative and antagonistic functions. Immunol Cell Biol. 2011;89(2):207.
14. Piper KP, Horlock C, Curnow SJ, Arrazi J, Nicholls S, Mahendra P, et al. CXCL10-CXCR3 interactions play an important role in the pathogenesis of acute graft-versus-host disease in the skin following allogeneic stem-cell transplantation. Blood. 2007;110(12):3827–32.
15. Clark RA, Watanabe R, Teague JE, Schlapbach C, Tawa MC, Adams N, et al. Skin effector memory T cells do not recirculate and provide immune protection in alemtuzumab-treated CTCL patients. Sci Transl Med. 2012;4(117):117ra7.
16. Ishida T, Utsunomiya A, Iida S, Inagaki H, Takatsuka Y, Kusumoto S, et al. Clinical significance of CCR4 expression in adult T-cell leukemia/lymphoma: its close association with skin involvement and unfavorable outcome. Clin Cancer Res Off J Am Assoc Cancer Res. 2003;9(10 Pt 1):3625–34.
17. Lu D, Duvic M, Medeiros LJ, Luthra R, Dorfman DM, Jones D. The T-cell chemokine receptor CXCR3 is expressed highly in low-grade mycosis fungoides. Am J Clin Pathol. 2001;115(3):413–21.
18. Kallinich T, Muche JM, Qin S, Sterry W, Audring H, Kroczek RA. Chemokine receptor expression on neoplastic and reactive T cells in the skin at different stages of mycosis fungoides. J Invest Dermatol. 2003;121(5):1045–52.

19. Kakinuma T, Sugaya M, Nakamura K, Kaneko F, Wakugawa M, Matsushima K, et al. Thymus and activation-regulated chemokine (TARC/CCL17) in mycosis fungoides: serum TARC levels reflect the disease activity of mycosis fungoides. J Am Acad Dermatol. 2003;48(1):23–30.
20. Ferenczi K, Fuhlbrigge RC, Pinkus J, Pinkus GS, Kupper TS. Increased CCR4 expression in cutaneous T cell lymphoma. J Invest Dermatol. 2002;119(6):1405–10.
21. Campbell JJ, Haraldsen G, Pan J, Rottman J, Qin S, Ponath P, et al. The chemokine receptor CCR4 in vascular recognition by cutaneous but not intestinal memory T cells. Nature. 1999;400(6746):776–80.
22. Berger CL, Hanlon D, Kanada D, Dhodapkar M, Lombillo V, Wang N, et al. The growth of cutaneous T-cell lymphoma is stimulated by immature dendritic cells. Blood. 2002;99(8):2929–39.
23. Hwang ST, Janik JE, Jaffe ES, Wilson WH. Mycosis fungoides and Sezary syndrome. Lancet (London, England). 2008;371(9616):945–57.
24. Eriksen KW, Kaltoft K, Mikkelsen G, Nielsen M, Zhang Q, Geisler C, et al. Constitutive STAT3-activation in Sezary syndrome: tyrphostin AG490 inhibits STAT3-activation, interleukin-2 receptor expression and growth of leukemic Sezary cells. Leukemia. 2001;15(5):787–93.
25. Zhang Q, Nowak I, Vonderheid EC, Rook AH, Kadin ME, Nowell PC, et al. Activation of Jak/STAT proteins involved in signal transduction pathway mediated by receptor for interleukin 2 in malignant T lymphocytes derived from cutaneous anaplastic large T-cell lymphoma and Sezary syndrome. Proc Natl Acad Sci U S A. 1996;93(17):9148–53.
26. Nielsen M, Kaltoft K, Nordahl M, Ropke C, Geisler C, Mustelin T, et al. Constitutive activation of a slowly migrating isoform of Stat3 in mycosis fungoides: tyrphostin AG490 inhibits Stat3 activation and growth of mycosis fungoides tumor cell lines. Proc Natl Acad Sci U S A. 1997;94(13):6764–9.
27. Wu J, Nihal M, Siddiqui J, Vonderheid EC, Wood GS. Low FAS/CD95 expression by CTCL correlates with reduced sensitivity to apoptosis that can be restored by FAS upregulation. J Invest Dermatol. 2009;129(5):1165–73.
28. Choi J, Goh G, Walradt T, Hong BS, Bunick CG, Chen K, et al. Genomic landscape of cutaneous T cell lymphoma. Nat Genet. 2015;47(9):1011–9.
29. Mao X, Lillington D, Scarisbrick JJ, Mitchell T, Czepulkowski B, Russell-Jones R, et al. Molecular cytogenetic analysis of cutaneous T-cell lymphomas: identification of common genetic alterations in Sezary syndrome and mycosis fungoides. Br J Dermatol. 2002;147(3):464–75.
30. van Doorn R, Zoutman WH, Dijkman R, de Menezes RX, Commandeur S, Mulder AA, et al. Epigenetic profiling of cutaneous T-cell lymphoma: promoter hypermethylation of multiple tumor suppressor genes including BCL7a, PTPRG, and p73. J Clin Oncol Off J Am Soc Clin Oncol. 2005;23(17):3886–96.
31. Lin WM, Lewis JM, Filler RB, Modi BG, Carlson KR, Reddy S, et al. Characterization of the DNA copy-number genome in the blood of cutaneous T-cell lymphoma patients. J Invest Dermatol. 2012;132(1):188–97.
32. (NCCN) NCCN. Clinical practice guidelines in oncology: T cell lymphomas (Version 1.2017) 2017. Available from: https://www.nccn.org/professionals/physician_gls/recently_updated.asp.
33. Olsen E, Vonderheid E, Pimpinelli N, Willemze R, Kim Y, Knobler R, et al. Revisions to the staging and classification of mycosis fungoides and Sezary syndrome: a proposal of the International Society for Cutaneous Lymphomas (ISCL) and the cutaneous lymphoma task force of the European Organization of Research and Treatment of cancer (EORTC). Blood. 2007;110(6):1713–22.
34. Bernengo MG, Novelli M, Quaglino P, Lisa F, De Matteis A, Savoia P, et al. The relevance of the CD4+ CD26- subset in the identification of circulating Sezary cells. Br J Dermatol. 2001;144(1):125–35.
35. Olsen EA, Whittaker S, Kim YH, Duvic M, Prince HM, Lessin SR, et al. Clinical end points and response criteria in mycosis fungoides and Sezary syndrome: a consensus statement of the

International Society for Cutaneous Lymphomas, the United States cutaneous lymphoma consortium, and the cutaneous lymphoma task force of the European Organisation for Research and Treatment of Cancer. J Clin Oncol Off J Am Soc Clin Oncol. 2011;29(18):2598–607.

36. Kim YH, Willemze R, Pimpinelli N, Whittaker S, Olsen EA, Ranki A, et al. TNM classification system for primary cutaneous lymphomas other than mycosis fungoides and Sezary syndrome: a proposal of the International Society for Cutaneous Lymphomas (ISCL) and the cutaneous lymphoma task force of the European Organization of Research and Treatment of Cancer (EORTC). Blood. 2007;110(2):479–84.

37. Jones D, Dang NH, Duvic M, Washington LT, Huh YO. Absence of CD26 expression is a useful marker for diagnosis of T-cell lymphoma in peripheral blood. Am J Clin Pathol. 2001;115(6):885–92.

38. Borowitz MJ, Weidner A, Olsen EA, Picker LJ. Abnormalities of circulating T-cell subpopulations in patients with cutaneous T-cell lymphoma: cutaneous lymphocyte-associated antigen expression on T cells correlates with extent of disease. Leukemia. 1993;7(6):859–63.

39. Kuchnio M, Sausville EA, Jaffe ES, Greiner T, Foss FM, McClanahan J, et al. Flow cytometric detection of neoplastic T cells in patients with mycosis fungoides based on levels of T-cell receptor expression. Am J Clin Pathol. 1994;102(6):856–60.

40. Abel EA, Lindae ML, Hoppe RT, Wood GS. Benign and malignant forms of erythroderma: cutaneous immunophenotypic characteristics. J Am Acad Dermatol. 1988;19(6):1089–95.

41. Harmon CB, Witzig TE, Katzmann JA, Pittelkow MR. Detection of circulating T cells with CD4+CD7- immunophenotype in patients with benign and malignant lymphoproliferative dermatoses. J Am Acad Dermatol. 1996;35(3 Pt 1):404–10.

42. Vonderheid EC, Bernengo MG, Burg G, Duvic M, Heald P, Laroche L, et al. Update on erythrodermic cutaneous T-cell lymphoma: report of the International Society for Cutaneous Lymphomas. J Am Acad Dermatol. 2002;46(1):95–106.

43. Robson A. The pathology of cutaneous T-cell lymphoma. Oncology (Williston Park, NY). 2007;21(2 Suppl 1):9–12.

44. Salhany KE, Cousar JB, Greer JP, Casey TT, Fields JP, Collins RD. Transformation of cutaneous T cell lymphoma to large cell lymphoma. A clinicopathologic and immunologic study. Am J Pathol. 1988;132(2):265–77.

45. Cotta AC, Cintra ML, de Souza EM, Chagas CA, Magna LA, Fleury RN, et al. Diagnosis of mycosis fungoides: a comparative immunohistochemical study of T-cell markers using a novel anti-CD7 antibody. Appl Immunohistochem Mol Morphol AIMM. 2006;14(3):291–5.

46. Campbell SM, Peters SB, Zirwas MJ, Wong HK. Immunophenotypic diagnosis of primary cutaneous lymphomas: a review for the practicing dermatologist. J Clin Aesthetic Dermatol. 2010;3(10):21–5.

47. Gerami P, Guitart J. The spectrum of histopathologic and immunohistochemical findings in folliculotropic mycosis fungoides. Am J Surg Pathol. 2007;31(9):1430–8.

48. Gerami P, Rosen S, Kuzel T, Boone SL, Guitart J. Folliculotropic mycosis fungoides: an aggressive variant of cutaneous T-cell lymphoma. Arch Dermatol. 2008;144(6):738–46.

49. Hale C. Woringer-Kolopp disease: Pathology Outlines; 2016, updated October 10, 2016. Available from: http://www.pathologyoutlines.com/topic/skintumornonmelanocyticworingerkolopp.html.

50. Tsang WY, Chan JK, Loo KT, Wong KF, Lee AW. Granulomatous slack skin. Histopathology. 1994;25(1):49–55.

51. Werner B, Brown S, Ackerman AB. "Hypopigmented mycosis fungoides" is not always mycosis fungoides! Am J Dermatopathol. 2005;27(1):56–67.

52. Poszepczynska-Guigne E, Schiavon V, D'Incan M, Echchakir H, Musette P, Ortonne N, et al. CD158k/KIR3DL2 is a new phenotypic marker of Sezary cells: relevance for the diagnosis and follow-up of Sezary syndrome. J Invest Dermatol. 2004;122(3):820–3.

53. Karube K, Aoki R, Nomura Y, Yamamoto K, Shimizu K, Yoshida S, et al. Usefulness of flow cytometry for differential diagnosis of precursor and peripheral T-cell and NK-cell lymphomas: analysis of 490 cases. Pathol Int. 2008;58(2):89–97.

54. Wood GS, Tung RM, Haeffner AC, Crooks CF, Liao S, Orozco R, et al. Detection of clonal T-cell receptor gamma gene rearrangements in early mycosis fungoides/Sezary syndrome by polymerase chain reaction and denaturing gradient gel electrophoresis (PCR/DGGE). J Invest Dermatol. 1994;103(1):34–41.

55. Kim YH. Clinical issues in cutaneous T-cell lymphoma. American Academy of Dermatology annual meeting, Miami Beach; 2013.

56. Zhang B, Beck AH, Taube JM, Kohler S, Seo K, Zwerner J, et al. Combined use of PCR-based TCRG and TCRB clonality tests on paraffin-embedded skin tissue in the differential diagnosis of mycosis fungoides and inflammatory dermatoses. J Mol Diag JMD. 2010;12(3):320–7.

57. Thurber SE, Zhang B, Kim YH, Schrijver I, Zehnder J, Kohler S. T-cell clonality analysis in biopsy specimens from two different skin sites shows high specificity in the diagnosis of patients with suggested mycosis fungoides. J Am Acad Dermatol. 2007;57(5):782–90.

58. Kirsch IR, Watanabe R, O'Malley JT, Williamson DW, Scott LL, Elco CP, et al. TCR sequencing facilitates diagnosis and identifies mature T cells as the cell of origin in CTCL. Sci Transl Med. 2015;7(308):308ra158.

59. Ralfkiaer U, Hagedorn PH, Bangsgaard N, Lovendorf MB, Ahler CB, Svensson L, et al. Diagnostic microRNA profiling in cutaneous T-cell lymphoma (CTCL). Blood. 2011;118(22):5891–900.

60. Agar NS, Wedgeworth E, Crichton S, Mitchell TJ, Cox M, Ferreira S, et al. Survival outcomes and prognostic factors in mycosis fungoides/Sezary syndrome: validation of the revised International Society for Cutaneous Lymphomas/European Organisation for Research and Treatment of Cancer staging proposal. J Clin Oncol Off J Am Soc Clin Oncol. 2010;28(31):4730–9.

61. Scarisbrick JJ, Prince HM, Vermeer MH, Quaglino P, Horwitz S, Porcu P, et al. Cutaneous lymphoma international consortium study of outcome in advanced stages of mycosis Fungoides and Sezary syndrome: effect of specific prognostic markers on survival and development of a prognostic model. J Clin Oncol Off J Am Soc Clin Oncol. 2015;33(32):3766–73.

62. Sun G, Berthelot C, Li Y, Glass DA 2nd, George D, Pandya A, et al. Poor prognosis in non-Caucasian patients with early-onset mycosis fungoides. J Am Acad Dermatol. 2009;60(2):231–5.

63. Talpur R, Singh L, Daulat S, Liu P, Seyfer S, Trynosky T, et al. Long-term outcomes of 1,263 patients with mycosis fungoides and Sezary syndrome from 1982 to 2009. Clin Cancer Res Off J Am Assoc Cancer Res. 2012;18(18):5051–60.

64. Vidulich KA, Talpur R, Bassett RL, Duvic M. Overall survival in erythrodermic cutaneous T-cell lymphoma: an analysis of prognostic factors in a cohort of patients with erythrodermic cutaneous T-cell lymphoma. Int J Dermatol. 2009;48(3):243–52.

65. Diamandidou E, Colome M, Fayad L, Duvic M, Kurzrock R. Prognostic factor analysis in mycosis fungoides/Sezary syndrome. J Am Acad Dermatol. 1999;40(6 Pt 1):914–24.

66. Arulogun SO, Prince HM, Ng J, Lade S, Ryan GF, Blewitt O, et al. Long-term outcomes of patients with advanced-stage cutaneous T-cell lymphoma and large cell transformation. Blood. 2008;112(8):3082–7.

67. Siegel RS, Pandolfino T, Guitart J, Rosen S, Kuzel TM. Primary cutaneous T-cell lymphoma: review and current concepts. J Clin Oncol Off J Am Soc Clin Oncol. 2000;18(15):2908–25.

68. Kural YB, Su O, Onsun N, Uras AR. Atopy, IgE and eosinophilic cationic protein concentration, specific IgE positivity, eosinophil count in cutaneous T cell lymphoma. Int J Dermatol. 2010;49(4):390–5.

69. Rook AH, Vowels BR, Jaworsky C, Singh A, Lessin SR. The immunopathogenesis of cutaneous T-cell lymphoma. Abnormal cytokine production by Sezary T cells. Arch Dermatol. 1993;129(4):486–9.

70. Kadin ME, Pavlov IY, Delgado JC, Vonderheid EC. High soluble CD30, CD25, and IL-6 may identify patients with worse survival in CD30+ cutaneous lymphomas and early mycosis fungoides. J Invest Dermatol. 2012;132(3 Pt 1):703–10.

71. Berti E, Tomasini D, Vermeer MH, Meijer CJ, Alessi E, Willemze R. Primary cutaneous CD8-positive epidermotropic cytotoxic T cell lymphomas. A distinct clinicopathological entity with an aggressive clinical behavior. Am J Pathol. 1999;155(2):483–92.

72. Edinger JT, Clark BZ, Pucevich BE, Geskin LJ, Swerdlow SH. CD30 expression and proliferative fraction in nontransformed mycosis fungoides. Am J Surg Pathol. 2009;33(12):1860–8.
73. Wasik MA, Vonderheid EC, Bigler RD, Marti R, Lessin SR, Polansky M, et al. Increased serum concentration of the soluble interleukin-2 receptor in cutaneous T-cell lymphoma. Clinical and prognostic implications. Arch Dermatol. 1996;132(1):42–7.
74. Hassel JC, Meier R, Joller-Jemelka H, Burg G, Dummer R. Serological immunomarkers in cutaneous T cell lymphoma. Dermatology (Basel, Switzerland). 2004;209(4):296–300.
75. Talpur R, Jones DM, Alencar AJ, Apisarnthanarax N, Herne KL, Yang Y, et al. CD25 expression is correlated with histological grade and response to denileukin diftitox in cutaneous T-cell lymphoma. J Invest Dermatol. 2006;126(3):575–83.
76. Horie R, Watanabe T. CD30: expression and function in health and disease. Semin Immunol. 1998;10(6):457–70.
77. Nadali G, Vinante F, Ambrosetti A, Todeschini G, Veneri D, Zanotti R, et al. Serum levels of soluble CD30 are elevated in the majority of untreated patients with Hodgkin's disease and correlate with clinical features and prognosis. J Clin Oncol Off J Am Soc Clin Oncol. 1994;12(4):793–7.
78. Hoppe RT, Medeiros LJ, Warnke RA, Wood GS. CD8-positive tumor-infiltrating lymphocytes influence the long-term survival of patients with mycosis fungoides. J Am Acad Dermatol. 1995;32(3):448–53.
79. Gjerdrum LM, Woetmann A, Odum N, Burton CM, Rossen K, Skovgaard GL, et al. FOXP3+ regulatory T cells in cutaneous T-cell lymphomas: association with disease stage and survival. Leukemia. 2007;21(12):2512–8.
80. Li S, Ross DT, Kadin ME, Brown PO, Wasik MA. Comparative genome-scale analysis of gene expression profiles in T cell lymphoma cells during malignant progression using a complementary DNA microarray. Am J Pathol. 2001;158(4):1231–7.
81. Shin J, Monti S, Aires DJ, Duvic M, Golub T, Jones DA, et al. Lesional gene expression profiling in cutaneous T-cell lymphoma reveals natural clusters associated with disease outcome. Blood. 2007;110(8):3015–27.
82. Tracey L, Villuendas R, Dotor AM, Spiteri I, Ortiz P, Garcia JF, et al. Mycosis fungoides shows concurrent deregulation of multiple genes involved in the TNF signaling pathway: an expression profile study. Blood. 2003;102(3):1042–50.
83. Martinez-Escala ME, Gonzalez BR, Guitart J. Mycosis Fungoides Variants. Surg Pathol Clin. 2014;7(2):169–89.
84. Talpur R, Bassett R, Duvic M. Prevalence and treatment of staphylococcus aureus colonization in patients with mycosis fungoides and Sezary syndrome. Br J Dermatol. 2008;159(1):105–12.
85. Kim YH, Jensen RA, Watanabe GL, Varghese A, Hoppe RT. Clinical stage IA (limited patch and plaque) mycosis fungoides. A long-term outcome analysis. Arch Dermatol. 1996;132(11):1309–13.
86. Gathers RC, Scherschun L, Malick F, Fivenson DP, Lim HW. Narrowband UVB phototherapy for early-stage mycosis fungoides. J Am Acad Dermatol. 2002;47(2):191–7.
87. Querfeld C, Rosen ST, Kuzel TM, Kirby KA, Roenigk HH Jr, Prinz BM, et al. Long-term follow-up of patients with early-stage cutaneous T-cell lymphoma who achieved complete remission with psoralen plus UV-A monotherapy. Arch Dermatol. 2005;141(3):305–11.
88. Kim YH, Martinez G, Varghese A, Hoppe RT. Topical nitrogen mustard in the management of mycosis fungoides: update of the Stanford experience. Arch Dermatol. 2003;139(2):165–73.
89. Deeths MJ, Chapman JT, Dellavalle RP, Zeng C, Aeling JL. Treatment of patch and plaque stage mycosis fungoides with imiquimod 5% cream. J Am Acad Dermatol. 2005;52(2):275–80.
90. Hoppe RT, Harrison C, Tavallaee M, Bashey S, Sundram U, Li S, et al. Low-dose total skin electron beam therapy as an effective modality to reduce disease burden in patients with mycosis fungoides: results of a pooled analysis from 3 phase-II clinical trials. J Am Acad Dermatol. 2015;72(2):286–92.

91. Hughes CF, Khot A, McCormack C, Lade S, Westerman DA, Twigger R, et al. Lack of durable disease control with chemotherapy for mycosis fungoides and Sezary syndrome: a comparative study of systemic therapy. Blood. 2015;125(1):71–81.

92. Duarte RF, Boumendil A, Onida F, Gabriel I, Arranz R, Arcese W, et al. Long-term outcome of allogeneic hematopoietic cell transplantation for patients with mycosis Fungoides and Sézary syndrome: a European Society for Blood and Marrow Transplantation Lymphoma Working Party Extended Analysis. J Clin Oncol. 2014;32(29):3347–8.

93. Wu PA, Kim YH, Lavori PW, Hoppe RT, Stockerl-Goldstein KE. A meta-analysis of patients receiving allogeneic or autologous hematopoietic stem cell transplant in mycosis fungoides and Sezary syndrome. Biol Blood Marrow Transpl J Am Soc Blood Marrow Transpl. 2009;15(8):982–90.

94. Watanabe R, Teague JE, Fisher DC, Kupper TS, Clark RA. Alemtuzumab therapy for leukemic cutaneous T-cell lymphoma: diffuse erythema as a positive predictor of complete remission. JAMA Dermatol. 2014;150(7):776–9.

95. Latkowski JA, Heald P. Strategies for treating cutaneous T-cell lymphoma: part 1: remission. J Clin Aesthetic Dermatol. 2009;2(6):22–7.

96. Dalton JA, Yag-Howard C, Messina JL, Glass LF. Cutaneous T-cell lymphoma. Int J Dermatol. 1997;36(11):801–9.

97. Axelrod PI, Lorber B, Vonderheid EC. Infections complicating mycosis fungoides and Sezary syndrome. JAMA. 1992;267(10):1354–8.

98. Drake LA, Cohen L, Gillies R, Flood JG, Riordan AT, Phillips SB, et al. Pharmacokinetics of doxepin in subjects with pruritic atopic dermatitis. J Am Acad Dermatol. 1999;41(2 Pt 1):209–14.

99. Demierre MF, Taverna J. Mirtazapine and gabapentin for reducing pruritus in cutaneous T-cell lymphoma. J Am Acad Dermatol. 2006;55(3):543–4.

100. Duval A, Dubertret L. Aprepitant as an antipruritic agent? N Engl J Med. 2009;361(14):1415–6.

101. Sugaya M, Morimura S, Suga H, Kawaguchi M, Miyagaki T, Ohmatsu H, et al. CCR4 is expressed on infiltrating cells in lesional skin of early mycosis fungoides and atopic dermatitis. J Dermatol. 2015;42(6):613–5.

102. Ito A, Ishida T, Yano H, Inagaki A, Suzuki S, Sato F, et al. Defucosylated anti-CCR4 monoclonal antibody exercises potent ADCC-mediated antitumor effect in the novel tumor-bearing humanized NOD/Shi-scid, IL-2Rgamma(null) mouse model. Cancer Immunol Immunother CII. 2009;58(8):1195–206.

103. Duvic M, Evans M, Wang C. Mogamulizumab for the treatment of cutaneous T-cell lymphoma: recent advances and clinical potential. Ther Adv Hematol. 2016;7(3):171–4.

104. Duvic M, Pinter-Brown LC, Foss FM, Sokol L, Jorgensen JL, Challagundla P, et al. Phase 1/2 study of mogamulizumab, a defucosylated anti-CCR4 antibody, in previously treated patients with cutaneous T-cell lymphoma. Blood. 2015;125(12):1883–9.

105. Ogura M, Ishida T, Hatake K, Taniwaki M, Ando K, Tobinai K, et al. Multicenter phase II study of mogamulizumab (KW-0761), a defucosylated anti-cc chemokine receptor 4 antibody, in patients with relapsed peripheral T-cell lymphoma and cutaneous T-cell lymphoma. J Clin Oncol Off J Am Soc Clin Oncol. 2014;32(11):1157–63.

106. Kantekure K, Yang Y, Raghunath P, Schaffer A, Woetmann A, Zhang Q, et al. Expression patterns of the immunosuppressive proteins PD-1/CD279 and PD-L1/CD274 at different stages of cutaneous T-cell lymphoma/mycosis fungoides. Am J Dermatopathol. 2012;34(1):126–8.

107. Samimi S, Benoit B, Evans K, et al. Increased programmed death-1 expression on cd4+ t cells in cutaneous t-cell lymphoma: implications for immune suppression. Arch Dermatol. 2010;146(12):1382–8.

108. Kim YH. A phase 2 study of pembrolizumab for the treatment of relapsed/refractory MF/SS. T-cell lymphoma forum 2016; January 28, 2016; San Francisco; 2016.

109. Khodadoust M RA, Porcu P, Foss FM, Moskowitz AJ, Shustov AR, Shanbhag S, Sokol L, Shine R, Fling SP, Li S, Rabhar Z, Kim J, Yang Y, Yearley J, Chartash EK, Townson SM,

Subrahmanyam PB, Maecker H, Alizadeh AA, Dai J, Horwitz SM, Sharon E, Kohrt H, Cheever MA, Kim YH. Pembrolizumab for treatment of relapsed/refractory mycosis fungoides and Sezary syndrome: clinical efficacy in a CITN multicenter phase 2 study. 3rd World Congress of Cutaneous Lymphomas; October 28, 2016.

110. S T, editor. T cell symposium and USCLC meeting highlights United States Cutaneous Lymphoma Consortium (USCLC) cutaneous lymphoma workshop; 2016; Washington, DC.

111. Rozati S, Kim YH. Experimental treatment strategies in primary cutaneous T-cell lymphomas. Curr Opin Oncol. 2016;28(2):166–71.

112. Marie-Cardine A, Viaud N, Thonnart N, Joly R, Chanteux S, Gauthier L, et al. IPH4102, a humanized KIR3DL2 antibody with potent activity against cutaneous T-cell lymphoma. Cancer Res. 2014;74(21):6060–70.

113. Querfeld C, Pacheco T, Foss FM, Halwani AS, Porcu P, Seto AG, Ruckman J, Landry ML, Jackson AL, Pestano LA, Dickinson BA, Sanseverino M, Rodman DM, Gordon G, Marshall W. Preliminary results of a phase 1 trial evaluating MRG-106, a synthetic microRNA antagonist (LNA antimiR) of microRNA-155, in patients with CTCL. Cancer. 2016;118(23):5830–9.

114. Frankel AE, Woo JH, Ahn C, Foss FM, Duvic M, Neville PH, et al. Resimmune, an anti-CD3epsilon recombinant immunotoxin, induces durable remissions in patients with cutaneous T-cell lymphoma. Haematologica. 2015;100(6):794–800.

115. Kim YH. A phase 1b study in cutaneous T-cell lymphoma (CTCL) with the novel topically applied skin-restricted histone deacetylase inhibitor (HDAC-i) SHP-141. American Society of Clinical Oncology (ASCO); Chicago; 2014.

116. Rook AH, Wood GS, Duvic M, Vonderheid EC, Tobia A, Cabana B. A phase II placebo-controlled study of photodynamic therapy with topical hypericin and visible light irradiation in the treatment of cutaneous T-cell lymphoma and psoriasis. J Am Acad Dermatol. 2010;63(6):984–90.

117. Rook AH, Gelfand JM, Wysocka M, Troxel AB, Benoit B, Surber C, et al. Topical resiquimod can induce disease regression and enhance T-cell effector functions in cutaneous T-cell lymphoma. Blood. 2015;126(12):1452–61.

118. Duvic M, Kuzel T, Dang N, et al. A dose finding lead-in study of E777 (diphtheria toxin fragment-interleukin-2 fusion protein) in persistent or recurrent cutaneous T-cell lymphoma (CTCL). Blood. 2014;124(21):3097.

119. Schlaak M, Theurich S, Pickenhain J, Skoetz N, Kurschat P, von Bergwelt-Baildon M. Allogeneic stem cell transplantation for advanced primary cutaneous T-cell lymphoma: a systematic review. Crit Rev Oncol Hematol. 2013;85(1):21–31.

120. Foss FM, Sausville EA. Prognosis and staging of cutaneous T-cell lymphoma. Hematol Oncol Clin North Am. 1995;9(5):1011–9.

121. Senff NJ, Hoefnagel JJ, Jansen PM, Vermeer MH, van Baarlen J, Blokx WA, et al. Reclassification of 300 primary cutaneous B-cell lymphomas according to the new WHO-EORTC classification for cutaneous lymphomas: comparison with previous classifications and identification of prognostic markers. J Clin Oncol Off J Am Soc Clin Oncol. 2007;25(12):1581–7.

122. Massone C, Fink-Puches R, Laimer M, Rutten A, Vale E, Cerroni L. Miliary and agminated-type primary cutaneous follicle center lymphoma: report of 18 cases. J Am Acad Dermatol. 2011;65(4):749–55.

123. Hamilton SN, Wai ES, Tan K, Alexander C, Gascoyne RD, Connors JM. Treatment and outcomes in patients with primary cutaneous B-cell lymphoma: the BC Cancer Agency experience. Int J Radiat Oncol Biol Phys. 2013;87(4):719–25.

124. Cerroni L, Kerl H. Primary cutaneous follicle center cell lymphoma. Leuk Lymphoma. 2001;42(5):891–900.

125. Swerdlow SH, Quintanilla-Martinez L, Willemze R, Kinney MC. Cutaneous B-cell lymphoproliferative disorders: report of the 2011 Society for Hematopathology/European Association for Haematopathology workshop. Am J Clin Pathol. 2013;139(4):515–35.

126. Willemze R, Kerl H, Sterry W, Berti E, Cerroni L, Chimenti S, et al. EORTC classification for primary cutaneous lymphomas: a proposal from the Cutaneous Lymphoma Study Group of the European Organization for Research and Treatment of Cancer. Blood. 1997;90(1):354–71.

127. Harris NL, Jaffe ES, Stein H, Banks PM, Chan JK, Cleary ML, et al. A revised European-American classification of lymphoid neoplasms: a proposal from the international lymphoma study group. Blood. 1994;84(5):1361–92.

128. Gulia A, Saggini A, Wiesner T, Fink-Puches R, Argenyi Z, Ferrara G, et al. Clinicopathologic features of early lesions of primary cutaneous follicle center lymphoma, diffuse type: implications for early diagnosis and treatment. J Am Acad Dermatol. 2011;65(5):991–1000.

129. Hoefnagel JJ, Vermeer MH, Jansen PM, Heule F, van Voorst Vader PC, Sanders CJ, et al. Primary cutaneous marginal zone B-cell lymphoma: clinical and therapeutic features in 50 cases. Arch Dermatol. 2005;141(9):1139–45.

130. Xie X, Sundram U, Natkunam Y, Kohler S, Hoppe RT, Kim YH, et al. Expression of HGAL in primary cutaneous large B-cell lymphomas: evidence for germinal center derivation of primary cutaneous follicular lymphoma. Modern Pathol Off J United States Can Acad Pathol Inc. 2008;21(6):653–9.

131. Li C, Inagaki H, Kuo TT, Hu S, Okabe M, Eimoto T. Primary cutaneous marginal zone B-cell lymphoma: a molecular and clinicopathologic study of 24 asian cases. Am J Surg Pathol. 2003;27(8):1061–9.

132. Connors JM, Hsi ED, Foss FM. Lymphoma of the skin. Hematol Am Soc Hematol Educ Program. 2002;1:263–82.

133. Swerdlow SH, Campo E, Pileri SA, Harris NL, Stein H, Siebert R, et al. The 2016 revision of the World Health Organization classification of lymphoid neoplasms. Blood. 2016;127(20):2375–90.

134. Grange F, Hedelin G, Joly P, Beylot-Barry M, D'Incan M, Delaunay M, et al. Prognostic factors in primary cutaneous lymphomas other than mycosis fungoides and the Sezary syndrome. The French study group on cutaneous lymphomas. Blood. 1999;93(11):3637–42.

135. Koens L, Vermeer MH, Willemze R, Jansen PM. IgM expression on paraffin sections distinguishes primary cutaneous large B-cell lymphoma, leg type from primary cutaneous follicle center lymphoma. Am J Surg Pathol. 2010;34(7):1043–8.

136. Demirkesen C, Tuzuner N, Esen T, Lebe B, Ozkal S. The expression of IgM is helpful in the differentiation of primary cutaneous diffuse large B cell lymphoma and follicle center lymphoma. Leuk Res. 2011;35(9):1269–72.

137. Grange F, Petrella T, Beylot-Barry M, Joly P, D'Incan M, Delaunay M, et al. Bcl-2 protein expression is the strongest independent prognostic factor of survival in primary cutaneous large B-cell lymphomas. Blood. 2004;103(10):3662–8.

138. Hallermann C, Niermann C, Fischer RJ, Schulze HJ. New prognostic relevant factors in primary cutaneous diffuse large B-cell lymphomas. J Am Acad Dermatol. 2007;56(4):588–97.

139. Koens L, Senff NJ, Vermeer MH, Willemze R, Jansen PM. Methotrexate-associated B-cell lymphoproliferative disorders presenting in the skin: a clinicopathologic and immunophenotypical study of 10 cases. Am J Surg Pathol. 2014;38(7):999–1006.

140. Geelen FA, Vermeer MH, Meijer CJ, Van der Putte SC, Kerkhof E, Kluin PM, et al. bcl-2 protein expression in primary cutaneous large B-cell lymphoma is site-related. J Clin Oncol Off J Am Soc Clin Oncol. 1998;16(6):2080–5.

141. Senff NJ, Noordijk EM, Kim YH, Bagot M, Berti E, Cerroni L, et al. European Organization for Research and Treatment of Cancer and International Society for Cutaneous Lymphoma consensus recommendations for the management of cutaneous B-cell lymphomas. Blood. 2008;112(5):1600–9.

142. Grange F, Beylot-Barry M, Courville P, Maubec E, Bagot M, Vergier B, et al. Primary cutaneous diffuse large B-cell lymphoma, leg type: clinicopathologic features and prognostic analysis in 60 cases. Arch Dermatol. 2007;143(9):1144–50.

143. Gupta E, Accurso J, Sluzevich J, Menke DM, Tun HW. Excellent outcome of immunomodulation or Bruton's tyrosine kinase inhibition in highly refractory primary cutaneous diffuse large B-cell lymphoma, leg type. Rare Tumors. 2015;7(4):6067.

144. Bekkenk MW, Geelen FA, van Voorst Vader PC, Heule F, Geerts ML, van Vloten WA, et al. Primary and secondary cutaneous CD30(+) lymphoproliferative disorders: a report from the

Dutch Cutaneous Lymphoma Group on the long-term follow-up data of 219 patients and guidelines for diagnosis and treatment. Blood. 2000;95(12):3653–61.

145. Kempf W, Pfaltz K, Vermeer MH, Cozzio A, Ortiz-Romero PL, Bagot M, et al. EORTC, ISCL, and USCLC consensus recommendations for the treatment of primary cutaneous CD30-positive lymphoproliferative disorders: lymphomatoid papulosis and primary cutaneous anaplastic large-cell lymphoma. Blood. 2011;118(15):4024–35.

146. Willemze R, Beljaards RC. Spectrum of primary cutaneous CD30 (Ki-1)-positive lymphoprolioerative disorders. A proposal for classification and guidelines for management and treatment. J Am Acad Dermatol. 1993;28(6):973–80.

147. Cerroni L. Lymphomatoid papulosis, pityriasis lichenoides et varioliformis acuta, and anaplastic large-cell (Ki-1+) lymphoma. J Am Acad Dermatol. 1997;37(2 Pt 1):287.

148. Brosens DA, Thulliez A. Histio-monocytic reticulosis and mycosis fungoides; four case reports. Arch Belg Dermatol Syphiligr. 1956;12(3):263–72.

149. Macaulay WL. Lymphomatoid papulosis. A continuing self-healing eruption, clinically benign – histologically malignant. Arch Dermatol. 1968;97(1):23–30.

150. Willemze R, Meyer CJ, Van Vloten WA, Scheffer E. The clinical and histological spectrum of lymphomatoid papulosis. Br J Dermatol. 1982;107(2):131–44.

151. Cardoso J, Duhra P, Thway Y, Calonje E. Lymphomatoid papulosis type D: a newly described variant easily confused with cutaneous aggressive CD8-positive cytotoxic T-cell lymphoma. Am J Dermatopathol. 2012;34(7):762–5.

152. Kempf W, Kazakov DV, Baumgartner HP, Kutzner H. Follicular lymphomatoid papulosis revisited: a study of 11 cases, with new histopathological findings. J Am Acad Dermatol. 2013;68(5):809–16.

153. Karai LJ, Kadin ME, Hsi ED, Sluzevich JC, Ketterling RP, Knudson RA, et al. Chromosomal rearrangements of 6p25.3 define a new subtype of lymphomatoid papulosis. Am J Surg Pathol. 2013;37(8):1173–81.

154. Kaudewitz P, Stein H, Dallenbach F, Eckert F, Bieber K, Burg G, et al. Primary and secondary cutaneous Ki-1+ (CD30+) anaplastic large cell lymphomas. Morphologic, immunohistologic, and clinical-characteristics. Am J Pathol. 1989;135(2):359–67.

155. Delsol G, Al Saati T, Gatter KC, Gerdes J, Schwarting R, Caveriviere P, et al. Coexpression of epithelial membrane antigen (EMA), Ki-1, and interleukin-2 receptor by anaplastic large cell lymphomas. Diagnostic value in so-called malignant histiocytosis. Am J Pathol. 1988;130(1):59–70.

156. Krenacs L, Wellmann A, Sorbara L, Himmelmann AW, Bagdi E, Jaffe ES, et al. Cytotoxic cell antigen expression in anaplastic large cell lymphomas of T- and null-cell type and Hodgkin's disease: evidence for distinct cellular origin. Blood. 1997;89(3):980–9.

157. Wilson MS, Weiss LM, Gatter KC, Mason DY, Dorfman RF, Warnke RA. Malignant histiocytosis. A reassessment of cases previously reported in 1975 based on paraffin section immunophcnotyping studies. Cancer. 1990;66(3):530–6.

Chapter 9
Fibrohistiocytic Skin Cancers: Dermatofibrosarcoma Protuberans, Atypical Fibroxanthoma, and Undifferentiated Pleomorphic Sarcoma

Kavita Mariwalla and Allison Hanlon

Abstract As a group, atypical fibroxanthoma, undifferentiated pleomorphic sarcoma, and dermatofibrosarcoma protuberans (DFSP) are rare cutaneous neoplasms with the potential for significant local destruction. In DFSP, delayed diagnosis is common as the clinical presentation can appear benign. Tissue stains are key for diagnosis of dermatofibrosarcoma protuberans from the benign histologic mimicker dermatofibroma. Debate exists regarding the relationship between atypical fibroxanthoma and undifferentiated pleomorphic sarcoma. The preferred treatment for fibrohistiocytic tumors is Mohs micrographic surgery. Since close monitoring for recurrence is critical, repair options for these commonly large postsurgical defects must be carefully planned. In all cases, preoperative planning and management of patient expectation is paramount to successful therapy.

Keywords Atypical fibroxanthoma · Undifferentiated pleomorphic sarcoma · Malignant fibrous histiocytoma · Dermatofibroma · Dermatofibrosarcoma protuberans · Sarcoma

K. Mariwalla
Mariwalla Dermatology, West Islip, NY, USA

A. Hanlon (✉)
Department of Medicine, Division of Dermatology, Vanderbilt University Medical Center, Nashville, TN, USA
e-mail: allison.m.hanlon@vanderbilt.edu

© Springer International Publishing AG, part of Springer Nature 2018
A. Hanlon (ed.), *A Practical Guide to Skin Cancer*,
https://doi.org/10.1007/978-3-319-74903-7_9

189

Introduction

Fibrohistiocytic skin tumors are rare neoplasms originating from dermal spindle cells. Malignancies typically included in the fibrohistiocytic skin tumor category are dermatofibrosarcoma protuberans, atypical fibroxanthoma, and undifferentiated pleomorphic sarcoma.

Dermatofibrosarcoma protuberans (DFSP) is a rare, low-grade malignancy that presents most commonly on the trunk. Because of its indolent course and rather benign appearance, there is often a delay in diagnosing DFSP. Complicating matters is that DFSP can have significant subclinical spread making definitive treatment challenging. While metastasis is rare, recurrence is common. DFSP fibrosarcoma, an aggressive variant of DFSP, can metastasize to the lung. Differentiating between DFSP and DFSP fibrosarcoma requires histologic evaluation and discerning between the two based on cellular features.

Atypical fibroxanthoma (AFX) is a rare skin cancer that presents on actinically damaged, sun-exposed skin. AFX is a low-grade skin cancer often successfully treated with Mohs micrographic surgery. AFX rarely metastasizes. Histologically, it is a well-defined, spindle cell neoplasm localized to the upper dermis. Undifferentiated pleomorphic sarcoma (UPS), previously known as malignant fibrous histiocytoma (MFH), is identical to AFX histologically. The two tumors differ in their depth of invasion with AFX remaining localized to the dermis, while UPS infiltrates deeply into subcutaneous tissue. UPS is an aggressive skin cancer with metastatic potential. Differentiating between AFX and UPS remains a diagnostic challenge.

Dermatofibrosarcoma Protuberans

Dermatofibrosarcoma protuberans is a rare, locally infiltrative cutaneous soft tissue sarcoma. DFSP most commonly presents on the trunk as an ill-defined plaque or nodule. The incidence of DFSP in the United States is 0.8–4.5 cases per million persons per year [1]. Women are more likely to develop DFSP than men. Black patients have an increased incidence almost two times greater than Caucasian patients [2]. Bednar tumor, a pigmented DFSP variant, is more common in black patients. DFSP can present at any age but most often presents in 30-year-old adults. DFSP fibrosarcoma (DFSP-FS) variant is an aggressive tumor with metastatic potential. DFSP-FS presents in older patients and has a worse prognosis [3].

DFSP presents as an asymptomatic, firm plaque that can vary in color from flesh colored to hyperpigmented or can be pink, yellow, or red (Fig. 9.1). Bednar tumors have dark brown pigmentation. The clinical appearance can be subtle during the early plaque stage, and in general, DFSP is slow growing. With time, the tumor will infiltrate subcutaneous structures making it more fixed, nodular, and possibly painful. Mature tumors may ulcerate and bleed. Due to the subtle, early clinical presentation, DFSP is often late to diagnosis. The clinical differential diagnosis includes

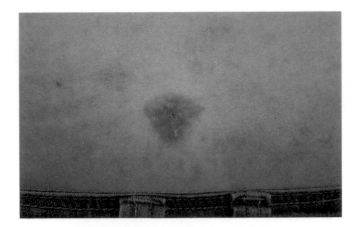

Fig. 9.1 Dermatofibrosarcoma protuberans

Fig. 9.2 Pigmented dermatofibroma

benign dermatofibroma (Fig. 9.2), pigmented basal cell carcinoma, hypertrophic scar, keloid, sarcoid, and soft tissue sarcomas. There is no clinical difference between DFSP and DFSP-FS.

Lesions suspicious for DFSP are biopsied via punch, incisional, or excisional techniques. Shave biopsy can be utilized, but does not examine deeper subcutaneous structures helpful in diagnosing DFSP. A shave biopsy may show a grenz zone, or narrow tumor-free margin, between the epidermis and dermal tumor present in DFSP. Histologically, DFSP is composed of monomorphic spindle cells in a whorled or storiform pattern [4] (Fig. 9.3). The spindle cells appear benign with minimal mitotic activity. DFSP invades subcutaneous tissues and often has subclinical expansion with peripheral tentacle-like extensions. This tentacle-like growth pattern makes obtaining clear histologic margins challenging. The pigmented Bednar tumors have melanin-containing dendritic cells along with the spindle cells. Rarely,

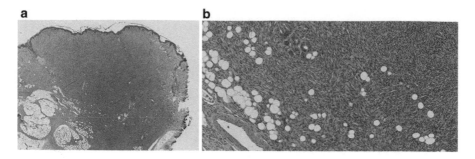

Fig. 9.3 Dermatofibrosarcoma protuberans (Photo courtesy of Jeffrey Zwerner, MD, PhD)

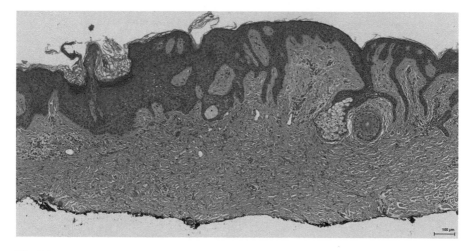

Fig. 9.4 Dermatofibroma (Photo courtesy of Jeffrey Zwerner, MD, PhD)

DFSP has sarcoma-like changes with cellular and nuclear pleomorphism. These tumors have metastatic potential and are known as the DFSP-FS variant [5]. Differentiating among DF (Fig. 9.4), DFSP, and DFSP-FS can be a histologic challenge. Immunohistochemistry aids in diagnosis with DFSP staining positive for CD34 and negative for factor XIIIa, while dermatofibroma (DF) is CD34 negative and factor XIIIa positive [6]. Poorly differentiated DFSP-FS can have loss of CD34 expression making it an unreliable marker. Hyaluronate and CD44 may help in differentiating a dermatofibroma from DFSP. CD44 is a cell membrane glycoprotein that binds to hyaluronate in the extracellular matrix. CD44 expression is significantly reduced or absent in DFSP but present in DF. In contrast, the DFSP tumor stroma stains strongly for hyaluronate, while the DF stroma shows a weak staining pattern [7].

Advances in molecular techniques have aided in the understanding and diagnosis of DFSP. DSFP has a characteristic unbalanced translocation t(17;22) (q22;q13) that leads to a unique fusion gene for platelet-derived growth factor beta polypeptide

(PDGFB gene) with collagen type 1A1 (COL1A1) gene [8]. Once fused, the normally regulated PDGFB gene is constitutively activated by the COL1A1 gene. Unregulated, the PDGFB/COL1A1 fusion protein leads to continuous activation of the tyrosine kinase PDGF receptor b and tumorigenesis [9]. Fluorescence in situ hybridization (FISH) assays can detect the PDGFB/COL1A1 fusion transcript [10]. Most often, FISH studies are not needed for tumor diagnosis.

DFSP has an infiltrative growth pattern with subclinical extension and tentacle-like projections into the surrounding collagen, fat, fascia, and muscle. Physical examination of patients includes assaying whether the DFSP is fixed to underlying structures. When a fixed, recurrent, or DFSP-FS tumor is present, magnetic resonance imaging (MRI) studies are recommended. The patient's lymph nodes are assessed clinically, but staging imaging studies are not recommended due to rare metastasis. In patients with the DFSP-FS variant or an advanced, recurrent tumor, a preoperative chest CT is recommended for lung metastasis evaluation.

The skin surrounding the tumor is palpated for subcutaneous firmness consistent with tumor extension. Scouting biopsies around the primary tumor can be performed to help delineate the tumor margins prior to surgical treatment.

Surgery is the first-line treatment of DFSP. The tumor's asymmetric, invasive fingerlike projections make surgical treatment challenging. Wide local excision (WLE) allows for a small percentage of the tumor's margins to be examined histologically. The rate of recurrence after wide local excision varies and depends upon the resection margins [11–13]. With wider surgical margins, the risk of recurrence declines. A retrospective review showed that tumors treated with surgical margins less than 3 cm recurred 47% of the time, while tumors treated with 3–5 cm margins recurred 7%. Margins greater than 5 cm were associated with the lowest recurrence rate (<5%) [14]. The National Comprehensive Cancer Network (NCCN) recommends margins of 2–4 cm with dissection to the underlying muscle or periosteum. Often, these recommendations cannot be followed due to tumor location.

Mohs micrographic surgery (MMS) is the preferred surgical treatment for DFSP. During MMS, the resected tissue's entire peripheral margin is examined. Through frozen section analysis, the surgeon/pathologist identifies where the margins are positive including the asymmetric tumor projections lost in specimen bread loafing with wide local excision. Preoperatively, surveillance biopsies are recommended, and most Mohs surgeons start their first layer at least 1 cm from the palpable margins of the tumor on gross exam. Intraoperative CD34 immunostains may aid the physician in identifying the tumor, which is a challenge with frozen sections. Examination of the complete margin allows for resection only in the sites with positive margins. Thus, tumor-free margins are obtained while conserving normal tissue. The DFSP recurrence rate after MMS is lower than WLE. In a systematic review of 23 nonrandomized trials, the local recurrence rate was 1.11% after MMS versus 6.32% after WLE [15]. MMS has limitations. Deeply penetrating tumors to fascia, muscle, and bone as well as recurrent tumors are not optimally treated with MMS. Local anesthesia may be difficult to obtain in deeper structures such as periosteum and bone. Due to its inherent growth pattern, DFSP that recurs cannot be mapped histologically since the Mohs technique relies on tumors growing in a contiguous fashion. The interpretation of frozen histology for DFSP can be challenging, with or without immunostaining. A final permanent histologic layer or margin can confirm an intraoperative negative frozen margin.

It should be noted that DFSP is a radiosensitive tumor, and surgical excision is not the only option for it. Radiation can be used as a primary treatment for inoperable tumors or in patients unable to tolerate surgical resection. The data is limited for radiation as the primary DFSP treatment. In patients with incomplete surgical margins, radiotherapy may be beneficial. Local recurrence after adjuvant radiation was 14.2% in patients with close or positive margins and none in patients with negative margins [16]. Sarcomatous DFSP tumors do not necessitate adjuvant radiation as it is unclear whether radiation is beneficial.

Molecular targeted therapies can treat metastatic and locally advanced tumors. Imatinib, a small molecular tyrosine kinase inhibitor that blocks the PDGF receptor, is FDA approved in the United States for the treatment of unresectable, recurrent, and/or metastatic DFSP. Imatinib can be used as a neoadjuvant to shrink tumors prior to surgical excision. Mohs micrographic surgery following imatinib therapy showed discontiguous tumor due to partial treatment.

Locally advanced, recurrent, or rare metastatic tumors may require nonsurgical therapy. A multidisciplinary approach is recommended for patients with advanced or aggressive tumors. Recurrent tumors are more likely to metastasize and deeply invade muscle and/or bone with increased surgical morbidity. Lymphadenectomy is recommended in patients with localized lymph node metastasis. Multiple metastases are not conducive to surgery.

The prognosis of DFSP is good with a 10-year survival of 99.1%. [17]. Higher mortality is associated with increased cellularity, high mitotic rate, male sex, black race, and head or limb location. While patients rarely die from DFSP, morbidity is high due to the risk of local recurrence. Most recurrences occur within the first 3 years posttreatment [18]. Recurrence is highest in patients initially treated with incomplete surgical margins. Age greater than 50 is associated with higher recurrence and decreased survival. Importantly, older patients are more likely to develop the DFSP-FS variant. Fatalities have been described in patients with incompletely resected DFSP-FS variant [19].

Close clinical monitoring is recommended with skin exams every 6 months for the first 3 years and annually for life. The skin exam includes inspection and palpation of the surgical scar. Any clinically suspicious lesions are biopsied via incisional or punch biopsy techniques. Lymph node palpation is performed with the skin exam. If lymphadenopathy is identified, radiographic imaging is recommended. Radiographic surveillance is not recommended if there are no concerning clinical findings. If a recurrence is detected, imaging is recommended. Because surveillance postoperatively is important and recurrence rate is high, most surgeons opt out of flap repairs over DFSP sites instead opting for linear closures or split thickness skin grafts to allow for better visualization of any recurrent masses.

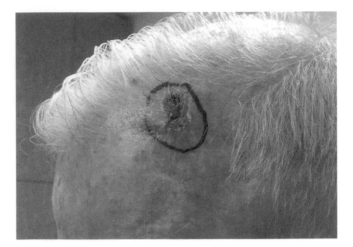

Fig. 9.5 Atypical fibroxanthoma

Atypical Fibroxanthoma

Atypical fibroxanthoma (AFX) is a rare skin cancer most commonly presenting as an asymptomatic pink papule or nodule on sun-damaged skin (Fig. 9.5). AFX frequently presents on the head and neck of fair-skinned, elderly men. The clinical differential diagnosis includes squamous cell carcinoma, sarcoma, amelanotic melanoma, and undifferentiated pleomorphic sarcoma (UPS).

First described by Helwig, AFX is a pleomorphic tumor with spindled and epithelioid cells localized to the dermis [20]. Severe cellular pleomorphism, atypical mitosis, and multinucleated giant cells are noted. Distinguishing AFX from other poorly differentiated tumors is necessary for both diagnostic and therapeutic purposes. Unfortunately, the distinction is often not straightforward. Immunohistochemistry stains aid in differentiating AFX from other spindled cell neoplasms including squamous cell carcinoma, desmoplastic melanoma, and leiomyosarcoma. AFX and undifferentiated pleomorphic sarcoma, formerly known as malignant fibrous histiocytoma (Fig. 9.6), share an immunophenotype. Previous immunohistochemistry studies have not shown a significant distinction between AFX and UPS [21–24]. Comparative genomic hybridization studies pointed at differences in the RAS pathway and p53 mutations, but these markers have not been recapitulated in full genomic sequencing [25]. Presently, distinguishing AFX from UPS rests on tumor location with AFX localized to the dermis, while UPS invades deeply through the subcutaneous fat and underlying structures (Fig. 9.7) [26]. Often, a superficial shave biopsy is performed for diagnosis. Differentiating between AFX and UPS is impossible without visualization of the subcutaneous fat. A shave biopsy with tumor at the deep margin may lead to a histologic description of a pleomorphic tumor consistent with

Fig. 9.6 Undifferentiated
pleomorphic sarcoma

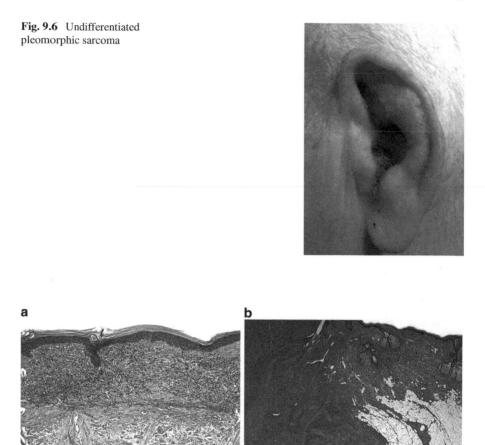

Fig. 9.7 Histology of AFX and UPS. 7A) AFX is a pleomorphic tumor with spindled and epithe-
loid cells localized to the dermis. 7B) UPS has similar pleomorphic and epitheloid histology but
deeply penetrates the dermis and subcutaneous fat (Source: Hanlon, Allison; MD, PhD; Stasko,
Thomas; Christiansen, Dan; Cyrus, Nika; Galan, Anjela, Dermatologic Surgery, LN2, CD10, and
Ezrin Do Not Distinguish Between Atypical Fibroxanthoma and Undifferentiated Pleomorphic
Sarcoma or Predict Clinical Outcome, Mar 1, 2017, Vol 43, Issue 3, with kind permission from
Wolters Kluwer Health, Inc.)

both AFX and UPS. The clinician can perform a second, deeper biopsy for further
histology review or proceed with surgical treatment, the first-line therapy for both
tumors.

AFX is treated surgically either with wide local excision or Mohs micrographic
surgery [27]. Wide local excision is associated with recurrence rates ranging from
0% to 20% [28, 29]. Positive margins are associated with an increased risk of recurrence. The risk of AFX recurrence following Mohs micrographic surgery (MMS) is
low.

In the largest retrospective review of 169 tumors treated with MMS and followed for a median of 21.7 months, 1% of patients had a local recurrence [21]. In a smaller study of 58 tumors treated with MMS and followed for a median of 4.5 years, no recurrences were reported [27]. The Mohs technique allows for visualization of the complete tumor margin likely resulting in decreased recurrence rates. In the Mohs technique, the central portion of the tumor is not examined for depth of subcutaneous invasion. If the margins are clear in the first or second Mohs stage, the tumor's depth of invasion – localized to the dermis versus the subcutaneous fat – may not be clear. Submitting the first stage or tumor debulking for permanent sections may be considered if there is concern that the tumor is more consistent with a UPS.

Radiation therapy is rarely used for AFX treatment. There are no randomized, controlled trials to guide care. Radiation is reserved for patients with recurrent, metastatic, or inoperable tumors.

Metastatic AFX is extraordinarily rare. Radiographic staging and sentinel lymph node biopsy are not indicated in the AFX patient evaluation. The metastatic rate ranges from 0.5% to 4% depending upon the retrospective review [21, 27, 30]. Immunosuppression was implicated as a possible risk factor for metastatic AFX, but large retrospective studies have not supported this relationship [31]. If an AFX tumor metastasizes, the primary tumor should be reexamined for features suggestive of UPS. Case reports, series, and retrospective reviews have described metastatic AFX that with further histologic review was better classified as UPS.

Debate surrounds whether UPS is a separate entity or a more aggressive variant of AFX. In 2002, the World Health Organization addressed the evolving classification of sarcomas. Malignant fibrous histiocytoma was a diagnosis of exclusion and contained multiple different sarcoma tumors, including fibrosarcoma and leiomyosarcoma. With advances in immunohistochemistry and electron microscopy, the sarcomas were further classified and MFH was renamed UPS [32]. Prior to reclassification, UPS contained a range of tumors with varying biologic behavior and potential for metastasis and recurrence. Examination of multiple retrospective studies reflects how, as the tumors became better classified, the risk of tumor recurrence and metastasis changed. The combined recurrence rate of MFH treated with MMS published before 1990 is 7.4%, with an average follow up of 41.7 months [33]. Prior to 2000, a mean recurrence rate of 37.5% was reported in seven cases with an average follow up of 41.7 months. The mean contemporary recurrence rate of UPS treated with MMS is 58.8%, significantly higher than the initial studies [29].

With the modern classification of UPS, the recommendations for treatment have advanced as well. Surgical treatment with sentinel lymph node and/or radiographic imaging of the lymph node basin is recommended. There are no studies comparing the efficacy of MMS versus wide local excision for the treatment of UPS. Close clinical monitoring after surgical treatment is necessary. Local recurrence and/or metastasis usually occurs within the first 2 years posttreatment [34]. Adjuvant radiation can be considered postsurgery for tumors with aggressive clinical behavior, but there are no recommendations to guide care.

Further study is needed to elucidate the relationship between AFX and UPS. The prognosis of AFX is excellent with low rate of recurrence and metastasis. In contrast,

UPS is an aggressive tumor with metastatic and life-threatening potential. Accurate, initial diagnosis is essential for determining patient's risk and the best therapeutic options.

References

1. Kreicher KL, Kurlander DE, Gittleman HR, Barnholtz-Sloan JS, Bordeaux JS. Incidence and survival of primary dermatofibrosarcoma protuberans in the United States. Dermatol Surg. 2016;42(1):24–31.
2. Rouhani P, Fletcher CD, Devesa SS, Toro JR. Cutaneous soft tissue sarcoma incidence patterns in the U.S. : an analysis of 12,114 cases. Cancer. 2008;113(3):616–27.
3. Connelly JH, Evans HL. Dermatofibrosarcoma protuberans. A clinicopathologic review with emphasis on fibrosarcomatous areas. Am J Surg Pathol. 1992;16(10):921–5.
4. Llombart B, Serra-Guillén C, Monteagudo C, López Guerrero JA, Sanmartín O. Dermatofibrosarcoma protuberans: a comprehensive review and update on diagnosis and management. Semin Diagn Pathol. 2013;30(1):13–28.
5. Goldblum JR, Reith JD, Weiss SW. Sarcomas arising in dermatofibrosarcoma protuberans: a reappraisal of biologic behavior in eighteen cases treated by wide local excision with extended clinical follow up. Am J Surg Pathol. 2000;24(8):1125–30.
6. Haycox CL, Odland PB, Olbricht SM, Piepkorn M. Immunohistochemical characterization of dermatofibrosarcoma protuberans with practical applications for diagnosis and treatment. J Am Acad Dermatol. 1997;37(3):438–44.
7. Calikoglu E, Augsburger E, Chavaz P, Saurat JH, Kaya G. CD44 and hyaluronate in the differential diagnosis of dermatofibroma and dermatofibrosarcoma protuberans. J Cutan Pathol. 2003;30(3):185–9.
8. Simon MP, Pedeutour F, Sirvent N, Grosgeorge J, et al. Deregulation of the platelet-derived growth factor B-chain gene via fusion with collagen gene COL1A1 in dermatofibrosarcoma protuberans and giant-cell fibroblastoma. Nat Genet. 1997;15(1):95–8.
9. Kiuru-Kuhlefelt S, El-Rifai W, Fanburg-Smith J, Kere J, Miettinen M, Knuutila S. Concomitant DNA copy number amplification at 17q and 22q in dermatofibrosarcoma protuberans. Cytogenet Cell Genet. 2001;92(3–4):192–5.
10. Patel KU, Szabo SS, Hernandez VS, Prieto VG, Abruzzo LV, Lazar AJ, López-Terrada D. Dermatofibrosarcoma protuberans COL1A1-PDGFB fusion is identified in virtually all dermatofibrosarcoma protuberans cases when investigated by newly developed multiplex reverse transcription polymerase chain reaction and fluorescence in situ hybridization assays. Human Pathol. 2008;39(2):184–93.
11. Fiore M, Miceli R, Mussi C, Lo Vullo S, Mariani L, Lozza L, Collini P, Olmi P, Casali PG, Gronchi A. Dermatofibrosarcoma protuberans treated at a single institution: a surgical disease with a high cure rate. J Clin Oncol. 2005;23(30):7669–75.
12. Stojadinovic A, Hoos A, Karpoff HM, Leung DH, Antonescu CR, Brennan MF, Lewis JJ. Soft tissue tumors of the abdominal wall: analysis of disease patterns and treatments. Arch Surg. 2001;136(1):70–9.
13. DuBay D, Cimmino V, Lowe L, Johnson TM, Sondak VK. Low recurrence rate after surgery for dermatofibrosarcoma protuberans: a multidisciplinary approach from a single institution. Cancer. 2004;100(5):1008–16.
14. Arnaud EJ, Perrault M, Revol M, Servant JM, Banzet P. Surgical treatment of dermatofibrosarcoma protuberans. Plast Reconstr Surg. 1997;100(4):884–95.
15. Foroozan M, Sei JF, Amini M, Beauchet A, Saiag P. Efficacy of Mohs micrographic surgery for the treatment of dermatofibrosarcoma protuberans: systematic review. Arch Dermatol. 2012;148(9):1055–63.

16. Haas RL, Keus RB, Loftus BM, Rutgers EJ, van Coevorden F, Bartelink H. The role of radiotherapy in the local management of dermatofibrosarcoma protuberans. Soft tissue tumours working group. Eur J Cancer. 1997;33(7):1055–60.
17. Kreicher KL, Kurlander DE, Gittleman HR, Barnholtz-Sloan JS, Bordeaux JS. Incidence and survival of primary dermatofibrosarcoma protuberans in the United States. Dermatol Surg. 2016;42(Suppl 1):S24–31.
18. Gloster HM Jr. Dermatofibrosarcoma protuberans. J Am Acad Dermatol. 1996;35(3):355–74.
19. Liang CA, Jambusaria-Pahlajani A, Karia PS, Elenitsas R, et al. A systematic review of outcome data for dermatofibrosarcoma protuberans with and without fibrosarcomatous change. J Am Acad Dermatol. 2014;71(4):781–6.
20. Helwig EB, May D. Atypical fibroxanthoma of the skin with metastasis. Cancer. 1986;57(2):368–76.
21. Hanlon A, et al. LN2, CD10, and Ezrin do not distinguish between atypical Fibroxanthoma and undifferentiated pleomorphic sarcoma or predict clinical outcome. Dermatol Surg. 2017;43(3):431–6.
22. Hollmig ST, Rieger KE, Henderson MT, West RB, Sundram UN. Reconsidering the diagnostic and prognostic utility of LN-2 for undifferentiated pleomorphic sarcoma and atypical fibroxanthoma. Am J Dermatopathol. 2013;35(2):176–9.
23. Wingard JR, Carter SL, Walsh JT, Kurtzberg J, Small TN, Gersten ID, et al. Results of a randomized, double-blind trial of fluconazole (FLU) vs voriconazole (VORI) for the prevention of invasive fungal infections (IFI) in 600 allogeneic blood and marrow transplant (BMT) patients (abstract). Blood (ASH Annual Meet Abstract). 2007;110:163.
24. Lazova R, Moynes R, May D, Scott G. LN-2 (CD74) a marker to distinguish atypical fibroxanthoma from malignant fibrous histiocytoma. Cancer. 1997;79(11):2115–24.
25. Mihic-Probst D, Zhao J, Saremasiani P, Baer A, Oehischlegel C, et al. CGH analysis shows genetic similarities and differences in atypical fibroxanthoma and undifferentiated high grade pleomorphic sarcoma. Anticancer Res. 2004;24(1):19–26.
26. McCalmont TH. AFX: what we now know. J Cutan Pathol. 2011;38(11):853–6.
27. Ang GC, Roenigk RK, Otley CC, Kim Phillips P, et al. *More than 2 decades of treating atypical fibroxanthoma at mayo clinic:what have we learned from 91 patients?* Dermatol Surg. 2009;35(5):765–72.
28. Love WE, Schmitt AR, Bordeaux JS. Managment of unusual cutaneous malignancies: atypical fibroxanthoma, malignant fibrous histiocytoma, sebaceous carcinoma, extramammary paget disease. Dermatol Clin. 2011;2(29):201–16.
29. Hollmig ST, et al. The evolving conception and management challenges of malignant fibrous histiocytoma. Dermatol Surg. 2012;38(12):1922–9.
30. Hueterh MJ, Zitelli JA, Brodland D. Mohs micrographic surgery for the treatment of spindle cell tumors of the skin. J Am Acad Dermatol. 2001;44(4):656–9.
31. McCoppin HH, et al. Clinical spectrum of atypical fibroxanthoma and undifferentiated pleomorphic sarcoma in solid organ transplant recipients: a collective experience. Dermatol Surg. 2012;38(2):230–9.
32. Fletcher CD. The evolving classification of soft tissue tumours: an update based on the new WHO classification. Histopathology. 2006;48(1):3–12.
33. Brown MD, Swanson NA. Treatment of malignant fibrous histiocytoma and atypical fibrous xanthoma with micrographic surgery. J Dermatol Surg Oncol. 1989;15(12):1287–92.
34. Withers AH, et al. Atypical fibroxanthoma and malignant fibrous histiocytoma. J Plast Reconstr Aesthet Surg. 2011;64(11):e273–8.

Chapter 10
Adnexal Carcinoma: Microcystic Adnexal Carcinoma and Sebaceous Carcinoma

Paul R. Massey, Anthony C. Soldano, and Matthew C. Fox

Abstract Microcystic adnexal carcinoma (MAC) and sebaceous carcinoma (SC) are rare adnexal neoplasms. MAC most commonly presents as a poorly defined, firm, skin-colored papule, nodule, or plaque on the head and neck. Although locally destructive, MAC does not typically metastasize. Rates of misdiagnosis are high, due to incomplete, superficial sampling. Resection techniques with meticulous margin control, including Mohs micrographic surgery (MMS), are recommended in the management of MAC.

Sebaceous carcinoma, originating from holocrine sebocytes, is often found on the head and neck and is among the most common eyelid neoplasms. SC commonly presents as a firm, subcutaneous nodule with a yellow hue. SC may masquerade as other neoplastic and inflammatory entities, delaying diagnosis. Patients with SC must be screened for Muir-Torre syndrome, a hereditary cancer syndrome. Treatment for SC is surgical. SC has metastatic potential, most commonly to draining lymph node basins. Radiation and chemotherapy play a role in the management of metastatic disease.

Keywords Microcystic adnexal carcinoma · Sebaceous carcinoma · Sebaceous neoplasm · Desmoplastic trichoepithelioma · Morpheaform basal cell carcinoma · Muir-Torre Syndrome · Sentinel lymph node biopsy · Mohs micrographic surgery

P. R. Massey (✉) · A. C. Soldano · M. C. Fox
Division of Dermatology, Dell Medical School,
University of Texas at Austin, Austin, TX, USA
e-mail: prmassey@seton.org

© Springer International Publishing AG, part of Springer Nature 2018   201
A. Hanlon (ed.), *A Practical Guide to Skin Cancer*,
https://doi.org/10.1007/978-3-319-74903-7_10

Microcystic Adnexal Carcinoma

Introduction

Microcystic adnexal carcinoma (MAC) is a rare skin tumor first described in a series of six patients presenting with indurated skin-colored plaques on the upper lip [1]. Goldstein et al. described MAC as a neoplasm exhibiting both follicular and sweat gland differentiation, a thesis that has been largely accepted over time [2–4].

Histologically, MAC demonstrates an infiltrative growth pattern. The tumor histology reflects its clinical behavior with local destruction to underlying structures, but rare metastasis [5, 6]. MAC most commonly presents on the head and neck of older female patients [7]. Despite the significant morbidity that tumors can cause, the 10-year survival for patients with MAC is approximately 97% [7]. Treatment of MAC is challenging, as it is prone to recur, likely due to its propensity for perineural invasion [8]. Resection techniques involving meticulous margin control such as Mohs micrographic surgery (MMS) are the gold standard for treatment, with recurrence rates ranging from 0% to 22% [8].

Epidemiology

MAC studies are limited by its low incidence. The largest series of patients with MAC reported to date illustrates the rarity of the condition, with a frequency of 0.16 to 0.65 per 1,000,000 persons [7]. While patients of all ages are susceptible, including two cases of congenital MAC reported in the literature [9, 10], the median age at diagnosis is 68 years [7].

Ninety percent of patients reported are Caucasian, with the remaining 10% African Americans, Asian/Pacific Islanders, and patients of other or unknown race. Case reports have confirmed the diagnosis of MAC in African Americans [10, 11], Japanese [12], and Chinese [13] patients, among several other ethnicities.

MAC has a tendency to affect female more than male patients [6, 7]. In a recent epidemiologic study of rare cutaneous tumors in Olmsted County, Minnesota, MAC and another sweat duct tumor, eccrine carcinoma, stood alone among a group of several rare neoplasms in demonstrating a female predominance [14].

Pathogenesis

Debate surrounds the cell of origin for MAC. In his initial report describing MAC, Goldstein et al. hypothesized the cell of origin to be a pluripotent keratinocyte "capable of both follicular and sweat gland differentiation" [1]. Immunohistochemical studies support the dual differentiation theory, as MAC stains with antibodies for sweat ducts, such as carcinoembryonic antigen (CEA) while simultaneously reacting with keratin stains [15]. Other studies support the classification of MAC as a principally eccrine differentiated tumor [16]. Leboit et al. report evidence of both sebaceous and apocrine differentiation in a series of MAC tumors, providing support for differentiation toward the pilosebaceous unit [17].

The risk factors for MAC include fair skin, radiation, UV exposure, immunosuppression, and genetic syndromes [18, 19]. Chiller et al. reported that American patients are more likely to develop MAC on the left side of their body, lending support to the role of ultraviolet radiation in tumor development [6]. The etiologic role of ultraviolet light in MAC development remains controversial, as UV-associated signature mutations in p53 are not found in the majority of MACs [20]. Similar to other cutaneous neoplasms, immunosuppressed MAC patients have developed regional or metastatic disease [18, 19]. The role of the immune system in surveilling and constraining the spread of MAC, however, remains uncertain [18]. Finally, there is a report of deletion of chromosome 6q in a case of MAC [21], significant in that chromosome 6q is frequently aberrant in salivary gland tumors [22].

There may be an association between MAC and Nicolau-Balus syndrome, a rare condition consisting of multiple syringomas, cysts, and atrophoderma vermiculatum [23]. In one case, a patient developed MAC while carrying a diagnosis of Nicolau-Balus syndrome [24]. Schaller described two cases of histologically "MAC-like" plaques in patients with atrophoderma vermiculatum arising in childhood, including a patient with a diagnosis of Nicolau-Balus syndrome [25]. In addition, a case of multiple MACs occurring in the same patient has been reported [26].

Clinical Features

MAC most commonly presents as a poorly defined, firm, skin-colored or yellow papule, nodule, or plaque [5, 27] (Fig. 10.1). Lesions do not ulcerate [5] and are commonly mistaken for a scar [28]. MAC most commonly presents on the upper cutaneous lip. Yu et al. reported that 74% of MACs in the SEER database were located in the head and neck, including the cutaneous lip [7]. Other well-represented body locations in the SEER database include the trunk (9%), upper extremities (9%), and lower extremities (5%) [7]. Lesions most commonly arise in sun-exposed skin [20].

On presentation, patients are most often asymptomatic; however, complaints of paresthesia or numbness, possibly owing to the tumor's tendency for perineural invasion, may be reported [29]. Due to its often indolent course and relatively innocent appearance, diagnosis is often delayed [5]. Perhaps owing to its insidious presentation, MAC can be large at the time of diagnosis. Multiple studies have demonstrated an average approximate size at diagnosis of 2 cm [27, 29].

Clinically, MAC has a propensity for aggressive local behavior and invasion, but a limited capacity for systemic dissemination. This disease phenotype is reflected in the SEER database: at presentation, 74% of patients diagnosed with MAC had disease limited to the skin, while a small but important minority (16%) demonstrated local invasion, either into the subcutaneous tissue or into soft tissue, muscle, or bone [7]. Only 1.8% of patients with known lymph node status (either clinical or patho-

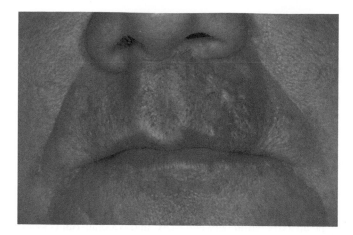

Fig. 10.1 Microcystic adnexal carcinoma. This tumor presents as a poorly defined, firm, pink plaque (From Rustemeyer J, Zwerger S, Pörksen M, et al. Oral Maxillofac Surg, 2013;17:141, Fig. 1, Springer Nature, under Creative Commons Attribution License)

logic) had evidence of regional metastatic disease, and 0.4% of patients presented with distant metastatic disease [7]. Death from MAC is extremely rare [30]. In fact, while overall survival of MAC patients is somewhat diminished, survival compared to the undiagnosed population is essentially unchanged [7].

Pathology

Histologically, MAC is a poorly circumscribed infiltrating tumor with ductal and follicular differentiation surrounded by a sclerotic stroma [31]. Goldstein et al. described a tumor with two seeming cell populations: in the high dermis, scattered aggregates of bland keratinocytes, several surrounding formed keratin-containing pseudo-horn cysts (Fig. 10.2), and a separate, deeper infiltrative cell population comprising strands and cords with occasional lumens (Fig. 10.3) [1]. Ducts are often thinly lined and may take on a "tadpole"-like shape as seen in syringomas (Fig. 10.4) [31]. Cell density diminishes as the tumor descends toward the subcutaneous tissue. The deeply infiltrative growth pattern of MAC belies its bland cytologic appearance, however, as mitotic figures or atypical cells are not frequently seen [5]. Perineural infiltration is characteristic (Fig. 10.5) [31], and frank invasion of nerve fibers can be seen [25].

Histologic misdiagnosis of MAC is quite common, ranging from 27% to 69% in some series, contributing to a delay in definitive diagnosis and treatment [6, 18].

The histologic differential diagnosis of MAC includes syringoma, desmoplastic trichoepithelioma (DTE), and morpheaform BCC. SCC [32], adenosquamous carcinoma, trichoadenoma, and metastatic adenocarcinoma may also be histologic confounders [33]. It is worth noting that the terminology describing what is now

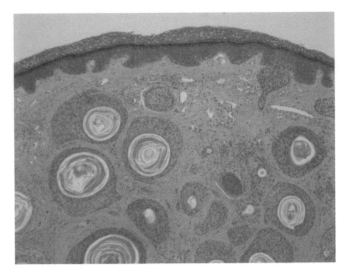

Fig. 10.2 Numerous keratocysts in the superficial portions of a MAC, 10× (Courtesy of Timothy F. Kolda, MD)

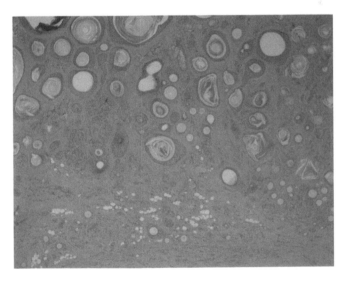

Fig. 10.3 Low-power view of MAC illustrates keratocysts in the superficial dermis beneath which are infiltrative cords embedded in a sclerotic stroma, 4× (Courtesy of Timothy F. Kolda, MD)

understood to be a MAC is quite confusing [34]. A number of terms are applied to infiltrative tumors of eccrine origin similar to MAC, including malignant syringoma, syringoid carcinoma [35], syringoid eccrine carcinoma, malignant sweat gland carcinoma, and syringomatous carcinoma [34]. Some authors have suggested the presence of small keratinaceous cysts in the high dermis (microcysts) confers

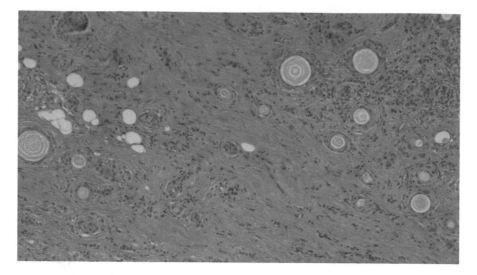

Fig. 10.4 Strands and cords with thinly lined lumens infiltrating the dermis, several in "tadpole" configuration simulating a syringoma, 20× (Courtesy of Timothy F. Kolda, MD)

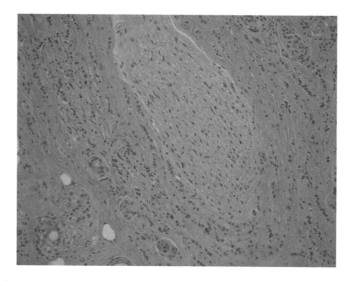

Fig. 10.5 Extensive perineural invasion, 20× (Courtesy of Timothy F. Kolda, MD)

specificity to MAC against other entities [36]. Often, however, a particular terminology is used in the literature without histologic explanation [34]. Some have suggested this group of lesions may be best viewed as a spectrum [37], and the term "locally aggressive adnexal carcinoma" has been suggested [20].

The distinction between MAC, DTE, and morpheaform BCC is critical as DTE is a benign lesion and misdiagnosis can lead to overtreatment and undue patient morbidity. These three entities share a number of histologic features, including presence on sun-damaged skin, sclerotic stroma, basaloid cells, and microcysts [38, 39]. Both MAC and DTE may demonstrate keratin cysts [40]. One useful clue on hematoxylin and eosin staining in discriminating MAC from DTE is the lack of ductal differentiation in DTE, which also typically has better-circumscribed architecture and the presence of a central dell [5, 38]. Likewise, morpheaform BCC will not typically demonstrate ductal differentiation and will often display clefting between tumor cells and the surrounding stroma.

There is a role for immunohistochemistry to elucidate a diagnosis of MAC when overlapping histologic features with DTE or morpheaform BCC are present [41]. MAC, DTE, and morpheaform BCC will react with pan-keratin stains (AE1/AE3). Carcinoembryonic antigen (CEA) and epithelial membrane antigen (EMA) are expressed in cells with ductal differentiation, as in MAC, and thus can be of use in differentiating MAC from DTE and morpheaform BCC [41, 42]. BerEP4, a reliable stain readily expressed in BCC, has been shown to effectively differentiate BCC and MAC [32, 43]. Cytokeratin 7, which is expressed in glandular tissue, is positive in MAC and negative in BCC and DTE [20]. While some authors have shown cytokeratin 20 to be helpful in differentiating MAC and DTE, as benign follicular neoplasms retain Merkel cells [44], others have not been able to replicate this association [20, 41]. The reliability of cytokeratin 15 staining in MAC has also demonstrated mixed results [32, 41].

Differential Diagnosis

The clinical differential diagnosis of MAC includes DTE, BCC, SCC, trichoadenoma, metastatic adenocarcinoma, and syringoma [27]. Syringomas are benign papules, usually multiple in number, with predilection for the orbits, especially in middle-aged women. Eruptive and familial variants have been described [45]. BCC may be pleomorphic in appearance, but is typically described as a pink or pearly papule or plaque, with a characteristic rolled border; in its morpheaform variant, an indurated sclerotic plaque is instead observed [46]. SCC affects sun-damaged skin and may be varied in clinical appearance; ulceration and hyperkeratosis may be present, and patients may present with a complaint of a wound that will not heal [47]. DTE presents as an indolent, firm, skin-colored plaque on the face, with a characteristic central dell and raised borders [48].

Differentiation between MAC, DTE, and morpheaform BCC is challenging clinically. Dermoscopy may be a useful adjunct. Shinohara et al. attempted to differentiate MAC from DTE on dermoscopy, noting that while both entities may demonstrate arborizing vessels or peripheral white dots, DTE is characterized by a central "structureless area" of presumptive scar, while MAC is not [40]. Similar to DTE, morpheaform BCC will also demonstrate arborizing vessels and telangiectasias with structureless hypopigmentation [49].

Evaluation and Treatment

The importance of appropriate biopsy technique and sampling cannot be overstated when there is clinical suspicion for MAC. Small and/or superficial biopsies contribute to misdiagnosis of this entity, such that when clinical suspicion exists, large specimens obtained via either incisional or excisional biopsy are optimal [17]. Because superficial shave biopsy may miss the deeply infiltrating, often perineural, ductal and basaloid cells which allow differentiation from other similar entities [41], this may be a suboptimal technique for evaluating a possibly malignant sclerotic plaque on sun-exposed skin.

Staging, Imaging

Routine imaging is not typically performed in MAC unless clinically indicated. When invasion of underlying deep tissue or bone is suspected, magnetic resonance imaging (MRI) [50, 51] and computerized tomography (CT) [52] have been used with success.

Surgical Treatment

The cornerstone for management of MAC is surgical extirpation. Due to high recurrence rates, wide local excision receives little support in the literature. While reported recurrence rates with wide local excision range from 30% to 50% [6, 53, 54], there is a clear lack of standardization about what surgical margins were selected [29]. In one retrospective study, tumor was present at the margins of 47% of standard excision specimens, and one patient required as many as four excisions for clearance [6]. Recurrences typically occur within 3 years of initial treatment and may be more aggressive than the original tumor presentation [6, 35]. Intrinsic tumor characteristics, such as perineural invasion [27] and subtle extension into the subcutis, likely contribute to high rates of recurrence.

MMS and excision with complete permanent section margin evaluation are well-suited treatment modalities. Published literature demonstrates a clear advantage to the use of MMS over standard excision in the treatment of MAC. Widely reported recurrence rates with MMS in primarily retrospective data range from 0% to 22% [8], with the latter figure based on a small cohort with a significant number of recurrent and likely more aggressive tumors [55]. In a meta-analysis of mostly retrospective case series, Diamantis et al. reported a total of 8 recurrences out of 146 cases of MAC treated by MMS (rate of approximately 5%) [8]. A recurrence rate of 5% was demonstrated in a prospective Australian study of 44 patients who underwent MMS for MAC [27]. Friedman et al. and Snow et al. reported zero recurrences in retrospective studies of 11 and 12 patients, respectively, after 5 years of follow-up [29]. Chiller et al. reported a mean of 2.6 stages to clear MAC via MMS [6]. Occasionally, resection with appropriate margin control is not possible due to size or location of the primary tumor [56, 57].

Nodal Management

Fine needle aspiration or lymphadenectomy may be performed for clinically suspicious enlarged lymph nodes [58]. There is insufficient evidence to suggest sentinel lymph node biopsy (SLNB) should be routinely performed in MAC [59], although there are rare reports of SLNB positivity in the literature [60].

Radiation and Chemotherapy

In rare cases, radiotherapy has been employed as both primary [61, 62] and adjuvant therapy [63]. Dosage and modality in these cases have been heterogeneous and results have been mixed. In some cases, there has been concern that radiation may have led to the onset of more aggressive disease [62, 64]. Much of the data on the use of radiotherapy is further limited by short follow-up times [63]. Baxi et al. reported on the use of wide local excision followed by radiation for MAC in a range of doses and modalities in a retrospective cohort of 16 patients, 11 of whom had positive margins after standard excision [63]. In this cohort, a 93% success rate was reported after a median of 5 years of follow-up, although post hoc confirmatory testing was not used. Radiation may be considered in non-resectable cases of MAC and in patients for whom surgery is not an option due to the morbidity of the procedure itself or underlying medical condition. Chemotherapy is not an accepted treatment modality for MAC.

Sebaceous Carcinoma

Introduction

Sebaceous carcinoma (SC) is a rare cutaneous neoplasm differentiated from holocrine sebocytes that favors sebaceous gland-rich sites on the head and neck. It is among the most common tumors of the eyelid [65]. SC has a propensity for locally aggressive behavior and can metastasize and contribute to mortality [66]. Delay in diagnosis is common both clinically and histologically [67]. Previously, the literature describing these tumors employed a heterogeneous terminology including sebaceous gland carcinoma, sebaceous cell carcinoma, and meibomian gland carcinoma, but SC is now generally accepted [65, 68]. SC is among the cutaneous neoplasms that are associated with Muir-Torre syndrome (MTS) [69, 70], an autosomal dominant genodermatosis characterized by elevated risk for visceral malignancies.

Traditional teaching held that extraocular SC is associated with a more favorable prognosis [71, 72]. However, Tripathi et al. recently demonstrated male sex, black race, and extraocular location are associated with higher mortality rates. There are likely differences in the etiology and the significance of SC as it pertains to periocular and extraocular location [70]. Surgery is the treatment of choice for SC, although, like MAC, standard excision has been associated with significant rates of recurrence [68]. MMS and surgical techniques that aim for complete histologic margin control are emerging as highly effective treatment options [73]. Radiation and chemotherapy are employed in select circumstances [68].

Epidemiology

SC is rare – the overall incidence is 2.3 cases per 1,000,000 person-years – but the incidence has increased significantly from 2000 to 2012 [66]. SC represents 1–5.5% of eyelid tumors in the United States [71, 74]. There is disagreement as to the proportion of SC among eyelid tumors in the United States, with reports of it being the second to fourth most common [71, 75–78]. BCC makes up the vast majority [71, 79–82], accounting for over 90% of eyelid tumors in one study [83].

Gender predilection data is conflicting in SC. Several recent analyses suggest males are more likely to develop SC than females [66, 84, 85], a departure from a previous reports that SC displays a female predominance [71, 79, 86–88]. It has been postulated that periocular SC is gender neutral, while extraocular SC is predominated by male patients [70].

SC is primarily a disease of advanced age, with nearly eight of ten of patients above the age of 60 and a mean age of onset at 73 years [66, 84]. Early onset (prior to the age of 40) has been reported, largely in patients with hereditary retinoblastoma who have received radiation [65, 89]. A patient as young as 8 years old with SC and hereditary retinoblastoma has been described [90].

White patients are disproportionately affected, comprising 84–86% of patients, with incidence rates of 2.0–2.3 cases per 1,000,000 person-years [66, 84], relative to 1.07 and 0.48 cases per 1,000,000 person-years for Asian and Black patients, respectively [66]. The former is of particular interest as historical data suggests that patients of Asian heritage may be more likely to develop SC than Caucasians [68, 80, 91]. While absolute rates appear lower than in Caucasians, SC appears to represent a disproportionate number of eyelid cancers among Asians. Of 512 eyelid tumors reported in a Chinese population, nearly 33% were SC [80].

Pathogenesis

Sebaceous glands are found throughout the body, typically in association with hair follicles. Around the eye, sebaceous glands are found in five locations: tarsal Meibomian glands, glands of Zeis, eyebrow and eyelid pilosebaceous units, and the caruncle [71]. SC commonly arises from tarsal Meibomian glands [74], but can arise from any location where sebaceous glands are found; SC may also be multifocal in origin [79, 82]. Once malignant transformation is underway, SC demonstrates a propensity for pagetoid, or superficial, extension [65, 82].

The role of UV radiation in SC is not established. Multiple studies failed to document UV signature mutations in p53 that are common in other nonmelanoma skin cancers (NMSC) [92, 93].

The role of p53 dysfunction in the development of SC, however, is accepted [94]. The prevalence of mutated p53 in SC is among the highest seen in human carcinomas [92]. The strong association between p53 and SC – especially periocular SC – as compared to other benign sebaceous neoplasms has been demonstrated [95]. Mutations in p53 may be associated with more aggressive behavior [96]. HPV does not seem to play a significant role in the development of SC [94, 97, 98]. HER2 overexpression [99] and CDKN2A hypermethylation have been associated with SC [100].

Other associations with SC include immune suppression [70, 101, 102], HIV [103], history of radiation [104–106], occurrence in nevus sebaceous [107], and history of hereditary retinoblastoma [90, 108–110], including among patients with hereditary retinoblastoma who have not received radiation [90].

Muir-Torre Syndrome

SC may occur sporadically but is often observed in patients with Muir-Torre syndrome (MTS). Recognized as a variant of hereditary nonpolyposis colon cancer (HNPCC) or Lynch syndrome, MTS is associated with mutations in mismatch repair (MMR) genes involved in DNA replication and repair [111]. MTS is associated with sebaceous neoplasms, cutaneous squamous cell carcinomas, keratoacanthomas, and visceral malignancies [70, 111–113]. As in other hereditary cancer syndromes, the MMR mutations are typically inherited as heterozygous germline mutations [114]. A second somatic event occurs in the normal allele, leading to protein loss and MMR errors. Without accurate DNA repair, normal errors in replication and some forms of DNA damage accumulate. Microsatellites, short tandem repeats found throughout the genome, are particularly prone to mutation. In the setting of MMR deficiency, these mutations accumulate and can be detected as microsatellite instability (MSI) [115]. Mutations in oncogenic proteins arise, and the malignant process is initiated. Mutations in MTS may be documented in MSH2, MSH6, MLH1, and PMS2, with MSH2/MSH6 mutations most common [114].

Patients with MTS develop, in order of decreasing frequency, sebaceous adenomas (68%), carcinomas (30%), and epitheliomas (27%) [116]. Keratoacanthomas and other NMSC may display sebaceous differentiation in patients with MTS [111]. Sebaceous hyperplasia does not appear related to MTS [117]. Cutaneous manifestations of MTS have been reported to be the earliest manifestation of the syndrome in 22% of patients [118, 119]. Current diagnostic criteria for MTS include at least one documented sebaceous neoplasm and at least one internal malignancy or multiple keratoacanthomas, multiple internal malignancies, and a family history of MTS [111, 120].

Clinical Features

The clinical appearance of SC is polymorphic, which may contribute to misdiagnosis and delay in diagnosis [65, 71]. It may have both nodular and pseudo-inflammatory presentations [65]. The classical finding is a firm subcutaneous nodule, typically less than 2 centimeters in size [121], on the eyelid with a yellow, lipidized appearance (Fig. 10.6) [65, 71, 74, 87]. Lesions may take on a pink or red hue and demonstrate telangiectatic vessels (Fig. 10.7) [122]. Overlying ulceration or skin breakdown may occur. The upper eyelid is affected two to three times more commonly than the lower [72, 79, 121], presumably due to the higher density of Meibomian glands on the upper lid. Both lids, however, may be affected [121]. A significant percentage of patients may have concomitant conjunctival or even corneal surface change [121]. The less common pseudo-inflammatory, or spreading, presentation may be even more insidious: the eyelid thickens diffusely and may take on a multinodular or yellow appearance, and the eyelids may be lost [65]. Involvement of the conjunctiva, cornea, and opposing lid may be seen [65, 82].

SC may be subdivided into periocular and extraocular variants, with the former traditionally believed to comprise 75% of cases [71, 87, 123]. Recent analyses have cast this breakdown of site presentation into question, with periocular sites ranging from 26 to 39% of cases [66, 84]. Of the extraocular tumors in one analysis, 93% presented on the head and neck [66]. Outside of the head and neck, the trunk is the next most common location for presentation [124].

The clinical behavior of SC is aggressive, with a capacity for local invasion, as well as metastasis to lymph nodes and internal organs [65]. Periocular SC can be locally invasive, infiltrating adjacent cutaneous epithelium, adjacent ocular epithelium, the lacrimal system, orbital soft tissue, and paranasal sinuses, and, rarely, may spread intracranially [65, 125]. Orbital invasion occurs in 6–17% of patients [88]. SC also displays true metastatic potential. In 1989 a nodal metastatic rate in periocular SC of 17–28% was reported [125]; a more recent report demonstrated a nodal metastatic rate of 8%, with preauricular nodes most commonly involved [126]. In a small Taiwanese series, a 16% rate of metastasis at 5 years was recorded [127]. When metastatic beyond lymphatics, SC tends to spread to the lung, liver, bone, and brain [88, 127, 128].

Fig. 10.6 Clinical photo of SC of the lower eyelid, #1. Sub-centimeter pink-yellow papule on the lower eyelid with focal eyelid hyperemia and edema (Courtesy of Vikram Durairaj, MD)

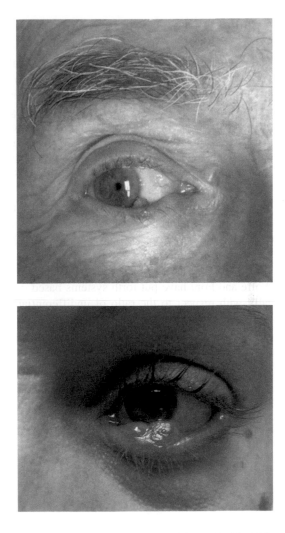

Fig. 10.7 Clinical photo of SC of the lower eyelid, #2. Pearly, telangiectatic multinodular plaque on the lower eyelid with diffuse surrounding eyelid hyperemia and edema (Courtesy of Vikram Durairaj, MD)

Reported historical mortality rates for SC range from 3% to 30% [79, 80, 121, 129, 130], with many older studies associated with higher mortality rates. More recently, a 10-year overall relative survival rate of 87% was reported, a rate that falls to 65% when regional metastatic disease is present [66]. Traditionally, periocular SC was felt to be more aggressive [79, 131–133]; however, a recent large analysis demonstrated a significantly lower rate of survival in extraocular cases of SC than in periocular [66].

Pathology

The histologic diagnosis of SC is particularly challenging, and rates of initial histologic misdiagnosis of SC are high, ranging from 40% to 75% [65]. Tumor characteristics depend strongly on the level of differentiation. The tumor is predominantly dermally based but may appear invasive, forming cords and trabeculae [87]. Well-differentiated tumors will attempt to recapitulate the sebaceous lobule (Fig. 10.8) [87]. To varying degrees, vacuolated, lipid-containing sebocytes with foamy cytoplasm are located centrally; these cells tend to have angulated or "scalloped" nuclei and will react positively with staining for lipid (Fig. 10.9) [87, 134]. Recognition of these cells is central to the diagnosis of SC [75]. Undifferentiated basaloid "germinative" cells are found peripherally [87] and may predominate, becoming hyperchromatic, pleomorphic, and mitotically active [134], obfuscating to varying degrees centrally located sebocytes (Fig. 10.10). SC may demonstrate squamous and basal cell differentiation [87].

A variety of histologic classification systems exist for SC [71, 79, 80, 86, 135]. Wolfe and Font have put forth systems based on degree of differentiation, specifically with respect to the ratio of undifferentiated germinative cells to sebaceous cells [86, 135], while Rao and Ni classify these tumors according to their growth pattern [79, 80]. Poorly differentiated tumors appear to be associated with a higher risk of metastasis and worse prognosis [79, 121, 136].

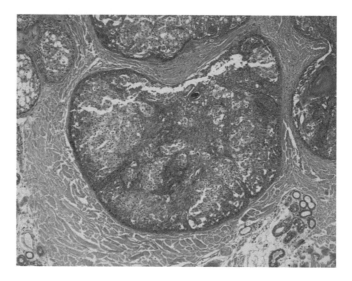

Fig. 10.8 Recapitulation of the sebaceous lobule with peripheral basaloid germinative cells and centrally located vacuolated sebocytes in a moderately differentiated SC, 10× (Courtesy of Anthony C. Soldano, MD)

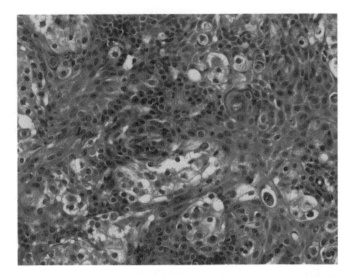

Fig. 10.9 Identification of these vacuolated, lipid-containing sebocytes with angulated or "scalloped" nuclei and foamy cytoplasm are critical for diagnosis of SC, 40× (Courtesy of Anthony C. Soldano, MD)

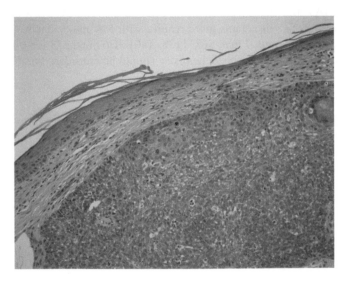

Fig. 10.10 Proliferation of basaloid germinative cells without apparent sebocytes in poorly differentiated SC demonstrating marked nuclear pleomorphism and increased mitotic activity, 20× (Courtesy of Anthony C. Soldano, MD)

In high-grade or poorly differentiated SC, vacuolated sebocytes may be rare, necrosis may be present, and stroma may be desmoplastic [36]. High-grade tumors also will demonstrate intraepithelial, or "pagetoid," spread and may be reminiscent histologically of either extramammary Paget's or Bowen's disease [75, 87]. This high-grade feature is present in approximately half of cases of SC [126] and may delay correct diagnosis due to its similarity with other cutaneous tumors. The disease's capacity for local superficial extension, including onto the conjunctival epithelium, may be attributed to this tendency for intraepithelial spread [71].

The histologic differential diagnosis of SC is myriad and includes other sebaceous neoplasms including sebaceous adenoma and sebaceous epithelioma, as well as BCC with sebaceous differentiation [68]. When pagetoid spread is present, SCC, extramammary Paget's, melanoma, and conjunctival carcinoma in situ must be considered [71, 137]. The vacuolated cells that are seen in SC also may evoke a differential diagnosis that includes entities with clear cells or clear cell change, such as clear cell SCC or BCC, eccrine carcinoma, and metastatic clear cell sarcoma, and clear cell carcinoma of the kidney and thyroid [36]. The differentiation from BCC, especially BCC with sebaceous differentiation, may be especially problematic. SC is typically more pleomorphic and mitotically active [75], and BCC does not demonstrate pagetoid spread [36].

Especially as poorly differentiated SC may lack apparent vacuolated sebocytes altogether, immunohistochemistry may be helpful in differentiating SC from other neoplastic conditions. While lipid detecting Oil Red O and Sudan stain may aid in elucidating sebaceous differentiation, the use of this technique is limited by the need for fresh tissue [71]. EMA and Ber-EP4 may help differentiate SC from BCC and SCC (Figs. 10.11 and 10.12), with the following immunohistochemical profiles: SC (EMA+, Ber-EP4 +), SCC (EMA+, Ber-EP4 -), and BCC (EMA-, Ber-EP4 +) [36, 138–140]. SC also stains more readily with low molecular weight keratin (CAM5.2) and cytokeratin 7 than SCC [138, 140]. Ki67 and p53 are often overexpressed [68]. Finally, immunohistochemistry should be considered in the setting of

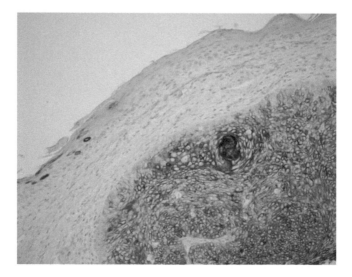

Fig. 10.11 Poorly differentiated SC showing positive staining for EMA, 20× (Courtesy of Anthony C. Soldano, MD)

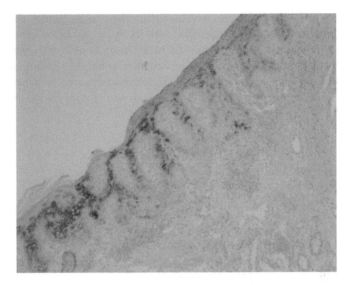

Fig. 10.12 EMA highlights the overlying intraepithelial (in situ) component seen above the tumor in Fig. 10, 20× (Courtesy of Anthony C. Soldano, MD)

SC to screen for patients at risk for MTS; the loss of MLH1 or MSH2 is particularly indicative [36, 111].

Differential Diagnosis

The clinical presentation of SC is varied and may mimic a number of other entities, both inflammatory and neoplastic [65]. In a series of 43 patients referred to specialty care with SC, the initial favored clinical diagnosis was correct in only 19% of patients [121]. Of inflammatory disorders, SC must be differentiated from chalazion, blepharitis, conjunctivitis, keratoconjunctivitis, and cicatricial pemphigoid [65, 126]. Especially challenging is the fact that SC will often induce an inflammatory state in the conjunctiva and eyelid and may even extend locally onto the conjunctiva via pagetoid growth [65]. Most inflammatory conditions will be bilateral in nature and will not cause loss of eyelid cilia as with SC. Chalazion, however, is often unilateral and particularly problematic for clinicians seeking to differentiate from SC [65, 77, 126]; in fact, 44% of misdiagnoses in one series ultimately confirmed as SC were originally diagnosed clinically as chalazion [121].

SC – especially the nodular variant – must also be differentiated from other neoplasms, such as BCC, SCC, conjunctival intraepithelial carcinoma, amelanotic melanoma, Merkel cell carcinoma, lymphoma, and other adnexal tumors [65]. Location may serve as a clue. While neoplasms strongly associated with sun exposure will typically occur on the lower eyelid, SC has a predilection for the upper eyelid. BCC will often be pink or pearly in color with a characteristic rolled border and will most often occur on the lower eyelid [65]. SCC will likely occur on the lower eyelid as well and will be marked by hyperkeratosis in the context of heavily sun-damaged skin [76]. Amelanotic melanoma, Merkel cell carcinoma, and lymphoma tend to lack the yellow hue of a sebaceous tumor [65]. Dermoscopy may be a useful clinical adjunct and with SC will often show polymorphous neovascularization and a yellow background [78].

Evaluation and Treatment

Muir-Torre Syndrome

A diagnosis of SC, as with any sebaceous neoplasm, should arouse suspicion for MTS. A detailed personal and family malignancy history should be obtained, and immunohistochemistry for MMR gene products should be considered [111, 134]. MSH2 mutations in particular appear to be tightly correlated to MTS, with an incidence of 61–93% [119]. The combination of the loss of MLH1 and MSH6, as well as MLH1, MSH2, and MSH6, has a positive predictive value for diagnosis of MTS of 100% [111]. These mutations are not found in sporadic SC [141]. When loss of MMR gene products is found, polymerase chain reaction testing for microsatellite instability (MSI) may then be considered [111]. It is important to note, however, that the loss of MMR gene products and positive testing for MSI does not confirm a diagnosis of MTS. A diagnosis requires a documented sebaceous neoplasm (with or without loss of MMR) and at least one internal malignancy or multiple keratoacanthomas, multiple internal malignancies, and a family history of MTS [111, 118]. Interestingly, SC associated with MTS tends to be less aggressive than those with sporadic occurrence [113, 142].

The diagnosis of SC should prompt a systemic evaluation for malignancy associated with MTS, beginning with a detailed history, physical exam, and review of systems. Many recommendations regarding screening in MTS are based on those developed for patients with HNPCC [69]. Investigation with upper and lower endoscopy in addition to genitourinary tract surveillance has been recommended [111], as has CT of the abdomen and pelvis on 2–5-year intervals [69]. Additional testing with urine cytology, carcinoembryonic antigen levels, cervical smear, chest radiography, mammography, and endometrial biopsy may also be undertaken [116]. Routine annual dermatologic exams are critical [69] (Fig. 10.13).

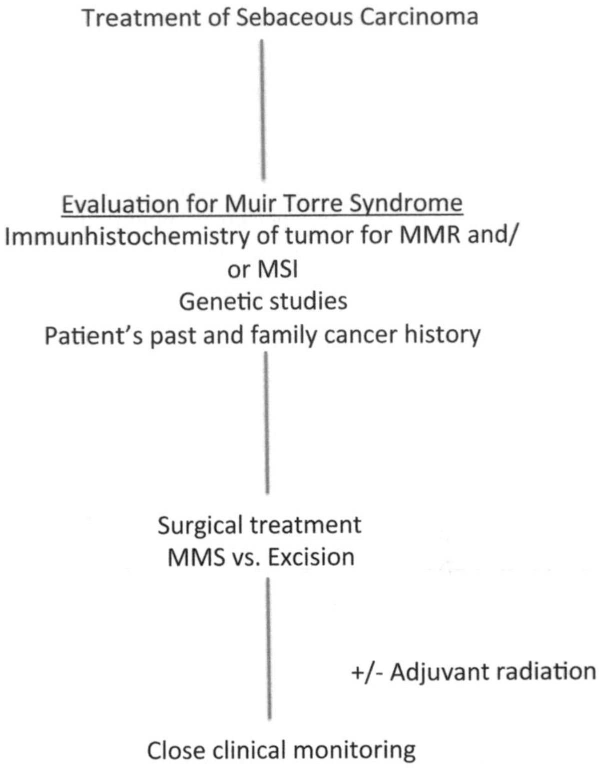

Fig. 10.13 Clinical
management of sebaceous
carcinoma

Treatment of Sebaceous Carcinoma

Evaluation for Muir Torre Syndrome
Immunhistochemistry of tumor for MMR and/
or MSI
Genetic studies
Patient's past and family cancer history

Surgical treatment
MMS vs. Excision

+/- Adjuvant radiation

Close clinical monitoring

Staging

Staging for SC is divergent according to whether the lesion arises in the periocular or extraocular skin. Periocular SC is staged according to the AJCC TNM classification for eyelid carcinoma [143], while SC of extraocular skin is typically staged within the AJCC TNM classification for cutaneous carcinoma [133, 144]. Staging for periocular SC differs from extraocular SC in its specificity for eye-specific structures, such as the tarsal plate and eyelid margin, as well as the type of treatment involved in clearing the tumor, whether it be enucleation, exenteration, or bone resection [68]. Cutaneous carcinoma staging depends primarily on size, the presence of certain high-risk features, and invasion into underlying bony structures (68). The orbital carcinoma TNM classification has been validated in retrospective studies in SC, with increasing T stage positively correlated with nodal metastasis and poor patient outcome [143]. Higher T stage may be used to distinguish periocular SC patients at risk for nodal metastasis and in need of SLNB [143].

Imaging and Nodal Management

Owing to the relative rarity of the tumor, there are no clear guidelines regarding the use of imaging in the initial management of a patient with SC [68, 133]. Recommendations are sparse, generally limited to commentary provided by clinicians with expertise treating SC. Radiologic staging may be employed for tumor with aggressive features or when concerning findings are noted upon physical exam or review of systems, such as palpable lymphadenopathy or symptoms concerning for disseminated disease [68]. As lymph nodes are the most common initial site of metastatic disease [126], imaging is typically directed to draining regional lymph node basins. Ultrasound or CT of regional lymph nodes at diagnosis and in follow-up for patients with high-risk features has been recommended [136].

There are limited reports supporting the use of MRI as well as 18F–fluorodeoxy-glucose positron emission tomography (PET) to detect locoregional disease and to direct further therapy [145–147]. In a retrospective study of PET/CT in periocular malignancies, of which 40% were SC, PET/CT was significantly more sensitive than CT for detection of lymph node metastases [148]. This may have been due to a significant number of false negatives with CT when imaging soft tissues of the neck [148]. In one report, imaging with PET/CT changed the plan of care for half of patients under study [148].

Lymph nodes are the most common site of metastatic involvement in SC, and reported rates of nodal metastases, including to the parotid gland, in periocular tumors range from 8 to 33% [88, 126, 130, 149, 150]. Rates of nodal metastasis among patients with extraocular SC range from 0% to as high as 21% [150, 151]. One large analysis reported rates of regional metastasis to be higher in periocular SC than extraocular SC [152].

Certain factors have been shown to increase the risk of lymph node involvement, such as AJCC TNM staging T2b or higher, as well as poor differentiation on histology [143, 152]. Nevertheless, reports of SLNB positivity in SC are rare, and the role of SLNB in SC, particularly in extraocular SC, is unclear [153–155]. In a series of ten patients with periocular SC who underwent SLNB, two false negatives were reported, while a third patient developed distant metastasis without lymph node involvement [153].

Nevertheless, the detection of metastatic tumor in regional lymph nodes may provide prognostic and staging information. When suspicious lymph nodes are discovered clinically or with imaging, fine needle aspiration may be performed [156]. Lymph node metastasis is treated with dissection and/or radiotherapy (see below) [88, 157].

Surgical Treatment

Surgical resection is the standard of care for management of SC, but its effectiveness is limited by the tendency of SC to recur. Wide local excision (WLE), with permanent or frozen sections for margin control, is often employed, with margins typically consisting of 5–6 mm of healthy tissue [158–161]. Recurrence rates with WLE range from 4% to 37% [68, 80, 87], with a median rate of 21% [68]; however, these data are limited by generally small series and disproportionate representation of periocular SC. When recurrences do occur, they typically do so within 5 years [71].

There is intrinsic appeal to the use of a tissue-conserving technique such as MMS in a disease with a propensity to affect the periocular skin. While much of the data on MMS for SC is favorable compared with WLE, most studies are in general retrospective and non-randomized. Recurrence rates of 11% in patients with SC treated with MMS have been reported, with nodal metastatic rates of 6–8% [73, 158, 162]. Recently, a retrospective single-institution series of 37 patients treated with MMS demonstrated zero recurrences with an average follow-up of 3.6 years [73]. In a rare study providing a head-to-head single institutional comparison between WLE and MMS, no significant difference in the rate of recurrence between the two modalities was observed [124].

There are features unique to SC that make successful resection via MMS a challenge. Some authors caution against reliance on frozen section margins in a disease with a high propensity for pagetoid spread [67] [162]. Furthermore, MMS relies upon contiguous tumor growth, and SC may show multicentric origin and skip lesions [163].

Radiation

The role of radiotherapy in SC has been limited primarily to patients who cannot tolerate surgery, for whom comorbid procedures such as exenteration are unacceptable [150] or in the adjuvant setting for high-risk or metastatic disease [156]. Historically, SC was viewed as a radioresistant process, and earlier studies reported significant treatment failures when radiotherapy was employed as a primary modality [164, 165]. However, low total radiation doses may be to blame for these treatment failures [166, 167]. In a recent series of 13 patients with periocular SC treated with radiotherapy (an average of 60 Gy total dose), 5 of whom were treated with RT as definitive therapy, 5-year progression-free and disease-free survival rates of 100% and 89%, respectively, were reported [166].

Radiotherapy has been employed in the adjuvant setting with modest success. Pardo et al. reported no evidence of disease in 2–7 years of follow-up in six patients with locally metastatic periocular SC treated with postoperative adjuvant radiotherapy to the ipsilateral parotid bed and lymph node basins [168]. While most patients who receive radiotherapy to the orbit develop conjunctivitis or keratitis, overall treatment tends to be well tolerated [166].

Ultimately, surgical resection is the mainstay of treatment for SC. Radiation is typically employed as definitive treatment only for select patients who are unable to undergo excision. There may be a role for adjuvant radiotherapy for high-risk tumors. More data is needed to better define the role of radiotherapy in this rare skin cancer.

Chemotherapy

Chemotherapy has been employed in metastatic SC in neoadjuvant, adjuvant, or palliative roles, but no consensus exists as to its use. Most of the knowledge about the use of chemotherapy in SC is limited to a few case reports [169]. A variety of regimens have been reported, most of them including the dipyrimidine 5-fluorouracil [169–174], along with cisplatin, carboplatin, and doxorubicin, among others. Complete and partial responses to these regimens have been reported, although clinical scenarios and time to follow-up are heterogeneous.

References

1. Goldstein DJ, Barr RJ, Santa Cruz DJ. Microcystic adnexal carcinoma: a distinct clinico-pathologic entity. Cancer. 1982;50(3):566–72.
2. Pujol RM, LeBoit PE, Su WP. Microcystic adnexal carcinoma with extensive sebaceous differentiation. Am J Dermatopathol. 1997;19(4):358–62.
3. Nickoloff BJ, Fleischmann HE, Carmel J, Wood CC, Roth RJ. Microcystic adnexal carcinoma. Immunohistologic observations suggesting dual (pilar and eccrine) differentiation. Arch Dermatol. 1986;122(3):290–4.
4. Boos MD, Elenitsas R, Seykora J, Lehrer MS, Miller CJ, Sobanko J. Benign subclinical syringomatous proliferations adjacent to a microcystic adnexal carcinoma: a tumor mimic with significant patient implications. Am J Dermatopathol. 2014;36(2):174–8.
5. Cardoso JC, Calonje E. Malignant sweat gland tumours: an update. Histopathology. 2015;67(5):589–606.
6. Chiller K, Passaro D, Scheuller M, Singer M, McCalmont T, Grekin RC. Microcystic adnexal carcinoma: forty-eight cases, their treatment, and their outcome. Arch Dermatol. 2000;136(11):1355–9.
7. Yu JB, Blitzblau RC, Patel SC, Decker RH, Wilson LD. Surveillance, Epidemiology, and End Results (SEER) database analysis of microcystic adnexal carcinoma (sclerosing sweat duct carcinoma) of the skin. Am J Clin Oncol. 2010;33(2):125–7.
8. Diamantis SA, Marks VJ. Mohs micrographic surgery in the treatment of microcystic adnexal carcinoma. Dermatol Clin. 2011;29(2):185–90. viii.
9. Fu T, Clark FL, Lorenz HP, Bruckner AL. Congenital microcystic adnexal carcinoma. Arch Dermatol. 2011;147(2):256–7.
10. Peterson CM, Ratz JL, Sangueza OP. Microcystic adnexal carcinoma: first reported case in an African American man. J Am Acad Dermatol. 2001;45(2):283–5.

11. Nadiminti H, Nadiminti U, Washington C. Microcystic adnexal carcinoma in African-Americans. Dermatol Surg. 2007;33(11):1384–7.
12. Ohtsuka H, Nagamatsu S. Microcystic adnexal carcinoma: review of 51 Japanese patients. Dermatology. 2002;204(3):190–3.
13. Chen J, Yang S, Liao T, Deng W, Li W. Microcystic adnexal carcinoma in a non-Caucasian patient: a case report and review of the literature. Oncol Lett. 2016;11(4):2471–4.
14. Tolkachjov SN, Schmitt AR, Muzic JG, Weaver AL, Baum CL. Incidence and clinical features of rare cutaneous malignancies in Olmsted County, Minnesota, 2000 to 2010. Dermatol Surg. 2017;43(1):116–24.
15. Wick MR, Cooper PH, Swanson PE, Kaye VN, Sun TT. Microcystic adnexal carcinoma. An immunohistochemical comparison with other cutaneous appendage tumors. Arch Dermatol. 1990;126(2):189–94.
16. Avraham JB, Villines D, Maker VK, August C, Maker AV. Survival after resection of cutaneous adnexal carcinomas with eccrine differentiation: risk factors and trends in outcomes. J Surg Oncol. 2013;108(1):57–62.
17. LeBoit PE, Sexton M. Microcystic adnexal carcinoma of the skin. A reappraisal of the differentiation and differential diagnosis of an underrecognized neoplasm. J Am Acad Dermatol. 1993;29(4):609–18.
18. Snow S, Madjar DD, Hardy S, Bentz M, Lucarelli MJ, Bechard R, et al. Microcystic adnexal carcinoma: report of 13 cases and review of the literature. Dermatol Surg. 2001;27(4):401–8.
19. Carroll P, Goldstein GD, Brown CW. Metastatic microcystic adnexal carcinoma in an immunocompromised patient. Dermatol Surg. 2000;26(6):531–4.
20. Smith KJ, Williams J, Corbett D, Skelton H. Microcystic adnexal carcinoma: an immunohistochemical study including markers of proliferation and apoptosis. Am J Surg Pathol. 2001;25(4):464–71.
21. Wohlfahrt C, Ternesten A, Sahlin P, Islam Q, Stenman G. Cytogenetic and fluorescence in situ hybridization analyses of a microcystic adnexal carcinoma with del(6)(q23q25). Cancer Genet Cytogenet. 1997;98(2):106–10.
22. Kishi M, Nakamura M, Nishimine M, Ishida E, Shimada K, Kirita T, et al. Loss of heterozygosity on chromosome 6q correlates with decreased thrombospondin-2 expression in human salivary gland carcinomas. Cancer Sci. 2003;94(6):530–5.
23. Dupré A, Carrère S, Bonafé JL, Christol B, Lassère J, Touron P. Eruptive generalized syringomas, milium and atrophoderma vermiculata. Nicolau and Balus' syndrome (author's transl). Dermatologica. 1981;162(4):281–6.
24. Ranasinghe AR, Batchelor J, Ha T. Nicolau Balus syndrome with microcystic adnexal carcinoma. J Am Acad Dermatol. 2013;68(4):AB56.
25. Schaller J, Rytina E, Rütten A, Hendricks C, Ha T, Requena L. Sweat duct proliferation associated with aggregates of elastic tissue and atrophodermia vermiculata: a simulator of microcystic adnexal carcinoma. Report of two cases. J Cutan Pathol. 2010;37(9):1002–9.
26. Page RN, Hanggi MC, King R, Googe PB. Multiple microcystic adnexal carcinomas. Cutis. 2007;79(4):299–303.
27. Leibovitch I, Huilgol SC, Selva D, Lun K, Richards S, Paver R. Microcystic adnexal carcinoma: treatment with Mohs micrographic surgery. J Am Acad Dermatol. 2005;52(2):295–300.
28. Connolly KL, Nehal KS, Disa JJ. Evidence-based medicine: cutaneous facial malignancies: nonmelanoma skin cancer. Plast Reconstr Surg. 2017;139(1):181e–90e.
29. Friedman PM, Friedman RH, Jiang SB, Nouri K, Amonette R, Robins P. Microcystic adnexal carcinoma: collaborative series review and update. J Am Acad Dermatol. 1999;41(2 Pt 1):225–31.
30. Yugueros P, Kane WJ, Goellner JR. Sweat gland carcinoma: a clinicopathologic analysis of an expanded series in a single institution. Plast Reconstr Surg. 1998;102(3):705–10.
31. Obaidat NA, Alsaad KO, Ghazarian D. Skin adnexal neoplasms--part 2: an approach to tumours of cutaneous sweat glands. J Clin Pathol. 2007;60(2):145–59.

32. Sellheyer K, Nelson P, Kutzner H, Patel RM. The immunohistochemical differential diagnosis of microcystic adnexal carcinoma, desmoplastic trichoepithelioma and morpheaform basal cell carcinoma using BerEP4 and stem cell markers. J Cutan Pathol. 2013;40(4):363–70.
33. Fu JM, McCalmont T, Yu SS. Adenosquamous carcinoma of the skin: a case series. Arch Dermatol. 2009;145(10):1152–8.
34. Frouin E, Vignon-Pennamen MD, Balme B, Cavelier-Balloy B, Zimmermann U, Ortonne N, et al. Anatomoclinical study of 30 cases of sclerosing sweat duct carcinomas (microcystic adnexal carcinoma, syringomatous carcinoma and squamoid eccrine ductal carcinoma). J Eur Acad Dermatol Venereol. 2015;29(10):1978–94.
35. Sebastien TS, Nelson BR, Lowe L, Baker S, Johnson TM. Microcystic adnexal carcinoma. J Am Acad Dermatol. 1993;29(5 Pt 2):840–5.
36. Crowson AN, Magro CM, Mihm MC. Malignant adnexal neoplasms. Mod Pathol. 2006;19(Suppl 2):S93–S126.
37. Urso C, Bondi R, Paglierani M, Salvadori A, Anichini C, Giannini A. Carcinomas of sweat glands: report of 60 cases. Arch Pathol Lab Med. 2001;125(4):498–505.
38. Merritt BG, Snow SN, Longley BJ. Desmoplastic trichoepithelioma, infiltrative/morpheaform BCC, and microcystic adnexal carcinoma: differentiation by immunohistochemistry and determining the need for Mohs micrographic surgery. Cutis. 2010;85(5):254–8.
39. Costache M, Bresch M, Böer A. Desmoplastic trichoepithelioma versus morpheic basal cell carcinoma: a critical reappraisal of histomorphological and immunohistochemical criteria for differentiation. Histopathology. 2008;52(7):865–76.
40. Shinohara R, Ansai S, Ogita A, Matsuda H, Saeki H, Tanaka M. Dermoscopic findings of microcystic adnexal carcinoma. Eur J Dermatol. 2015;25(5):516–8.
41. Hoang MP, Dresser KA, Kapur P, High WA, Mahalingam M. Microcystic adnexal carcinoma: an immunohistochemical reappraisal. Mod Pathol. 2008;21(2):178–85.
42. Nagatsuka H, Rivera RS, Gunduz M, Siar CH, Tamamura R, Mizukawa N, et al. Microcystic adnexal carcinoma with mandibular bone marrow involvement: a case report with immunohistochemistry. Am J Dermatopathol. 2006;28(6):518–22.
43. Krahl D, Sellheyer K. Monoclonal antibody Ber-EP4 reliably discriminates between microcystic adnexal carcinoma and basal cell carcinoma. J Cutan Pathol. 2007;34(10):782–7.
44. Abesamis-Cubillan E, El-Shabrawi-Caelen L, PE LB. Merked cells and sclerosing epithelial neoplasms. Am J Dermatopathol. 2000;22(4):311–5.
45. Patrizi A, Neri I, Marzaduri S, Varotti E, Passarini B. Syringoma: a review of twenty-nine cases. Acta Derm Venereol. 1998;78(6):460–2.
46. Salasche SJ, Amonette RA. Morpheaform basal-cell epitheliomas. A study of subclinical extensions in a series of 51 cases. J Dermatol Surg Oncol. 1981;7(5):387–94.
47. Alam M, Ratner D. Cutaneous squamous-cell carcinoma. N Engl J Med. 2001;344(13):975–83.
48. Wang Q, Ghimire D, Wang J, Luo S, Li Z, Wang H, et al. Desmoplastic trichoepithelioma: a clinicopathological study of three cases and a review of the literature. Oncol Lett. 2015;10(4):2468–76.
49. Popadić M. Dermoscopy of aggressive basal cell carcinomas. Indian J Dermatol Venereol Leprol. 2015;81(6):608–10.
50. Tawfik AM, Kreft A, Wagner W, Vogl TJ. MRI of a microcystic adnexal carcinoma of the skin mimicking a fibrous tumour: case report and literature review. Br J Radiol. 2011;84(1002):e114–7.
51. Gomez-Maestra MJ, España-Gregori E, Aviñó-Martinez JA, Mancheño-Franch N, Peña S. Brainstem and cavernous sinus metastases arising from a microcystic adnexal carcinoma of the eyebrow by perineural spreading. Can J Ophthalmol. 2009;44(3):e17–8.
52. Beltramini GA, Baj A, Moneghini L, Poli T, Combi VA, Giannì AB. Microcystic adnexal carcinoma of the centrofacial region: a case report. Acta Otorhinolaryngol Ital. 2010;30(4):213.
53. Cooper PH, Mills SE, Leonard DD, Santa Cruz DJ, Headington JT, Barr RJ, et al. Sclerosing sweat duct (syringomatous) carcinoma. Am J Surg Pathol. 1985;9(6):422–33.

54. Abbate M, Zeitouni NC, Seyler M, Hicks W, Loree T, Cheney RT. Clinical course, risk factors, and treatment of microcystic adnexal carcinoma: a short series report. Dermatol Surg. 2003;29(10):1035–8.
55. Palamaras I, McKenna JD, Robson A, Barlow RJ. Microcystic adnexal carcinoma: a case series treated with mohs micrographic surgery and identification of patients in whom paraffin sections may be preferable. Dermatol Surg. 2010;36(4):446–52.
56. Lopez M, Cole EL. Microcystic adnexal carcinoma: reconstruction of a large centrofacial defect. Plast Reconstr Surg Glob Open. 2014;2(11):e254.
57. Eisen DB, Zloty D. Microcystic adnexal carcinoma involving a large portion of the face: when is surgery not reasonable? Dermatol Surg. 2005;31(11 Pt 1):1472–7. discussion 8.
58. Rotter N, Wagner H, Fuchshuber S, Issing WJ. Cervical metastases of microcystic adnexal carcinoma in an otherwise healthy woman. Eur Arch Otorhinolaryngol. 2003;260(5):254–7.
59. Green M, Mitchum M, Marquart J, Bowden LP, Bingham J. Microcystic adnexal carcinoma in the axilla of an 18-year-old woman. Pediatr Dermatol. 2014;31(6):e145–8.
60. Ban M, Sugie S, Kamiya H, Kitajima Y. Microcystic adnexal carcinoma with lymph node metastasis. Dermatology. 2003;207(4):395–7.
61. Gulmen S, Pullon PA. Sweat gland carcinoma of the lips. Oral Surg Oral Med Oral Pathol. 1976;41(5):643–9.
62. Stein JM, Ormsby A, Esclamado R, Bailin P. The effect of radiation therapy on microcystic adnexal carcinoma: a case report. Head Neck. 2003;25(3):251–4.
63. Baxi S, Deb S, Weedon D, Baumann K, Poulsen M. Microcystic adnexal carcinoma of the skin: the role of adjuvant radiotherapy. J Med Imaging Radiat Oncol. 2010;54(5):477–82.
64. Yuh WT, Engelken JD, Whitaker DC, Dolan KD. Bone marrow invasion of microcystic adnexal carcinoma. Ann Otol Rhinol Laryngol. 1991;100(7):601–3.
65. Shields JA, Demirci H, Marr BP, Eagle RC, Shields CL. Sebaceous carcinoma of the ocular region: a review. Surv Ophthalmol. 2005;50(2):103–22.
66. Tripathi R, Chen Z, Li L, Bordeaux JS. Incidence and survival of sebaceous carcinoma in the United States. J Am Acad Dermatol. 2016;75(6):1210–5.
67. Doxanas MT, Green WR. Sebaceous gland carcinoma. Review of 40 cases. Arch Ophthalmol. 1984;102(2):245–9.
68. Kyllo RL, Brady KL, Hurst EA. Sebaceous carcinoma: review of the literature. Dermatol Surg. 2015;41(1):1–15.
69. Ponti G, Ponz de Leon M. Muir-Torre syndrome. Lancet Oncol. 2005;6(12):980–7.
70. Dores GM, Curtis RE, Toro JR, Devesa SS, Fraumeni JF. Incidence of cutaneous sebaceous carcinoma and risk of associated neoplasms: insight into Muir-Torre syndrome. Cancer. 2008;113(12):3372–81.
71. Nelson BR, Hamlet KR, Gillard M, Railan D, Johnson TM. Sebaceous carcinoma. J Am Acad Dermatol. 1995;33(1):1–15. quiz 6-8.
72. Natarajan K, Rai R, Pillai SB. Extra ocular sebaceous carcinoma: a rare case report. Indian Dermatol Online J. 2011;2(2):91–3.
73. Brady KL, Hurst EA. Sebaceous carcinoma treated with Mohs micrographic surgery. Dermatol Surg. 2017;43(2):281–6.
74. Slutsky JB, Jones EC. Periocular cutaneous malignancies: a review of the literature. Dermatol Surg. 2012;38(4):552–69.
75. Pereira PR, Odashiro AN, Rodrigues-Reyes AA, Correa ZM, de Souza Filho JP, Burnier MN. Histopathological review of sebaceous carcinoma of the eyelid. J Cutan Pathol. 2005;32(7):496–501.
76. Reifler DM, Hornblass A. Squamous cell carcinoma of the eyelid. Surv Ophthalmol. 1986;30(6):349–65.
77. Nemoto Y, Arita R, Mizota A, Sasajima Y. Differentiation between chalazion and sebaceous carcinoma by noninvasive meibography. Clin Ophthalmol. 2014;8:1869–75.
78. Coates D, Bowling J, Haskett M. Dermoscopic features of extraocular sebaceous carcinoma. Australas J Dermatol. 2011;52(3):212–3.

79. Rao NA, Hidayat AA, McLean IW, Zimmerman LE. Sebaceous carcinomas of the ocular adnexa: a clinicopathologic study of 104 cases, with five-year follow-up data. Hum Pathol. 1982;13(2):113–22.
80. Ni C, Searl SS, Kuo PK, Chu FR, Chong CS, Albert DM. Sebaceous cell carcinomas of the ocular adnexa. Int Ophthalmol Clin. 1982;22(1):23–61.
81. Yin VT, Merritt HA, Sniegowski M, Esmaeli B. Eyelid and ocular surface carcinoma: diagnosis and management. Clin Dermatol. 2015;33(2):159–69.
82. Wali UK, Al-Mujaini A. Sebaceous gland carcinoma of the eyelid. Oman J Ophthalmol. 2010;3(3):117–21.
83. Cook BE, Bartley GB. Epidemiologic characteristics and clinical course of patients with malignant eyelid tumors in an incidence cohort in Olmsted County, Minnesota. Ophthalmology. 1999;106(4):746–50.
84. Dasgupta T, Wilson LD, Yu JB. A retrospective review of 1349 cases of sebaceous carcinoma. Cancer. 2009;115(1):158–65.
85. Blake PW, Bradford PT, Devesa SS, Toro JR. Cutaneous appendageal carcinoma incidence and survival patterns in the United States: a population-based study. Arch Dermatol. 2010;146(6):625–32.
86. Wolfe JT, Yeatts RP, Wick MR, Campbell RJ, Waller RR. Sebaceous carcinoma of the eyelid. Errors in clinical and pathologic diagnosis. Am J Surg Pathol. 1984;8(8):597–606.
87. Dowd MB, Kumar RJ, Sharma R, Murali R. Diagnosis and management of sebaceous carcinoma: an Australian experience. ANZ J Surg. 2008;78(3):158–63.
88. Kass LG, Hornblass A. Sebaceous carcinoma of the ocular adnexa. Surv Ophthalmol. 1989;33(6):477–90.
89. Sung D, Kaltreider SA, Gonzalez-Fernandez F. Early onset sebaceous carcinoma. Diagn Pathol. 2011;6:81.
90. Kivelä T, Asko-Seljavaara S, Pihkala U, Hovi L, Heikkonen J. Sebaceous carcinoma of the eyelid associated with retinoblastoma. Ophthalmology. 2001;108(6):1124–8.
91. Abdi U, Tyagi N, Maheshwari V, Gogi R, Tyagi SP. Tumours of eyelid: a clinicopathologic study. J Indian Med Assoc. 1996;94(11):405. -9, 16, 18.
92. Kiyosaki K, Nakada C, Hijiya N, Tsukamoto Y, Matsuura K, Nakatsuka K, et al. Analysis of p53 mutations and the expression of p53 and p21WAF1/CIP1 protein in 15 cases of sebaceous carcinoma of the eyelid. Invest Ophthalmol Vis Sci. 2010;51(1):7–11.
93. Hussain RM, Matthews JL, Dubovy SR, Thompson JM, Wang G. UV-independent p53 mutations in sebaceous carcinoma of the eyelid. Ophthal Plast Reconstr Surg. 2014;30(5):392–5.
94. Gonzalez-Fernandez F, Kaltreider SA, Patnaik BD, Retief JD, Bao Y, Newman S, et al. Sebaceous carcinoma. Tumor progression through mutational inactivation of p53. Ophthalmology. 1998;105(3):497–506.
95. Shalin SC, Sakharpe A, Lyle S, Lev D, Calonje E, Lazar AJ. p53 staining correlates with tumor type and location in sebaceous neoplasms. Am J Dermatopathol. 2012;34(2):129–35. quiz 36-8.
96. Hayashi N, Furihata M, Ohtsuki Y, Ueno H. Search for accumulation of p53 protein and detection of human papillomavirus genomes in sebaceous gland carcinoma of the eyelid. Virchows Arch. 1994;424(5):503–9.
97. Cho KJ, Khang SK, Koh JS, Chung JH, Lee SS. Sebaceous carcinoma of the eyelids: frequent expression of c-erbB-2 oncoprotein. J Korean Med Sci. 2000;15(5):545–50.
98. Stagner AM, Afrogheh AH, Jakobiec FA, Iacob CE, Grossniklaus HE, Deshpande V, et al. p16 expression is not a surrogate marker for high-risk human papillomavirus infection in periocular sebaceous carcinoma. Am J Ophthalmol. 2016;170:168–75.
99. Kwon MJ, Shin HS, Nam ES, Cho SJ, Lee MJ, Lee S, et al. Comparison of HER2 gene amplification and KRAS alteration in eyelid sebaceous carcinomas with that in other eyelid tumors. Pathol Res Pract. 2015;211(5):349–55.
100. Liau JY, Liao SL, Hsiao CH, Lin MC, Chang HC, Kuo KT. Hypermethylation of the CDKN2A gene promoter is a frequent epigenetic change in periocular sebaceous carcinoma and is associated with younger patient age. Hum Pathol. 2014;45(3):533–9.

101. Landis MN, Davis CL, Bellus GA, Wolverton SE. Immunosuppression and sebaceous tumors: a confirmed diagnosis of Muir-Torre syndrome unmasked by immunosuppressive therapy. J Am Acad Dermatol. 2011;65(5):1054–8.e1.
102. Hoss E, Nelson SA, Sharma A. Sebaceous carcinoma in solid organ transplant recipients. Int J Dermatol. 2017;56:746.
103. Yen MT, Tse DT. Sebaceous cell carcinoma of the eyelid and the human immunodeficiency virus. Ophthal Plast Reconstr Surg. 2000;16(3):206–10.
104. Rumelt S, Hogan NR, Rubin PA, Jakobiec FA. Four-eyelid sebaceous cell carcinoma following irradiation. Arch Ophthalmol. 1998;116(12):1670–2.
105. Hood IC, Qizilbash AH, Salama SS, Young JE, Archibald SD. Sebaceous carcinoma of the face following irradiation. Am J Dermatopathol. 1986;8(6):505–8.
106. Schlernitzauer DA, Font RL. Sebaceous gland carcinoma of the eyelid. Arch Ophthalmol. 1976;94(9):1523–5.
107. Izumi M, Tang X, Chiu CS, Nagai T, Matsubayashi J, Iwaya K, et al. Ten cases of sebaceous carcinoma arising in nevus sebaceus. J Dermatol. 2008;35(11):704–11.
108. Wenzel CT, Halperin EC, Fisher SR. Second malignant neoplasms of the head and neck in survivors of retinoblastoma. Ear Nose Throat J. 2001;80(2):106, 9–12.
109. Lemos LB, Santa Cruz DJ, Baba N. Sebaceous carcinoma of the eyelid following radiation therapy. Am J Surg Pathol. 1978;2(3):305–11.
110. Howrey RP, Lipham WJ, Schultz WH, Buckley EG, Dutton JJ, Klintworth GK, et al. Sebaceous gland carcinoma: a subtle second malignancy following radiation therapy in patients with bilateral retinoblastoma. Cancer. 1998;83(4):767–71.
111. John AM, Schwartz RA. Muir-Torre syndrome (MTS): an update and approach to diagnosis and management. J Am Acad Dermatol. 2016;74(3):558–66.
112. Mahalingam M. MSH6, past and present and Muir-Torre syndrome-connecting the dots. Am J Dermatopathol. 2017;39(4):239–49.
113. Schwartz RA, Torre DP. The Muir-Torre syndrome: a 25-year retrospect. J Am Acad Dermatol. 1995;33(1):90–104.
114. Jessup CJ, Redston M, Tilton E, Reimann JD. Importance of universal mismatch repair protein immunohistochemistry in patients with sebaceous neoplasia as an initial screening tool for Muir-Torre syndrome. Hum Pathol. 2016;49:1–9.
115. Sinicrope FA, Sargent DJ. Molecular pathways: microsatellite instability in colorectal cancer: prognostic, predictive, and therapeutic implications. Clin Cancer Res. 2012;18(6):1506–12.
116. Cohen PR, Kohn SR, Kurzrock R. Association of sebaceous gland tumors and internal malignancy: the Muir-Torre syndrome. Am J Med. 1991;90(5):606–13.
117. Lazar AJ, Lyle S, Calonje E. Sebaceous neoplasia and Torre-Muir syndrome. Curr Diagn Pathol. 2007;13(4):301–19.
118. Bhaijee F, Brown AS. Muir-Torre syndrome. Arch Pathol Lab Med. 2014;138(12):1685–9.
119. Grob A, Feser C, Grekin S. Muir-torre syndrome:a case associated with an infrequent gene mutation. J Clin Aesthet Dermatol. 2016;9(1):56–9.
120. Singh RS, Grayson W, Redston M, Diwan AH, Warneke CL, McKee PH, et al. Site and tumor type predicts DNA mismatch repair status in cutaneous sebaceous neoplasia. Am J Surg Pathol. 2008;32(6):936–42.
121. Zürcher M, Hintschich CR, Garner A, Bunce C, Collin JR. Sebaceous carcinoma of the eyelid: a clinicopathological study. Br J Ophthalmol. 1998;82(9):1049–55.
122. Demirci H, Nelson CC, Shields CL, Eagle RC, Shields JA. Eyelid sebaceous carcinoma associated with Muir-Torre syndrome in two cases. Ophthal Plast Reconstr Surg. 2007;23(1):77–9.
123. Wick MR, Goellner JR, Wolfe JT, Su WP. Adnexal carcinomas of the skin. II. Extraocular sebaceous carcinomas. Cancer. 1985;56(5):1163–72.
124. Hou JL, Killian JM, Baum CL, Otley CC, Roenigk RK, Arpey CJ, et al. Characteristics of sebaceous carcinoma and early outcomes of treatment using Mohs micrographic surgery versus wide local excision: an update of the Mayo Clinic experience over the past 2 decades. Dermatol Surg. 2014;40(3):241–6.

125. Cook BE, Bartley GB. Treatment options and future prospects for the management of eyelid malignancies: an evidence-based update. Ophthalmology. 2001;108(11):2088–98; quiz 99–100, 121.

126. Shields JA, Demirci H, Marr BP, Eagle RC, Shields CL. Sebaceous carcinoma of the eyelids: personal experience with 60 cases. Ophthalmology. 2004;111(12):2151–7.

127. Wang JK, Liao SL, Jou JR, Lai PC, Kao SC, Hou PK, et al. Malignant eyelid tumours in Taiwan. Eye (Lond). 2003;17(2):216–20.

128. Husain A, Blumenschein G, Esmaeli B. Treatment and outcomes for metastatic sebaceous cell carcinoma of the eyelid. Int J Dermatol. 2008;47(3):276–9.

129. Muqit MM, Roberts F, Lee WR, Kemp E. Improved survival rates in sebaceous carcinoma of the eyelid. Eye (Lond). 2004;18(1):49–53.

130. Boniuk M, Zimmerman LE. Sebaceous carcinoma of the eyelid, eyebrow, caruncle, and orbit. Trans Am Acad Ophthalmol Otolaryngol. 1968;72(4):619–42.

131. Sawyer AR, McGoldrick RB, Mackey S, Powell B, Pohl M. Should extraocular sebaceous carcinoma be investigated using sentinel node biopsy? Dermatol Surg. 2009;35(4):704–8.

132. Rulon DB, Helwig EB. Cutaneous sebaceous neoplasms. Cancer. 1974;33(1):82–102.

133. Chang AY, Miller CJ, Elenitsas R, Newman JG, Sobanko JF. Management considerations in extraocular sebaceous carcinoma. Dermatol Surg. 2016;42(Suppl 1):S57–65.

134. Shalin SC, Lyle S, Calonje E, Lazar AJ. Sebaceous neoplasia and the Muir-Torre syndrome: important connections with clinical implications. Histopathology. 2010;56(1):133–47.

135. Font R. Eyelids and lacrimal drainage system. In: Spencer WH, editor. Ophthalmic pathology: an atlas and textbook. 3rd ed. Philadelphia: WB Saunders; 1986. p. 2169–214.

136. Pfeiffer ML, Yin VT, Myers J, Esmaeli B. Regional nodal recurrence of sebaceous carcinoma of the caruncle 11 years after primary tumor resection. JAMA Ophthalmol. 2013;131(8):1091–2.

137. Kohler S, Rouse RV, Smoller BR. The differential diagnosis of pagetoid cells in the epidermis. Mod Pathol. 1998;11(1):79–92.

138. Sramek B, Lisle A, Loy T. Immunohistochemistry in ocular carcinomas. J Cutan Pathol. 2008;35(7):641–6.

139. Beer TW, Shepherd P, Theaker JM. Ber EP4 and epithelial membrane antigen aid distinction of basal cell, squamous cell and basosquamous carcinomas of the skin. Histopathology. 2000;37(3):218–23.

140. Ansai SI. Topics in histopathology of sweat gland and sebaceous neoplasms. J Dermatol. 2017;44(3):315–26.

141. Rajan Kd A, Burris C, Iliff N, Grant M, Eshleman JR, Eberhart CG. DNA mismatch repair defects and microsatellite instability status in periocular sebaceous carcinoma. Am J Ophthalmol. 2014;157(3):640–7.e1–2.

142. Buitrago W, Joseph AK. Sebaceous carcinoma: the great masquerader: emerging concepts in diagnosis and treatment. Dermatol Ther. 2008;21(6):459–66.

143. Esmaeli B, Nasser QJ, Cruz H, Fellman M, Warneke CL, Ivan D. American joint committee on cancer T category for eyelid sebaceous carcinoma correlates with nodal metastasis and survival. Ophthalmology. 2012;119(5):1078–82.

144. American Joint Committee on Cancer. New York, NY: Springer; 2010.

145. Reina RS, Parry E. Aggressive extraocular sebaceous carcinoma in a 52-year-old man. Dermatol Surg. 2006;32(10):1283–6.

146. Orcurto A, Gay BE, Sozzi WJ, Gilliet M, Leyvraz S. Long-term remission of an aggressive sebaceous carcinoma following chemotherapy. Case Rep Dermatol. 2014;6(1):80–4.

147. Herceg D, Kusacić-Kuna S, Dotlić S, Petrović R, Bracić I, Horvatić Herceg G, et al. F-18 FDG PET evaluation of a rapidly growing extraocular sebaceous carcinoma. Clin Nucl Med. 2009;34(11):798–801.

148. Baek CH, Chung MK, Jeong HS, Son YI, Choi J, Kim YD, et al. The clinical usefulness of (18)F-FDG PET/CT for the evaluation of lymph node metastasis in periorbital malignancies. Korean J Radiol. 2009;10(1):1–7.

149. Ginsberg J. Present status of meibomian gland carcinoma. Arch Ophthalmol. 1965;73:271–7.
150. Erovic BM, Goldstein DP, Kim D, Al Habeeb A, Waldron J, Ghazarian D, et al. Sebaceous gland carcinoma of the head and neck: the Princess Margaret Hospital experience. Head Neck. 2013;35(3):316–20.
151. Bailet JW, Zimmerman MC, Arnstein DP, Wollman JS, Mickel RA. Sebaceous carcinoma of the head and neck. Case report and literature review. Arch Otolaryngol Head Neck Surg. 1992;118(11):1245–9.
152. Tryggvason G, Bayon R, Pagedar NA. Epidemiology of sebaceous carcinoma of the head and neck: implications for lymph node management. Head Neck. 2012;34(12):1765–8.
153. Ho VH, Ross MI, Prieto VG, Khaleeq A, Kim S, Esmaeli B. Sentinel lymph node biopsy for sebaceous cell carcinoma and melanoma of the ocular adnexa. Arch Otolaryngol Head Neck Surg. 2007;133(8):820–6.
154. Nijhawan N, Ross MI, Diba R, Ahmadi MA, Esmaeli B. Experience with sentinel lymph node biopsy for eyelid and conjunctival malignancies at a cancer center. Ophthal Plast Reconstr Surg. 2004;20(4):291–5.
155. Savar A, Oellers P, Myers J, Prieto VG, Torres-Cabala C, Frank SJ, et al. Positive sentinel node in sebaceous carcinoma of the eyelid. Ophthal Plast Reconstr Surg. 2011;27(1):e4–6.
156. Harrington CR, Egbert BM, Swetter SM. Extraocular sebaceous carcinoma in a patient with Muir-Torre syndrome. Dermatol Surg. 2004;30(5):817–9.
157. Pfeiffer ML, Savar A, Esmaeli B. Sentinel lymph node biopsy for eyelid and conjunctival tumors: what have we learned in the past decade? Ophthal Plast Reconstr Surg. 2013;29(1):57–62.
158. Spencer JM, Nossa R, Tse DT, Sequeira M. Sebaceous carcinoma of the eyelid treated with Mohs micrographic surgery. J Am Acad Dermatol. 2001;44(6):1004–9.
159. Grigoryan KV, Leithauser L, Gloster HM. Aggressive extraocular sebaceous carcinoma recurring after mohs micrographic surgery. Case Rep Oncol Med. 2015;2015:534176.
160. Callahan EF, Appert DL, Roenigk RK, Bartley GB. Sebaceous carcinoma of the eyelid: a review of 14 cases. Dermatol Surg. 2004;30(8):1164–8.
161. Dogru M, Matsuo H, Inoue M, Okubo K, Yamamoto M. Management of eyelid sebaceous carcinomas. Ophthalmologica. 1997;211(1):40–3.
162. Snow SN, Larson PO, Lucarelli MJ, Lemke BN, Madjar DD. Sebaceous carcinoma of the eyelids treated by mohs micrographic surgery: report of nine cases with review of the literature. Dermatol Surg. 2002;28(7):623–31.
163. Cavanagh HD, Green WR, Goldberg HK. Multicentric sebaceous adenocarcinoma of the meibomian gland. Am J Ophthalmol. 1974;77(3):326–32.
164. Nunery WR, Welsh MG, McCord CD. Recurrence of sebaceous carcinoma of the eyelid after radiation therapy. Am J Ophthalmol. 1983;96(1):10–5.
165. Hendley RL, Rieser JC, Cavanagh HD, Bodner BI, Waring GO. Primary radiation therapy for meibomian gland carcinoma. Am J Ophthalmol. 1979;87(2):206–9.
166. Hata M, Koike I, Omura M, Maegawa J, Ogino I, Inoue T. Noninvasive and curative radiation therapy for sebaceous carcinoma of the eyelid. Int J Radiat Oncol Biol Phys. 2012;82(2):605–11.
167. Yen MT, Tse DT, Wu X, Wolfson AH. Radiation therapy for local control of eyelid sebaceous cell carcinoma: report of two cases and review of the literature. Ophthal Plast Reconstr Surg. 2000;16(3):211–5.
168. Pardo FS, Wang CC, Albert D, Stracher MA. Sebaceous carcinoma of the ocular adnexa: radiotherapeutic management. Int J Radiat Oncol Biol Phys. 1989;17(3):643–7.
169. Jung YH, Woo IS, Kim MY, Han CW, Rha EY. Palliative 5-fluorouracil and cisplatin chemotherapy in recurrent metastatic sebaceous carcinoma: case report and literature review. Asia Pac J Clin Oncol. 2016;12(1):e189–93.
170. Murthy R, Honavar SG, Burman S, Vemuganti GK, Naik MN, Reddy VA. Neoadjuvant chemotherapy in the management of sebaceous gland carcinoma of the eyelid with regional lymph node metastasis. Ophthal Plast Reconstr Surg. 2005;21(4):307–9.

171. Priyadarshini O, Biswas G, Biswas S, Padhi R, Rath S. Neoadjuvant chemotherapy in recurrent sebaceous carcinoma of eyelid with orbital invasion and regional lymphadenopathy. Ophthal Plast Reconstr Surg. 2010;26(5):366–8.
172. Paschal BR, Bagley CS. Sebaceous land carcinoma of the eyelid: complete response to sequential combination chemotherapy. N C Med J. 1985;46(9):473–4.
173. el Nakadi B, Nouwynck C, Salhadin A. Combined therapeutic approach for extraorbital sebaceous carcinoma in a Torre's syndrome. Eur J Surg Oncol. 1995;21(3):321–2.
174. De Leo A, Innocenzi D, Onesti MG, Potenza C, Toscani M, Scuderi N. Extraocular sebaceous carcinoma in Muir Torre Syndrome with unfavorable prognosis. Cancer Chemother Pharmacol. 2006;58(6):842–4.

Chapter 11
Extramammary Paget's Disease

Nathalie C. Zeitouni and Jose A. Cervantes

Abstract Extramammary Paget's disease (EMPD) is a rare, slow-growing intraepithelial adenocarcinoma typically localized to areas of apocrine gland distribution outside the mammary glands. EMPD typically involves the vulva, perianal area, and male genitalia, with rare sites including the thighs, buttocks, axilla, eyelids, and external ear canal. The vulva remains the most frequently involved site with 65% of EMPD located in this area. Lesions appear as erythematous, brown or white, moist plaques that are well differentiated and often accompanied by subtle subjective symptoms of pruritus and pain. Its pathogenesis has been debated, but most cases are thought to arise as a primary intraepidermal neoplasm of glandular origin. A minority of disease appears to be intraepithelial spread of an underlying dermal adnexal malignancy or a regional neoplasm with contiguous epithelium. The diagnosis of EMPD is confirmed histologically by the presence of vacuolated Paget cells in the epidermis that stain for glandular cytokeratins, epithelial membrane antigen, and carcinoembryonic antigen. Treatment options which include surgical excision, Mohs micrographic surgery, radiotherapy, photodynamic therapy, topical imiquimod 5% cream, 5-fluorouracil, and systemic chemotherapy have also been used successfully. Recurrence is common, necessitating a close follow-up.

Keywords Extramammary Paget's disease · Genital disease · Perianal disease · Vulva · Vulvar neoplasia · Skin cancer · Imiquimod · Pruritic lesions · Paget cells

N. C. Zeitouni (✉)
Dermatology, St. Joseph's Hospital and Medical Center, Dignity Health, Phoenix, AZ, USA
e-mail: Nathaliezeitouni@email.arizona.edu

J. A. Cervantes
Tucson Hospital Medical Education Program, Tucson Medical Center, Tucson, AZ, USA

© Springer International Publishing AG, part of Springer Nature 2018   231
A. Hanlon (ed.), *A Practical Guide to Skin Cancer*,
https://doi.org/10.1007/978-3-319-74903-7_11

Introduction

In 1874, Sir James Paget described an eczema-like lesion on the nipple with an associated underlying breast malignancy, now called mammary Paget's disease (MPD). Extramammary Paget's disease (EMPD) was first described by Crocker in 1889 when he discussed an occurrence of Paget on the penis and scrotum [1]. This entity would further expand when perianal EMPD and Paget's disease of the vulva were subsequently described in 1893 and 1901, respectively [2].

EMPD is a rare, slow-growing intraepithelial adenocarcinoma typically localized to areas of apocrine gland distribution outside the mammary glands. EMPD typically involves the vulva, perianal area, and male genitalia, with rare sites including the thighs, buttocks, axilla, eyelids, and external ear canal [3, 4]. The vulva remains the most frequently involved site with 65% of EMPD located in this area [5].

Clinically, lesions appear as erythematous, brown or white, moist plaques that are well differentiated and often accompanied by subtle subjective symptoms of pruritus and pain. Its pathogenesis has been debated, but most cases are thought to arise as a primary intraepidermal neoplasm of glandular origin. A minority of the disease appears to be intraepithelial spread of an underlying dermal adnexal malignancy or a regional neoplasm with contiguous epithelium [6].

The diagnosis of EMPD is confirmed histologically by the presence of vacuolated Paget cells in the epidermis that stain for glandular cytokeratins, epithelial membrane antigen, and carcinoembryonic antigen [7]. Treatment generally involves surgical excision or Mohs micrographic surgery, although radiotherapy, photodynamic therapy, 5-fluorouracil, topical imiquimod 5% cream, and systemic chemotherapy have also been used successfully [8–10].

Epidemiology

EMPD is a rare condition with only a few hundred cases reported in the medical literature. Precise incidence is unknown. It is rarer than mammary Paget's disease (MPD), accounting for only 6.5% of all cases of Paget's disease [11, 12]. EMPD is a cutaneous malignancy that is frequently found in skin areas containing abundant apocrine glands such as the genitalia, the groin, and the axilla [13]. The most common location for EMPD is the vulva, yet the disease accounts for only 1–2% of all vulvar malignancies [2, 14–16]. Ectopic EMPD has been described in cutaneous areas devoid of apocrine glands but is exceedingly rare [4, 17].

EMPD most commonly affects individuals aged 50–80 years with a peak age of 65 and predilection toward women and Caucasians, although a male predominance seems to exist in certain parts of Asia [6, 13, 18]. Since the first report of familial EMPD was discovered in 1973 by Kuehn et al., only seven other cases have been reported in the literature [19–21]. Of these cases, all but the one recently reported in two Chinese brothers occurred in Japan [22]. Findings in these cases suggested a correlation between genetic abnormalities and a predisposition in cancers, especially in East Asian populations [13, 21–23].

Pathogenesis

The exact pathogenesis of EMPD is still not completely understood. Although EMPD is generally accepted to be an intraepithelial adenocarcinoma [24], cell origin remains debated because the condition is found in both apocrine and non-apocrine gland-bearing skin. Unlike mammary Paget's disease of the breast which is always associated with an underlying ductal carcinoma, the cause of EMPD is not always associated with malignancy. Recent literature suggests that EMPD is heterogeneous and can be divided into primary EMPD and secondary EMPD [2, 3, 14, 25].

Primary EMPD occurs more often than secondary EMPD, with figures showing that the primary type comprises roughly 75–96% of EMPD cases [2, 3, 26]. The primary or cutaneous form is thought to originate in the epidermis, the underlying apocrine sweat glands, or the epidermal basal cells [3, 26, 27]. Although this form is not associated with an underlying malignancy, in roughly 10–20% of all EMPD cases, the tumor has been documented to progress, infiltrate the underlying dermis, and even metastasize through the blood and lymphatic vessels [14, 25, 26]. Recently it has been suggested that Toker cells, which are present in both the vulvar epidermis and mammary tissue, may represent the benign precursors of the Paget cell [3, 28, 29].

The more rarely occurring secondary EMPD originates from epidermotropic spread of neoplastic cells from an underlying adenocarcinoma in the adjacent adnexal gland (25%) typically from apocrine origin or within a contiguous epithelium (10–15%) from visceral carcinoma, usually the rectum, bladder, urethra, cervix, prostate, perianal area, vulvar region, glans penis, or groin [2, 3, 6, 13, 30]. Secondary EMPD is known to commonly metastasize through the lymphatic system [3, 14, 26].

Lastly, a multicentric theory suggests that EMPD may arise from a common oncogenic stimulus resulting in the development of malignancies at different sites, where EMPD is found in conjunction with another malignancy with no direct anatomical relationship, e.g., EMPD of the scrotum and hepatocellular carcinoma, and the rare association between EMPD and MPD [13, 31].

Clinical Presentation

The onset of disease is often insidious with patients complaining most often of pruritus [6, 14, 32]. Additionally, patients may experience burning paresthesia, pain, edema, and bleeding [2, 26, 32]. EMPD most commonly arises from areas of high apocrine gland density. The anatomical location most commonly affected is the vulva, making up about 65% of all reported cases [5, 13, 25, 33]. In cases affecting the vulva, lesions typically arise from the labia majora, spread centrifugally toward the pubis, and frequently involve the inguinal folds, perineum, labia minora, vagina,

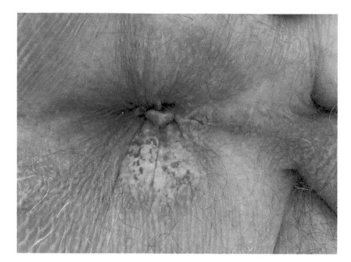

Fig. 11.1 Perianal EMPD

inner face of the thighs, buttocks, and axilla [25, 32–38]. In advanced disease, the entire anogenital region may be affected, making it impossible to distinguish the primary location of the tumor, which is significant given that primary tumors at certain locations are associated with specific types of internal malignancies [26, 32].

Secondary EMPD of the vulva is defined as involvement of the vulvar skin by a noncutaneous internal neoplasm, either by epidermotropic metastasis or by contiguous involvement. Adnexal carcinomas arising from underlying apocrine glands or from Bartholin's glands are involved in 4–17% and 1–20% and have distant or noncontiguous carcinoma of the endometrium, cervix, urethra, bladder, colon, rectum, ovary, liver, and gallbladder have all been described. Of these associated malignancies, anal and rectal adenocarcinoma involving the skin of the anogenital region are the most commonly implicated with secondary EMPD of the vulva [5, 25, 33, 39].

EMPD of the perianal region makes up about 20% of all reported cases. Clinically, it closely resembles vulvar EMPD, often originating adjacent to the anus and subsequently spreading to involve the perineum, gluteal folds, and genitalia [36]. Perianal EMPD is associated with an adnexal adenocarcinoma in 7% of cases and an internal malignancy in 14% of cases. Secondary perianal EMPD which makes up the majority of perianal cases (70–80%) is strongly associated with adenocarcinoma of the anus and colorectum [40]. Other malignancies that have been reported to cause secondary perianal EMPD are carcinoma of the stomach, breast, and ureter [41]. See Fig. 11.1.

EMPD of the male genitalia (penis and scrotum) makes up about 14% of all cases and is thought to be more frequently associated with internal malignancy; in particular, underlying neoplasms of the prostate, bladder, testicles, ureter, and kidney occur in up to 11% of cases [5, 37, 38, 42–44]. The lesions typically start on the scrotum, the penis, or the inguinal folds and subsequently may spread to involve the abdomen, with rare cases involving only the glans penis [45–47]. Patients may also exhibit inguinal lymph node involvement, with associated edema of the lower extremities [47].

Axillary EMPD may be primary or secondary, but carcinoma of the breast should be excluded prior to the diagnosis. It appears to affect men more frequently and most often presents unilaterally, although bilateral cases have been reported [48]. Cases have also been reported to follow genital EMPD [49, 50].

Ectopic EMPD appears in areas devoid of apocrine glands and has been reported to affect the external ear canal, cheek, eyelids, trunk (both abdomen and back), extremities, and umbilical region [5, 17, 18, 51–56]. There are also isolated reports of EMPD affecting various sites of the mucosa, including the tongue, bronchial tree, esophagus, and urethra, in association with prostatic and urinary bladder neoplasms [57–60].

Multiple EMPD is rare and includes simultaneous presentation of both mammary and extramammary disease or as EMPD at occurring at different sites such as anogenital and axillary involvement [39, 61]. Rare reports exist of EMPD associated with distant tumors arising in organs without a direct epithelial connection to the affected dermis. Examples include carcinoma of the ovaries, bile duct, liver, and kidneys [62, 63]. Although it is likely that these cases simply represent synchronous coincidental neoplasms, it has been suggested that a multicentric oncogenic stimulus exists that can induce distant adenocarcinoma, a theory supported by the occasional association between EMPD and MPD [13].

Depending on the site and duration of the lesion, EMPD can have a variable morphological presentation. The primary lesion may present as a macule, patch, or plaque, with color presentations varying from pink to light/dark red-brown. Larger lesions have been documented to present with a mixture of colors [35, 64]. Pigmentary changes may also be appreciated, more often hypopigmented than hyperpigmented [50, 65]. Although typically well demarcated, larger, more advanced lesions may be irregular with poorly defined borders [6, 25].

Depending on the anatomical location of the lesion, the surface of the lesion may have a pityriasis-like coarse, lamellar scale. The lesion may be eroded with or without leukoplakia-like keratosis, ulcerated with an associated crust, or cobblestone-like papules [11]. Rare morphological features include alopecia neoplastica, sclerodermiform maculae, and lichenoid papules [66, 67]. Infiltrative nodules, vegetative lesions, and regional lymphadenopathy may also be present. "Underpants-pattern erythema" is a particular clinical aspect of genital EMPD started within the groin and spreading peripherally to the areas covered by underwear. This particular presentation is a manifestation of lymphatic invasion and is associated with metastatic disease and a poor prognosis [68].

EMPD can resemble a variety of cutaneous conditions, which can delay the diagnosis. On average, the disease is not diagnosed for 2 years after the onset of symptoms [16, 26, 32, 69]. Given the vague presentation and subjective symptoms, the condition may be misdiagnosed as pruritus ani, fungal infection, contact dermatitis, lichen sclerosis, or intertrigo. A reasonable differential diagnosis may include contact or seborrheic eczema, psoriasis inversa, perianal streptogenic dermatitis, lichen sclerosis, candidal intertrigo, tinea corporis, histiocytosis, mycosis fungoides, Crohn disease, hidradenitis suppurativa, condyloma accuminata, leukoplakia, amelanotic melanoma, Bowen disease, and superficial basal cell carcinoma [2, 6, 13, 70]. Any nonhealing eczematous patch in the anogenital or axillary region not responding to topical steroids or antifungals should raise suspicion for EMPD and warrant a biopsy [6, 14, 45, 71].

Histopathology

The diagnosis of Paget's disease is confirmed by the presence of Paget cells. Histologically, it presents similarly to mammary Paget's disease [6, 14, 45]. Paget cells are usually about twice the size of surrounding keratinocytes. They are characterized as large cells with an abundant basophilic or amphophilic cytoplasm. The nucleus is usually large and centrally located with pleomorphic nuclei and a prominent nucleolus. Signet ring cells may be present and mitotic figures are common [40, 72]. See Fig. 11.2.

Paget cells may occur as solitary cells or in irregular clusters, nests, or glandular structures within the epidermis [26]. They may infiltrate the upper epidermis but are more commonly concentrated in the lower epidermis in the pilosebaceous apparatus, sweat gland, and excretory ducts [3, 13, 73]. Paget cells are distinguished from surrounding epithelial cells by a clear halo lacking intracellular bridges. Hyperkeratosis, acanthosis, and focal parakeratosis may be appreciated, along with an inflammatory infiltrate composed of lymphocytes, histiocytes, neutrophils, and plasma cells in the upper dermis [3, 6, 11].

The histological pattern of epidermal infiltration of Paget cell is often termed pagetoid spread to indicate a condition where the cells are distributed in a singly or

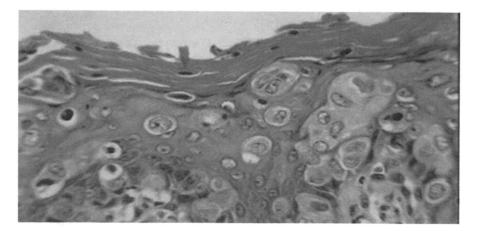

Fig. 11.2 Histological presentation of EMPD

small group pattern throughout the epithelial layer [2]. Conditions known to exhibit this particular pattern include malignant melanoma, Bowen disease, Langerhans cell histiocytosis, mycosis fungoides, Spitz nevus, and sebaceous carcinoma. Given that most of these conditions affect the skin in the same general areas as EMPD, it is reasonable that they be given consideration on your differential diagnosis [3, 74, 75].

Immunohistochemical staining may also help identify Paget cells and even differentiate between primary and secondary EMPD. When large mucin droplets present within the cell, the nucleus may be displaced to the periphery creating a signet ring. The presence of intracytoplasmic sialomucin accounts for the positivity of some histochemical stains such as periodic acid-Schiff, mucicarmine, Alcian blue, aldehyde-fuchsin toluidine blue, and colloidal iron which is often helpful in the diagnosis [13, 26, 76].

Minor variations in antigen expression exist between primary and secondary EMPD, particularly with regard to gross cystic disease fluid protein-15 (GCDFO-15) and cytokeratins (CK) 7 and 20. CK7 has a sensitivity ranging from 86% to 100% but is not specific for EMPD, whereas CK20 may be more specific for EMPD [77, 78]. Additionally, in perianal cases where CK20 was positive and GCDFP was negative, there appeared to be a stronger association with underlying carcinoma, whereas, when CK20 was negative and GCDFP was positive, the association was not present [79–81].

Differential staining pattern of mucin core proteins (MUC), specifically MUC5A2, appears to be associated with EMPD, particularly of the vulvar and male genitalia, and its absence is well correlated with more invasive disease [82–84]. An overexpression of p53 and of fatty acid synthase is correlated with invasive disease [85]. Carcinoembryonic antigen may also play a role in diagnosis as it has been found to be quite sensitive for EMPD, and its absence appears to have an association with underlying carcinomas [30, 77, 86]. Serum levels of RCAS1, a novel antigen, have also been reported to be sensitive to EMPD cells [87].

Among the hormonal receptors studied, androgen receptors are detected in more than 50% of EMPD cases, whereas there appears to be a consistent absence of positivity for both estrogen and progesterone receptors [84, 88, 89]. Overexpression of human epidermal growth factor receptor 2 (Her-2) protein, which is expressed in 30–50% of cases, was found to be associated with a higher recurrence following therapy and a potentially more aggressive disease course [90, 91].

Work-Up

Following any biopsy-proven diagnosis of EMPD, a thorough history of present illness, review of systems, and physical examination including a full cutaneous examination should be performed. In particular, one should carefully examine for enlarged lymph nodes around the affected area and hepatosplenomegaly, through breast and digital rectal examinations. Further work-up for EMPD should be directed at investigating for both invasive disease and an associated underlying malignancy, as the results of these investigations affect both the prognosis and subsequent therapy [6, 14].

A work-up for patients with disease affecting the vulva should include screening for gastrointestinal (GI) and genitourinary (GU) malignancies and breast disease. A reasonable approach would include a pelvic examination, to include a Pap smear and colposcopy, abdominopelvic ultrasound with or without a CT, colonoscopy, cystoscopy, intravenous pyelogram, hysteroscopy, mammogram, chest radiograph, and serum tumor markers CEA and CA-19 [6, 14, 92, 93].

In cases of perianal EMPD, a screen for GI and GU malignancy would be warranted. An investigation may include an upper endoscopy, rectal examination, colonoscopy, sigmoidoscopy or barium enema, cystoscopy with or without CT urogram, and if female a mammogram [2, 6, 30]. In men with genital involvement, screening for underlying GU malignancies should be completed and may include cystoscopy, with or without CT urogram [5, 38, 45]. Serum prostate-specific antigen may also be of some utility [94]. If dermal invasion is noted, a sentinel node biopsy may be considered to determine if there is nodal involvement [26]. A positron-emission tomography scan may also have some utility in evaluating for lymph node involvement and distant metastases [2, 26].

Course and Prognosis

The prognosis of primary cutaneous EMPD is often favorable when confined to the epidermis [3, 15, 34, 46]. Invasive disease, consisting of greater than 1 mm of invasion into the dermis, which is thought to occur in up to 20% of cases, significantly worsens the prognosis [40, 50]. Disease with lymphovascular invasion and metastasis to the regional lymph nodes is often fatal with some studies reporting a 0% survival at 5 years [3]. Serum CEA levels have also been used to predict the progression of disease with elevated levels indicating systemic metastases and an increased risk of death [50, 93]. Overall mortality rates have been reported to be as high as 46% with metastatic EMPD [5].

Prognosis of secondary EMPD is typically worse with the overall mortality rate dependent on the associated underlying internal malignancy. On average, the survival rate of secondary EMPD is reported to be 36 months [5, 26, 64].

Treatment and Follow-Up

Surgery is the most common modality used to treat EMPD. The surgical procedures commonly used include wide local excision and simple or radical vulvectomy [14, 32, 54, 95, 96].

Surgical removal requires that the excision be adequately wide and with sufficient depth so as to completely remove the lesion in its entirety. There appears to be a considerable variation between the accepted ideal surgical margins to be utilized in WLE, with most reports describing a 2–5 cm margin. Some evidence suggests that well-demarcated EMPD lesions may be adequately managed with 1 cm margin resection [97, 98]. It is however common for EMPD to be multifocal with irregular histological margins and subclinical extension [14, 32]. Depending on the anatomical location of the lesion, WLE has a reported recurrence rate of 22–60% [2, 6, 32, 71].

Several strategies have been employed to overcome the unreliable clinical examination, including preoperative mapping with scouting biopsies, a method that was recently found to be enhanced by handheld reflectance confocal microscopy with early results showing a reduction in the number of biopsies needed to render a correct diagnosis [99–101]. Upon review of this technique, several groups have reported minimal recurrence, with long-term follow-up [100, 102]. Beyond improved recurrence rates vs. WLE, this technique offers the added benefit of enhanced preoperative planning, patient education, reconstruction, and a reduction in repeat surgeries [102]. Another method of mapping with high sensitivity for Paget cells (99.8%) can be achieved with fluorescein visualization [32, 103]. Another preoperative mapping method that has demonstrated some utility is staged, square excisions used initially for lentigo maligna [32, 104]. Intraoperative staining with antibodies to CK-7 alone or in combination with CEA has also been reported to decrease recurrence rates [26, 45, 71, 77, 105]. Despite these techniques, recurrence rates are high, most likely stemming from false-negative biopsies, sampling errors, and the multicentric nature of the disease.

Intraoperative frozen sections are employed to confirm tumor-free margins. This technique has been widely utilized for lesions affecting the penoscrotal areas [106, 107]. Several retrospective studies have identified a high rate of false-negative margins (40%), and its use appears limited in its utility with multifocal disease [108, 109]. Routine frozen sections which sample about 0.1% of the surgical margin have yielded inconsistent results, with little effect on outcomes [32, 110, 111].

Alternatively, Mohs micrographic surgery (MMS) appears to be well suited for irregular but contiguous lesions and has demonstrated favorable long-term outcomes and been associated with a higher recurrence-free survival rate than fixed surgical margins [32, 98, 102, 112]. MMS involves examining all of the histological tumor margins, with the goal of obtaining complete tumor-free margins, while preserving unaffected tissue and reducing the need for repeated surgery [71, 98, 113]. When compared to WLE, Mohs has been widely reported to have lower recurrence rates for primary EMPD and recurrent disease [32, 98, 112, 114, 115]. In general, recurrence rates have been reported to be 8–27% for primary disease and 28–50% for recurrent disease [98, 112]. A reported 97% of MMS surgeries obtained tumor-free margins when utilizing a 5 cm margin [98, 107]. Additional supplements to the MMS have been suggested to decrease local recurrence. Photodynamic therapy and scouting biopsies have been described to improve the definitive treatment with MMS [71, 99].

In cases of invasive and secondary Paget's disease, more extensive surgeries such as radical vulvectomy, hemivulvectomy, and bilateral inguinal lymph node dissection have been documented to produce better recurrence rates than both MMS and WLE [14, 25, 96]. In general, radical vulvectomy and hemivulvectomy are associated with recurrence rates of 15% and 20%, respectively [6, 32, 116]. It should be noted that invasive surgery is associated with significantly higher morbidity and that the associated sequela from such procedures decreases function and quality of life [115].

Radiotherapy may be indicated in nonsurgical candidates, in patients seeking nonsurgical options, in adjuvant therapy, or for recurrent disease [96, 117, 118]. Although its efficacy was questioned during its early use, more recent literature suggests effectiveness as both a primary therapy and as an adjuvant to surgery [119, 120]. Its benefits have been demonstrated in both EMPD confined to the epidermis and invasive disease [121]. Radiotherapy has also been successfully used in cases of local recurrence and should be considered in cases where large lesions are deemed inoperable or if the patient's comorbidities necessitate nonsurgical options [69, 122, 123]. Described techniques including beam type, beam energy, and total doses are variable among different publications [124, 125]. Radiation changes to the skin can be a limiting factor for treatment duration and tolerance.

Photodynamic therapy (PDT) which involves the preferential accumulation of photosensitizer in target lesions is a highly selective tissue sparing therapy with the added benefit of stimulating the host immune response [126, 127]. Recent literature on its use indicates that PDT with systemic porfimer sodium and topical ALA may benefit a select group of patients with noninvasive, superficial lesions on cosmetically and functionally important areas and as an option for recurrence following surgery [127–130]. Its use on bulky and invasive disease has also been associated with high rate of recurrence and is currently not a suitable replacement for surgery when invasive disease is identified [26, 131]. There also appears to be a suitable role for PDT augmentation and MMS to optimize cosmesis and function while minimizing tissue excision [6, 32].

Laser therapy appears to be efficacious for superficial lesions. Its utility on deeper or invasive lesions is limited by the photon penetration which is only a few millimeters [32]. As a primary therapy, its use is associated with a high recurrence of disease and may be more efficacious in combination with WLE, when guided by photodynamic diagnosis with ALA-induced fluorescence [132, 133]. Postoperative pain has been noted to be high and reported to hinder subsequent therapy [134].

Topical therapies with cytotoxic agents 5-fluorouracil (5-FU) and bleomycin have been used to treat EMPD. Imiquimod 5% cream, an immunomodulator, has shown some promising results, with clinical and pathological clearance of EMPD frequently reported [135–139]. It can be used as an alternative to surgery, as an adjunct before and after surgery, and in combination with other therapies. In the largest literature review to date on the subject, which included both primary and recurrent disease, both men and women were found to have an overall cure rate of 87.5% with a 12–20% relapse rate at an average follow-up of 20 months. [140–143] 5-FU has been used preoperatively for cytoreduction, aiding with the surgical resection process by delineating surgical margins, and postoperative detection of early disease recurrence [6, 144, 145]. When used alone, 5-FU is not sufficient to appropriately treat EMPD that extends beyond the superficial layers of the epidermis (1–2 mm). Topical bleomycin has been used to treat patients with recurrent noninvasive primary vulvar EMPD but is currently not considered sufficient to treat EMPD as a sole agent [32, 146].

Systemic chemotherapy using carboplatin, epirubicin, adriamycin, docetaxel, vincristine, calcium folate, mitomycin-C, etoposide, and 5-FU has been used to treat EMPD. These agents are most often used in combination and as adjuncts to other therapies [147–153]. Systemic chemotherapy may be used in metastatic disease, to decrease tumor burden prior to excision decreasing the extent of surgical resection. Current recommendations support the use of systemic chemotherapy as a tertiary measure for nonsurgical candidates and those forgoing the use of radiotherapy [32, 149, 154, 155]. The detection of HER2/neu in a subgroup of EMPD patients has led to the use of trastuzumab, a monoclonal antibody directed against HER-2 [91, 156, 157].

Regardless of the treatment modality, long-term surveillance is recommended as recurrence has been reported up to 15 years following treatment [6, 115]. Although no current guidelines have been currently published, consensus among experts in the field recommends a biannual evaluation for 36 months, followed by an annual evaluation for the subsequent 10 years for noninvasive, primary cutaneous EMPD. In secondary or invasive EMPD, follow-up is necessary to exclude the development of associated internal malignancies. It is recommended that follow-up for perianal EMPD includes an annual examination, a proctosigmoidoscopy, and a colonoscopy every 2–3 years. Vulval EMPD may be similarly followed up with regular inspection of the vulva and the liberal use of regular pelvic ultrasound scans and hysteroscopy with a low threshold for biopsy of any newly appearing lesions [6, 13, 30].

References

1. Crocker HR. Paget's disease, affecting the scrotum and penis. Trans Path Soc Lond. 1889;40:187.
2. Love WE, Schmitt AR, Bordeaux JS. Management of unusual cutaneous malignancies: atypical fibroxanthoma, malignant fibrous histiocytoma, sebaceous carcinoma, extramammary Paget disease. Dermatol Clin. 2011;29(2):201–16. viii
3. Lloyd J, Flanagan AM. Mammary and extramammary Paget's disease. J Clin Pathol. 2000;53(10):742–9.
4. Heymann WR. Extramammary Paget's disease. Clin Dermatol. 1993;11(1):83–7.
5. Chanda JJ. Extramammary Paget's disease: prognosis and relationship to internal malignancy. J Am Acad Dermatol. 1985;13(6):1009–14.
6. Shepherd V, Davidson EJ, Davies-Humphreys J. Extramammary Paget's disease. BJOG. 2005;112(3):273–9.
7. Wojnarowska F, Cooper S. Anogenital (non-venereal) disease. Dermatology. Edinburgh: Mosby; 2003. p. 1099–113.

8. LEE KY, Roh MR, Chung WG, Chung KY. Comparison of Mohs micrographic surgery and wide excision for extramammary Paget's disease: Korean experience. Dermatol Surg. 2009;35(1):34–40.

9. Moreno-Arias G, Conill C, Sola-Casas M, Mascaro-Galy J, Grimalt R. Radiotherapy for in situ extramammary Paget disease of the vulva. J Dermatolog treat. 2003;14(2):119–23.

10. Brown R, McCormack M, Lankester K, Spittle M. Spontaneous apparent clinical resolution with histologic persistence of a case of extramammary Paget's disease: response to topical 5-fluorouracil. Cutis. 2000;66(6):454–5.

11. Wagner G, Sachse MM. Extramammary Paget disease–clinical appearance, pathogenesis, management. JDDG: Journal der Deutschen Dermatologischen Gesellschaft. 2011;9(6):448–54.

12. Fardal RW, Kierland RR, Clagett OT, Woolner LB. Prognosis in cutaneous Paget's disease. Postgrad Med. 1964;36(6):584–93.

13. Kanitakis J. Mammary and extramammary Paget's disease. J Eur Acad Dermatol Venereol. 2007;21(5):581–90.

14. Landay M, Satmary W, Memarzadeh S, Smith D, Barclay D. Premalignant & malignant disorders of the vulva & vagina. Current diagnosis & treatment obstetrics & gynecology. 10th ed. New York: McGraw-Hill; 2007. p. 822–7.

15. Kodama S, Kaneko T, Saito M, Yoshiya N, Honma S, Tanaka K. A clinicopathologic study of 30 patients with Paget's disease of the vulva. Gynecol Oncol. 1995;56(1):63–70.

16. Parker LP, Parker JR, Bodurka-Bevers D, Deavers M, Bevers MW, Shen-Gunther J, et al. Paget's disease of the vulva: pathology, pattern of involvement, and prognosis. Gynecol Oncol. 2000;77(1):183–9.

17. Sawada Y, Bito T, Kabashima R, Yoshiki R, Hino R, Nakamura M, et al. Ectopic extramammary Paget's disease: case report and literature review. Acta Derm Venereol. 2010;90(5):502–5.

18. Urabe A, Matsukuma A, Shimizu N, Nishimura M, Wada H, Hori Y. Extramammary Paget's disease: comparative histopathologic studies of intraductal carcinoma of the breast and apocrine adenocarcinoma. J Cutan Pathol. 1990;17(5):257–65.

19. Kuehn PG, Tennant R, Brenneman AR. Familial occurrence of extramammary Paget's disease. Cancer. 1973;31(1):145–8.

20. Demitsu T, Gonda K, Tanita M, Takahira K, Inoue T, Okada O, et al. Extramammary Paget's disease in two siblings. Br J Dermatol. 1999;141(5):951–3.

21. Inoue S, Aki T, Mihara M. Extramammary Paget's disease in siblings. Dermatology. 2000;201(2):178.

22. Zhang X, Jin W, Zhu H, Yu H. Extramammary Paget's disease in two brothers. Indian J Dermatol. 2015;60(4):423.

23. Kang Z, Xu F, Zhu Y, Fu P, Q-a Z, Hu T, et al. Genetic analysis of mismatch repair genes alterations in extramammary Paget disease. Am J Surg Pathol. 2016;40(11):1517–25.

24. Marchesa P, Fazio VW, Oliart S, Goldblum JR, Lavery IC, Milsom JW. Long-term outcome of patients with perianal Paget's disease. Ann Surg Oncol. 1997;4(6):475–80.

25. Fanning J, Lambert HL, Hale TM, Morris PC, Schuerch C. Paget's disease of the vulva: prevalence of associated vulvar adenocarcinoma, invasive Paget's disease, and recurrence after surgical excision. Am J Obstet Gynecol. 1999;180(1):24–7.

26. Neuhaus I, Grekin R. Mammary and extramammary Paget disease. Fitzpatrick's dermatology in general medicine. 7th ed. New York: McGraw-Hill; 2008. p. 1094–198.

27. Perrotto J, Abbott JJ, Ceilley RI, Ahmed I. The role of immunohistochemistry in discriminating primary from secondary extramammary Paget disease. Am J Dermatopathol. 2010;32(2):137–43.

28. Willman JH, Golitz LE, Fitzpatrick JE. Vulvar clear cells of Toker: precursors of extramammary Paget's disease. Am J Dermatopathol. 2005;27(3):185–8.

29. Belousova IE, Kazakov DV, Michal M, Suster S. Vulvar toker cells: the long-awaited missing link: a proposal for an origin-based histogenetic classification of extramammary paget disease. Am J Dermatopathol. 2006;28(1):84–6.

30. Lam C, Funaro D. Extramammary Paget's disease: summary of current knowledge. Dermatol Clin. 2010;28(4):807–26.
31. Li YC, Lu LY, Yang YT, Chang CC, Chen LM. Extramammary Paget's disease of the scrotum associated with hepatocellular carcinoma. J Chin Med Assoc. 2009;72(10):542–6.
32. Zollo J, Zeitouni N. The Roswell park cancer institute experience with extramammary Paget's disease. Br J Dermatol. 2000;142(1):59–65.
33. Goldblum JR, Hart WR. Vulvar Paget's disease: a clinicopathologic and immunohistochemical study of 19 cases. Am J Surg Pathol. 1997;21(10):1178–87.
34. Siesling S, Elferink MA, van Dijck JA, Pierie JP, Blokx WA. Epidemiology and treatment of extramammary Paget disease in the Netherlands. Eur J Surg Oncol. 2007;33(8):951–5.
35. Wilkinson EJ, Brown HM. Vulvar Paget disease of urothelial origin: a report of three cases and a proposed classification of vulvar Paget disease. Hum Pathol. 2002;33(5):549–54.
36. McCarter MD, Quan SH, Busam K, Paty PP, Wong D, Guillem JG. Long-term outcome of perianal Paget's disease. Dis Colon Rectum. 2003;46(5):612–6.
37. Salamanca J, Benito A, Garcia-Penalver C, Azorin D, Ballestin C, Rodriguez-Peralto JL. Paget's disease of the glans penis secondary to transitional cell carcinoma of the bladder: a report of two cases and review of the literature. J Cutan Pathol. 2004;31(4):341–5.
38. Lai YL, Yang WG, Tsay PK, Swei H, Chuang SS, Wen CJ. Penoscrotal extramammary Paget's disease: a review of 33 cases in a 20-year experience. Plast Reconstr Surg. 2003;112(4):1017–23.
39. Popiolek DA, Hajdu SI, Gal D. Synchronous Paget's disease of the vulva and breast. Gynecol Oncol. 1998;71(1):137–40.
40. Goldblum JR, Hart WR. Perianal Paget's disease: a histologic and immunohistochemical study of 11 cases with and without associated rectal adenocarcinoma. Am J Surg Pathol. 1998;22(2):170–9.
41. Sasaki M, Terada T, Nakanuma Y, Kono N, Kasahara Y, Watanabe K. Anorectal mucinous adenocarcinoma associated with latent perianal Paget's disease. Am J Gastroenterol. 1990;85(2):199–202.
42. Powell FC, Bjornsson J, Doyle JA, Cooper AJ. Genital Paget's disease and urinary tract malignancy. J Am Acad Dermatol. 1985;13(1):84–90.
43. Koga F, Gotoh S, Suzuki S. A case of invasive bladder cancer with Pagetoid skin lesion of the vulva and anogenital Paget's disease. Nihon Hinyokika Gakkai Zasshi. 1997;88(4):503–6.
44. Allan S, McLaren K, Aldridge R. Paget's disease of the scrotum: a case exhibiting positive prostate-specific antigen staining and associated prostatic adenocarcinoma. Br J Dermatol. 1998;138(4):689–91.
45. Yang WJ, Kim DS, Im YJ, Cho KS, Rha KH, Cho NH, et al. Extramammary Paget's disease of penis and scrotum. Urology. 2005;65(5):972–5.
46. Ekwueme KC, Zakhour HD, Parr NJ. Extramammary Paget's disease of the penis: a case report and review of the literature. J Med Case Reports. 2009;3(1):4.
47. Hoch WH. Adenocarcinoma of the scrotum (extramammary Paget's disease): case report and review of the literature. J Urol. 1984;132(1):137–9.
48. Hashimoto T, Inamoto N, Nakamura K. Triple extramammary Paget's disease. Immunohistochemical studies. Dermatologica. 1986;173(4):174–9.
49. Van Hamme C, Marot L, Dachelet C, Dumont M, Salamon E, Lachapelle JM. Paget's extramammary disease of the axillae and perineum. Ann Dermatol Venereol. 2002;129(5 Pt 1):717–9.
50. Hatta N, Yamada M, Hirano T, Fujimoto A, Morita R. Extramammary Paget's disease: treatment, prognostic factors and outcome in 76 patients. Br J Dermatol. 2008;158(2):313–8.
51. Gonzalez-Castro J, Iranzo P, Palou J, Mascaro J. Extramammary Paget's disease involving the external ear. Br J Dermatol. 1998;138(5):914–5.
52. Inada S, Kohno T, Sakai I. A case of extramammary Paget's disease on the back. Jpn J Clin Dermatol. 1985;39:685–91.

53. Chilukuri S, Page R, Reed JA, Friedman J, Orengo I. Ectopic extramammary Paget's disease arising on the cheek. Dermatol Surg. 2002;28(5):430–3.
54. Cohen MA, Hanly A, Poulos E, Goldstein GD. Extramammary Paget's disease presenting on the face. Dermatol Surg. 2004;30(10):1361–3.
55. Remond B, Aractingi S, Blanc F, Verola O, Vignon D, Dubertret L. Umbilical Paget's disease and prostatic carcinoma. Br J Dermatol. 1993;128(4):448–50.
56. Whorton CM, Patterson JB. Carcinoma of Moll's glands with extramammary Paget's disease of the eyelid. Cancer. 1955;8(5):1009–15.
57. Matsukuma S, Aida S, Shima S, Tamai S. Paget's disease of the esophagus. A case report with review of the literature. Am J Surg Pathol. 1995;19(8):948–55.
58. Higashiyama M, Doi O, Kodama K, Tateishi R, Kurokawa E. Extramammary Paget's disease of the bronchial epithelium. Arch Pathol Lab Med. 1991;115(2):185–8.
59. Changus GW, Yonan TN, Bartolome JS. Extramammary Paget's disease of the tongue. Laryngoscope. 1971;81(10):1621–5.
60. Pierie J-PE, Choudry U, Muzikansky A, Finkelstein DM, Ott MJ. Prognosis and management of extramammary Paget's disease and the association with secondary malignancies. J Am Coll Surg. 2003;196(1):45–50.
61. Koseki S, Mitsuhashi Y, Yoshikawa K, Kondo S. A case of triple extramammary Paget's disease. J Dermatol. 1997;24(8):535–8.
62. Hayashibara Y, Ikeda S. Extramammary Paget's disease with internal malignancies. Gan To Kagaku Ryoho. 1988;15(4 Pt 2–3):1569–75.
63. Nakano S, Narita R, Tabaru A, Ogami Y, Otsuki M. Bile duct cancer associated with extramammary Paget's disease. Am J Gastroenterol. 1995;90(3):507–8.
64. Balducci L, Crawford ED, Smith GF, Lambuth B, McGehee R, Hardy C. Extramammary Paget's disease: an annotated review. Cancer Invest. 1988;6(3):293–303.
65. Chen YH, Wong TW, Lee J. Depigmented genital extramammary Paget's disease: a possible histogenetic link to Toker's clear cells and clear cell papulosis. J Cutan Pathol. 2001;28(2):105–8.
66. Iwenofu OH, Samie FH, Ralston J, Cheney RT, Zeitouni NC. Extramammary Paget's disease presenting as alopecia neoplastica. J Cutan Pathol. 2008;35(8):761–4.
67. Bansal D, Bowman CA. Extramammary Paget's disease masquerading as lichen sclerosus. Int J STD AIDS. 2004;15(2):141–2.
68. Murata Y, Kumano K, Tani M. Underpants-pattern erythema: a previously unrecognized cutaneous manifestation of extramammary Paget's disease of the genitalia with advanced metastatic spread. J Am Acad Dermatol. 1999;40(6 Pt 1):949–56.
69. Shaco-Levy R, Bean SM, Vollmer RT, Jewell E, Jones EL, Valdes CL, et al. Paget disease of the vulva: a study of 56 cases. Eur J Obstet Gynecol Reprod Biol. 2010;149(1):86–91.
70. Wolff K, Johnson RA. Fitzpatrick's color atlas and synopsis of clinical dermatology. New York: McGraw Hill; 2009.
71. O'connor WJ, Lim KK, Zalla MJ, Gagnot M, Otley CC, Nguyen TH, et al. Comparison of Mohs micrographic surgery and wide excision for extramammary Paget's disease. Dermatol Surg. 2003;29(7):723–7.
72. Bhatia P, Ahuja A, Dey P, Suri V. Vulval intraepithelial neoplasia with extra mammary pagets disease: a rare association. J Clin Pathol. 2007;60(1):110–2.
73. Jones RE Jr, Austin C, Ackerman AB. Extramammary Paget's disease: a critical reexamination. Am J Dermatopathol. 1979;1(2):101–32.
74. Roth LM, Lee SC, Ehrlich CE. Paget's disease of the vulva. A histogenetic study of five cases including ultrastructural observations and review of the literature. Am J Surg Pathol. 1977;1(3):193–206.
75. Sitakalin C, Ackerman AB. Mammary and extramammary Paget's disease. Am J Dermatopathol. 1985;7(4):335–40.
76. Ishida-Yamamoto A, Sato K, Wada T, Takahashi H, Toyota N, Shibaki T, et al. Fibroepithelioma-like changes occurring in perianal Paget's disease with rectal mucinous

carcinoma: case report and review of 49 cases of extramammary Paget's disease. J Cutan Pathol. 2002;29(3):185–9.

77. Battles OE, Page DL, Johnson JE. Cytokeratins, CEA, and mucin histochemistry in the diagnosis and characterization of extramammary Paget's disease. Am J Clin Pathol. 1997;108(1):6–12.

78. Lundquist K, Kohler S, Rouse RV. Intraepidermal cytokeratin 7 expression is not restricted to Paget cells but is also seen in Toker cells and Merkel cells. Am J Surg Pathol. 1999;23(2):212–9.

79. Kohler S, Smoller BR. Gross cystic disease fluid protein-15 reactivity in extramammary Paget's disease with and without associated internal malignancy. Am J Dermatopathol. 1996;18(2):118–23.

80. Nowak MA, Guerriere-Kovach P, Pathan A, Campbell TE. Perianal Paget's disease: distinguishing primary and secondary lesions using immunohistochemical studies including gross cystic disease fluid protein-15 and cytokeratin 20 expression. Arch Pathol Lab Med. 1998;122(12):1077.

81. Mazoujian G, Pinkus GS, Haagensen DE Jr. Extramammary Paget's disease--evidence for an apocrine origin. An immunoperoxidase study of gross cystic disease fluid protein-15, carcinoembryonic antigen, and keratin proteins. Am J Surg Pathol. 1984;8(1):43–50.

82. Liegl B, Leibl S, Gogg-Kamerer M, Tessaro B, Horn LC, Moinfar F. Mammary and extramammary Paget's disease: an immunohistochemical study of 83 cases. Histopathology. 2007;50(4):439–47.

83. Kuan S-F, Montag AG, Hart J, Krausz T, Recant W. Differential expression of mucin genes in mammary and extramammary Paget's disease. Am J Surg Pathol. 2001;25(12):1469–77.

84. Yoshii N, Kitajima S, Yonezawa S, Matsukita S, Setoyama M, Kanzaki T. Expression of mucin core proteins in extramammary Paget's disease. Pathol Int. 2002;52(5–6):390–9.

85. Alo PL, Galati GM, Sebastiani V, Ricci F, Visca P, Mariani L, et al. Fatty acid synthase expression in Paget's disease of the vulva. Int J Gynecol Pathol. 2005;24(4):404–8.

86. Mori O, Hachisuka H, Sasai Y. Immunohistochemical demonstration of epithelial membrane antigen (EMA), carcinoembryonic antigen (CEA), and keratin on mammary and extramammary Paget's disease. Acta Histochem. 1989;85(1):93–100.

87. Enjoji M, Noguchi K, Watanabe H, Yoshida Y, Kotoh K, Nakashima M, et al. A novel tumour marker RCAS1 in a case of extramammary Paget's disease. Clin Exp Dermatol. 2003;28(2):211–3.

88. Liegl B, Horn LC, Moinfar F. Androgen receptors are frequently expressed in mammary and extramammary Paget's disease. Mod Pathol. 2005;18(10):1283–8.

89. Diaz de Leon E, Carcangiu ML, Prieto VG, McCue PA, Burchette JL, To G, et al. Extramammary Paget disease is characterized by the consistent lack of estrogen and progesterone receptors but frequently expresses androgen receptor. Am J Clin Pathol. 2000;113(4):572–5.

90. Plaza JA, Torres-Cabala C, Ivan D, Prieto VG. HER-2/neu expression in extramammary Paget disease: a clinicopathologic and immunohistochemistry study of 47 cases with and without underlying malignancy. J Cutan Pathol. 2009;36(7):729–33.

91. Ogawa T, Nagashima Y, Wada H, Akimoto K, Chiba Y, Nagatani T, et al. Extramammary Paget's disease: analysis of growth signal pathway from the human epidermal growth factor receptor 2 protein. Hum Pathol. 2005;36(12):1273–80.

92. Gu M, Ghafari S, Lin F. Pap smears of patients with extramammary Paget's disease of the vulva. Diagn Cytopathol. 2005;32(6):353–7.

93. Oji M, Furue M, Tamaki K. Serum carcinoembryonic antigen level in Paget's disease. Br J Dermatol. 1984;110(2):211–3.

94. Hammer A, Hager H, Steiniche T. Prostate-specific antigen-positive extramammary Paget's disease—association with prostate cancer. Apmis. 2008;116(1):81–8.

95. Petković S, Jeremić K, Vidakovic S, Jeremić J, Lazović G. Paget's disease of the vulva--a review of our experience. Eur J Gynaecol Oncol. 2005;27(6):611–2.

96. Tsutsumida A, Yamamoto Y, Minakawa H, Yoshida T, Kokubu I, Sugihara T. Indications for lymph node dissection in the treatment of extramammary Paget's disease. Dermatol Surg. 2003;29(1):21–4.
97. Murata Y, Kumano K. Extramammary Paget's disease of the genitalia with clinically clear margins can be adequately resected with 1 cm margin. Eur J Dermatol. 2005;15(3):168–70.
98. Hendi A, Brodland DG, Zitelli JA. Extramammary Paget's disease: surgical treatment with Mohs micrographic surgery. J Am Acad Dermatol. 2004;51(5):767–73.
99. Appert DL, Otley CC, Phillips PK, Roenigk RK. Role of multiple scouting biopsies before Mohs micrographic surgery for extramammary Paget's disease. Dermatol Surg. 2005;31(11):1417–22.
100. Kato T, Fujimoto N, Fujii N, Tanaka T. Mapping biopsy with punch biopsies to determine surgical margin in extramammary Paget's disease. J Dermatol. 2013;40(12):968–72.
101. Yelamos O, Hibler BP, Cordova M, Hollmann TJ, Kose K, Marchetti MA, et al. Handheld reflectance confocal microscopy for the detection of recurrent extramammary Paget disease. JAMA Dermatol. 2017.
102. Kim SJ, Thompson AK, Zubair AS, Otley CC, Arpey CJ, Baum CL, et al. Surgical treatment and outcomes of patients with extramammary paget disease: a cohort study. Dermatol Surg. 2017.
103. Misas JE, Cold CJ, Hall FW. Vulvar Paget disease: fluorescein-aided visualization of margins. Obstet Gynecol. 1991;77(1):156–9.
104. Johnson TM, Headington J, Baker SR, Lowe L. Usefulness of the staged excision for lentigo maligna and lentigo maligna melanoma: the "square" procedure. J Am Acad Dermatol. 1997;37(5:758–64.
105. Hendi A, Perdikis G, Snow JL. Unifocality of extramammary Paget disease. J Am Acad Dermatol. 2008;59(5):811–3.
106. Zhu Y, Ye DW, Chen ZW, Zhang SL, Qin XJ. Frozen section-guided wide local excision in the treatment of penoscrotal extramammary Paget's disease. BJU Int. 2007;100(6):1282–7.
107. Damavandy AA, Hendi A, Zitelli JA. Surgical treatment of cutaneous extramammary Paget's disease. Curr Dermatol Rep. 2016;5(3):166–71.
108. Fishman DA, Chambers SK, Schwartz PE, Kohorn EI, Chambers JT. Extramammary Paget's disease of the vulva. Gynecol Oncol. 1995;56(2):266–70.
109. Gunn RA, Gallager HS. Vulvar Paget's disease. A topographic study. Cancer. 1980;46(3):590–4.
110. Louis-Sylvestre C, Haddad B, Paniel BJ. Paget's disease of the vulva: results of different conservative treatments. Eur J Obstet Gynecol Reprod Biol. 2001;99(2):253–5.
111. Stacy D, Burrell MO, Franklin EW 3rd. Extramammary Paget's disease of the vulva and anus: use of intraoperative frozen-section margins. Am J Obstet Gynecol. 1986;155(3):519–23.
112. Bae JM, Choi YY, Kim H, Oh BH, Roh MR, Nam K, et al. Mohs micrographic surgery for extramammary Paget disease: a pooled analysis of individual patient data. J Am Acad Dermatol. 2013;68(4):632–7.
113. Thomas CJ, Wood GC, Marks VJ. Mohs micrographic surgery in the treatment of rare aggressive cutaneous tumors: the Geisinger experience. Dermatol Surg. 2007;33(3):333–9.
114. Abide JM, Nahai F, Bennett RG. The meaning of surgical margins. Plast Reconstr Surg. 1984;73(3):492–7.
115. Coldiron BM, Goldsmith BA, Robinson JK. Surgical treatment of extramammary Paget's disease. A report of six cases and a reexamination of Mohs micrographic surgery compared with conventional surgical excision. Cancer. 1991;67(4):933–8.
116. Bergen S, DiSaia PJ, Liao SY, Berman ML. Conservative management of extramammary Paget's disease of the vulva. Gynecol Oncol. 1989;33(2):151–6.
117. Guerrieri M, Back MF. Extramammary Paget's disease: role of radiation therapy. Australas Radiol. 2002;46(2):204–8.
118. Burrows NP, Jones DH, Hudson PM, Pye RJ. Treatment of extramammary Paget's disease by radiotherapy. Br J Dermatol. 1995;132(6):970–2.

119. Moreno-Arias G, Conill C, Castells-Mas A, Arenas M, Grimalt R. Radiotherapy for genital extramammary Paget's disease in situ. Dermatol Surg. 2001;27(6):587–90.
120. Yanagi T, Kato N, Yamane N, Osawa R. Radiotherapy for extramammary Paget's disease: histopathological findings after radiotherapy. Clin Exp Dermatol. 2007;32(5):506–8.
121. Besa P, Rich TA, Delclos L, Edwards CL, Ota DM, Wharton JT. Extramammary Paget's disease of the perineal skin: role of radiotherapy. Int J Radiat Oncol Biol Phys. 1992;24(1):73–8.
122. Luk N, Yu K, Yeung W, Choi C, Teo M. Extramammary Paget's disease: outcome of radiotherapy with curative intent. Clin Exp Dermatol. 2003;28(4):360–3.
123. Hata M, Koike I, Wada H, Miyagi E, Kasuya T, Kaizu H, et al. Radiation therapy for extramammary Paget's disease: treatment outcomes and prognostic factors. Ann Oncol. 2013;25(1):291–7. https://doi.org/10.1093/annonc/mdt478.
124. Brierley J, Stockdale A. Radiotherapy: an effective treatment for extramammary Paget's disease. Clin Oncol. 1991;3(1):3–5.
125. Kwan W, Teo P, Ngar Y, Yu K, Choi P. Perineal Paget's disease: effective treatment with fractionated high dose rate brachytherapy. Clin Oncol. 1995;7(6):400–1.
126. Korbelik M, Dougherty GJ. Photodynamic therapy-mediated immune response against subcutaneous mouse tumors. Cancer Res. 1999;59(8):1941–6.
127. Henta T, Itoh Y, Kobayashi M, Ninomiya Y, Ishibashi A. Photodynamic therapy for inoperable vulval Paget's disease using – aminolaevulinic acid: successful management of a large skin lesion. Br J Dermatol. 1999;141:347–9.
128. Shieh S, Dee A, Cheney R, Frawley N, Zeitouni N, Oseroff A. Photodynamic therapy for the treatment of extramammary Paget's disease. Br J Dermatol. 2002;146(6):1000–5.
129. Housel JP, Izikson L, Zeitouni NC. Noninvasive extramammary Paget's disease treated with photodynamic therapy: case series from the Roswell Park Cancer Institute. Dermatol Surg. 2010;36(11):1718–24.
130. Mikasa K, Watanabe D, Kondo C, Kobayashi M, Nakaseko H, Yokoo K, et al. 5-Aminolevulinic acid-based photodynamic therapy for the treatment of two patients with extramammary Paget's disease. J Dermatol. 2005;32(2):97–101.
131. Li Q, Gao T, Jiao B, Qi X, Long HA, Qiao H, et al. Long-term follow-up of in situ extramammary Paget's disease in Asian skin types IV/V treated with photodynamic therapy. Acta Derm Venereol. 2010;90(2):159–64.
132. Becker-Wegerich PM, Fritsch C, Schulte KW, Megahed M, Neuse W, Goerz G, et al. Carbon dioxide laser treatment of extramammary Paget's disease guided by photodynamic diagnosis. Br J Dermatol. 1998;138(1):169–72.
133. Ewing TL. Paget's disease of the vulva treated by combined surgery and laser. Gynecol Oncol. 1991;43(2):137–40.
134. Kurzl RG. Paget's disease. Semin Dermatol. 1996;15(1):60–6.
135. Zampogna JC, Flowers FP, Roth WI, Hassenein AM. Treatment of primary limited cutaneous extramammary Paget's disease with topical imiquimod monotherapy: two case reports. J Am Acad Dermatol. 2002;47(4):S229–S35.
136. Berman B, Spencer J, Villa A, Poochareon V, Elgart G. Successful treatment of extramammary Paget's disease of the scrotum with imiquimod 5% cream. Clin Exp Dermatol. 2003;28(s1):36–8.
137. Cohen PR, Schulze KE, Tschen JA, Hetherington GW, Nelson BR. Treatment of extramammary Paget disease with topical imiquimod cream: case report and literature review. South Med J. 2006;99(4):396–403.
138. Wang LC, Blanchard A, Judge DE, Lorincz AA, Medenica MM, Busbey S. Successful treatment of recurrent extramammary Paget's disease of the vulva with topical imiquimod 5% cream. J Am Acad Dermatol. 2003;49(4):769–71.
139. Luyten A, Sörgel P, Clad A, Gieseking F, Maass-Poppenhusen K, Lellé RJ, et al. Treatment of extramammary Paget disease of the vulva with imiquimod: a retrospective, multicenter study by the German Colposcopy Network. J Am Acad Dermatol. 2014;70(4):644–50.

140. Ye JN, Rhew DC, Yip F, Edelstein L. Extramammary Paget's disease resistant to surgery and imiquimod monotherapy but responsive to imiquimod combination topical chemotherapy with 5-fluorouracil and retinoic acid: a case report. Cutis. 2006;77(4):245–50.
141. Qian Z, Zeitoun N, Shieh S, Helm T, Oseroff A. Successful treatment of extramammary Paget's disease with imiquimod. J Drugs Dermatol JDD. 2003;2(1):73–6.
142. Vereecken P, Awada A, Ghanem G, da Costa CM, Larsimont D, Simoens C, et al. A therapeutic approach to perianal extramammary Paget's disease: topical imiquimod can be useful to prevent or defer surgery. Med Sci Monit. 2007;13(6):CS75–CS7.
143. Machida H, Moeini A, Roman LD, Matsuo K. Effects of imiquimod on vulvar Paget's disease: a systematic review of literature. Gynecol Oncol. 2015;139(1):165–71.
144. Eliezri YD, Silvers DN, Horan DB. Role of preoperative topical 5-fluorouracil in preparation for Mohs micrographic surgery of extramammary Paget's disease. J Am Acad Dermatol. 1987;17(3):497–505.
145. Del Castillo L, Garcia C, Schoendorff C, Garcia J, Torres L, Garcia AD. Spontaneous apparent clinical resolution with histologic persistence of a case of extramammary Paget's disease: response to topical 5-fluorouracil. Cutis. 2000;65(5):331–3.
146. Watring WG, Roberts JA, Lagasse LD, Berman ML, Ballon SC, Moore JG, et al. Treatment of recurrent Paget's disease of the vulva with topical bleomycin. Cancer. 1978;41(1):10–1.
147. Thirlby RC, Hammer CJ, Galagan KA, Travaglini JJ, Picozzi VJ. Perianal Paget's disease: successful treatment with combined chemoradiotherapy. Dis Colon Rectum. 1990;33(2):150–2.
148. Yamazaki N. Chemotherapy for advanced adenocarcinoma of the skin: experience with combination chemotherapy and a review of the literature. Gan to kagaku ryoho Cancer & chemotherapy. 1997;24(1):30–6.
149. Watanabe Y, Hoshiai H, Ueda H, Nakai H, Obata K, Noda K. Low-dose mitomycin C, etoposide, and cisplatin for invasive vulvar Paget's disease. Int J Gynecol Cancer. 2002;12(3):304–7.
150. Kariya K, Tsuji T, Schwartz RA. Trial of Low-dose 5-fluorouracil/cisplatin therapy for advanced extramammary Paget's disease. Dermatol Surg. 2004;30(s2):341–4.
151. Oguchi S, Kaneko M, Uhara H, Saida T. Docetaxel induced durable response in advanced extramammary Paget's disease: a case report. J Dermatol. 2002;29(1):33–7.
152. Kao SC-H, Yap ML, Berry M, Santos L, Lin M, Goldrick A. Metastatic extramammary paget's disease responding to cisplatin, 5-fluorouracil and radiotherapy-a case report. Asia Pac J Clin Oncol. 2009;1:3.
153. Beleznay K, Levesque M, Gill S. Response to 5-fluorouracil in metastatic extramammary Paget disease of the scrotum presenting as pancytopenia and back pain. Curr Oncol. 2009;16(5):81–3.
154. Fujisawa Y, Umebayashi Y, Otsuka F. Metastatic extramammary Paget's disease successfully controlled with tumour dormancy therapy using docetaxel. Br J Dermatol. 2006;154(2):375–6.
155. Mochitomi Y, Sakamoto R, Gushi A, Hashiguchi T, Mera K, Matsushita S, et al. Extramammary Paget's disease/carcinoma successfully treated with a combination chemotherapy: report of two cases. J Dermatol. 2005;32(8):632–7.
156. Tanskanen M, Jahkola T, Asko-Seljavaara S, Jalkanen J, Isola J. HER2 oncogene amplification in extramammary Paget's disease. Histopathology. 2003;42(6):575–9.
157. Takahagi S, Noda H, Kamegashira A, Madokoro N, Hori I, Shindo H, et al. Metastatic extramammary Paget's disease treated with paclitaxel and trastuzumab combination chemotherapy. J Dermatol. 2009;36(8):457–61.

Chapter 12
Procedures in the Diagnosis and Treatment of Skin Cancer

Sarah Yagerman and Mary L. Stevenson

Abstract Skin cancer is the most common type of cancer in the United States and constitutes a health burden to the population. Comprised predominately of basal cell carcinoma, cutaneous squamous cell carcinoma, and melanoma, skin cancer accounts for nearly 20,000 deaths annually. Early diagnosis and treatment of skin cancer are critical in limiting morbidity and mortality. Diagnosis is generally made based on close examination and biopsy of suspicious lesions. Appropriate treatment depends on the specific histopathologic diagnosis as well as other considerations including area and size of the lesion and comorbidities of the patient. Treatment modalities include superficial therapies, such as cryotherapy or topical treatment, electrodessication and curettage, and surgical therapies including standard excision and Mohs micrographic surgery. Additionally, for more advanced disease, treatment may require a multidisciplinary approach, often with involvement of medical and radiation oncologists, and may include the use of systemic agents or radiation therapy.

Keywords Biopsy · Excision · Melanoma · Atypical nevi · Non-melanoma skin cancer · Keratinocyte carcinoma · Basal cell carcinoma · Cutaneous squamous cell carcinoma · Mohs micrographic surgery

Introduction

Skin cancer is the most common cancer in the United States with one in five Americans developing some form in their lifetime [1]. The vast majority of these cancers are keratinocyte carcinomas (KCs), formerly known as non-melanoma skin cancers (NMSC), with 5.4 million cases treated in 3.3 million people in 2012 [2]. Basal cell carcinoma, a form of KC, is the most common skin cancer, followed

S. Yagerman · M. L. Stevenson (✉)
The Ronald O. Perelman Department of Dermatology,
NYU Langone Medical Center, New York, NY, USA
e-mail: mary.stevenson@nyumc.org

© Springer International Publishing AG, part of Springer Nature 2018
A. Hanlon (ed.), *A Practical Guide to Skin Cancer*,
https://doi.org/10.1007/978-3-319-74903-7_12

second by squamous cell carcinoma [2]. While rarer, melanoma contributes significant mortality claiming roughly 9,000 lives each year in the United States and accounts for the majority of skin cancer-related deaths [3, 4], though, in the Central and Southern United States, rates of death from cutaneous squamous cell carcinoma (CSCC) rival those of other cancers including melanoma [5]. Skin conditions collectively are fourth among all diseases globally in an assessment of years lost to disability. KC is second only to diabetic ulcers in the list of contributing skin conditions [6]. It is estimated that in the United States skin cancer treatment costs $8.1 billion per year [7].

Identification of suspicious lesions through routine total body skin exams is the first step in diagnosis and treatment of cutaneous malignancies. While the US Preventive Services Task Force has concluded there is insufficient evidence to recommend an annual skin examination by a physician [6], the American Academy of Dermatology and American Cancer Society encourage routine total body skin exams especially for those at high risk for skin cancer. A recent survey of US dermatologists showed that the majority screen patients at least every 2–3 years and those at higher risk for skin cancer were most often screened semiannually or annually [8]. Features to help identify a patient at risk include history of blistering sunburns as a teenager, red or blonde hair, marked freckling of the upper back, family history of melanoma, and intermittent high-intensity sun exposure [9, 10]. Additionally, patients with any history of skin cancer should have routine follow-up to assess for recurrence and new primary skin cancers.

After identification of a suspicious lesion on exam, the next step is to perform a biopsy, which will be discussed in detail below. The specimen will be submitted to a dermatopathology lab and processed for histopathologic evaluation. Depending on the subtype of skin cancer, treatment may range from surgical treatment, localized destruction, radiation, or in some cases topical therapy or systemic chemotherapy. In this chapter, the diagnosis and treatment of KCs will be discussed separately from atypical melanocytic neoplasms and malignant melanomas. And while the majority of skin cancers may be treated by a dermatologist or dermatologic surgeon, the treatment of specific types of skin cancer may rely on an interdisciplinary approach from the primary care physician, dermatologist, surgeons (including dermatologic surgeons, ENT surgeons, plastic surgeons, and surgical oncologists), and sometimes a radiation oncologist and/or medical oncologist.

Keratinocyte Carcinomas, Formerly Non-melanoma Skin Cancers

Keratinocyte carcinoma (KC) refers to any type of skin cancer whose cell of origin is a keratinocyte. Keratinocytes are found in the epidermis, and the two primary forms of KC are cutaneous squamous cell carcinoma (CSCC) and basal cell carcinoma (BCC). These types of carcinomas were formerly referred to as non-melanoma skin cancer; however, their rising incidence and implication in public health merit them with the more apt name of keratinocyte carcinoma [11]. These cancers are so common that they are not included in the Surveillance, Epidemiology, and End Results (SEER) program database making it difficult to ascertain their exact incidence. It is estimated that there are 700,000 cases of CSCC and two million cases of BCC per year in the United States [12, 13]. BCC is the single most common cancer in the United States, more common than all other cancers combined [14]. Aggressive forms of BCC which are at higher risk for recurrence are determined histologically and include morpheaform, infiltrating, metatypical, and micronodular BCC, as well as BCC with perineural invasion. Similarly, certain CSCCs are considered to be more aggressive, or high risk for recurrence and potential metastasis, with the most recognized high-risk features including location on the ear or lip, tumors deeper than 2 mm, diameter greater than or equal to 2 cm, poor cellular differentiation, and perineural invasion [15, 16]. Additionally, skin cancers occurring in the setting of a patient with immunosuppression may be considered high risk.

Biopsy

Lesions suspicious for KC include features of scale, redness, erosion, ulceration, bleeding, and persistence or a lesion that is non-healing [17]. Pigmented BCCs and CSCCs may be more difficult to identify with their clinical features sometimes overlapping with atypical melanocytic neoplasms which will be discussed further below. After identification of a suspicious lesion, the first diagnostic test is skin biopsy. A skin biopsy allows for a small sample of epidermis and dermis to be submitted and reviewed by a dermatopathologist for definitive diagnosis. Risks of skin biopsy include bleeding, infection, and scarring which should be disclosed to the patient. Determination of which type of cutaneous biopsy is appropriate will depend on the size of the neoplasm and the anatomic location. The most common types of biopsy include a punch biopsy, a shave biopsy, and an excisional biopsy. The latter will be discussed in further detail under melanocytic neoplasms. Execution of a biopsy requires a good setup of the necessary instruments (Table 12.1, Fig. 12.1).

Similar to any procedure, the clinician should have a checklist of all steps performed each time the skin is biopsied. Once the decision to biopsy is made, the reason for obtaining the biopsy and risks of the procedure should be discussed with the patient. Verbal and written consent should be obtained, and steps should be taken—whether it is photograph of the lesion, triangulation, or both such that if the lesion is identified as a skin cancer, it may be correctly identified and treated in the future. Triangulation measures the lesion of concern's location with respect to two or three additional anatomy landmarks on the patient. This will help the surgeon to identify the biopsy site, should definitive treatment be delayed to the point where the primary lesion is no longer visible, and to prevent wrong site procedures [19, 20].

Table 12.1 A comprehensive list of supplies to set up for a successful biopsy and their uses [18]

Supply	Function
Isopropyl alcohol, iodine, or chlorhexidine	Skin cleansing prep
Sterile gauze 4 × 4	Holding pressure for hemostasis, keeping a clean surgical field
Gloves- nitrile	Clean technique
Cloth or fenestrated drape	Creating a clean field to work on
Syringes 1 and 3 ml	Holding anesthetic
Needles: 18 G and 30 G	To draw up lidocaine and inject it, respectively
Lidocaine 1% with epinephrine 1:100,000	Numbing the patient
Size 15 surgical blade or punch 3, 4, or 6 mm	For obtaining the specimen
Tissue forceps	For shave or punch biopsy
Tissue scissors	For punch biopsy
Needle holder	For punch biopsy
20% aluminum chloride	For hemostasis in a shave biopsy
Sutures	For punch biopsy closure
Petrolatum and band aid or dressing	To dress wound
Formalin bottle	For specimen

From Skin biopsy techniques for the internist, Patrick C. Alguire, Jan 1, 1998, Volume 13, Issue 1, Table 2, with kind permission from SpringerNature and Patrick C. Alguire

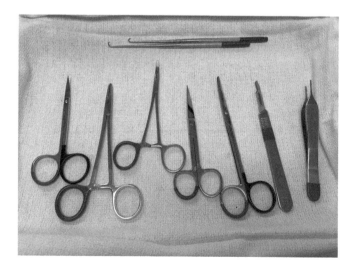

Fig. 12.1 Useful instruments which may be used for shave, punch, or excisional biopsy. From left to right: curved iris scissors, needle driver, hemostat, suture scissors, baby Metzenbaums, 15 blade and handle, and Addison forceps. Above are two skin hooks which may aid in skin stabilization and minimize trauma

Fig. 12.2 Demonstration of injection technique for numbing the skin. Notice the 30-gauge needle enters the skin at an acute angle, causing a bleb to form underneath the lesion of interest

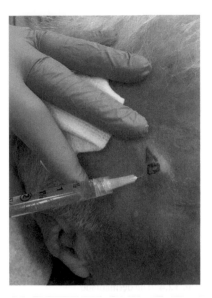

Shave Biopsy

The shave biopsy, generally the preferred method for sampling cutaneous neoplasms, does not require sutures. The area to be biopsied should be marked with a surgical marking pen prior to initiation, as injection with lidocaine may distort the primary cutaneous process. Then the skin should be prepped with alcohol, iodine, or chlorhexidine. Chlorhexidine has a longer duration of action but must not be used near the eyes or ears where it may cause keratitis or otitis, respectively [21]. Local anesthesia by subcutaneous injection is then performed. Use of 1% lidocaine with or without epinephrine is standard of care [14]. While the onset of lidocaine is extremely rapid, several minutes are needed for epinephrine to vasoconstrict the surrounding blood vessels, and procedures in highly vascular areas should allow several minutes between time of injection and time of biopsy. For patients with a true allergy to lidocaine, use of either ester-type local anesthetics, bacteriostatic normal saline, or 1% diphenhydramine is suggested as an alternative. In the pediatric population, premedication with topical lidocaine may be beneficial prior to injection. Lidocaine 1% generally with epinephrine 1:100,000 is injected with a 30-gauge needle at a 30-degree angle to the skin until desired anesthesia is obtained, generally not more than 1 cc for small biopsies, though doses up to 7 mg/kg are safe at this concentration (4.5 mg/kg if 1% plain lidocaine is used without epinephrine) (Fig. 12.2).

The shape and properties such as depth of resultant specimen depend on the technique of shave biopsy used. Commonly, a #15 blade, held like a pencil between the thumb and third digit with the index finger stabilizing the blade with pressure from above, may be used to score around the lesion, and then the belly of the blade is used in a horizontal pass to come under the specimen and remove it (Fig. 12.3).

Fig. 12.3 A shave biopsy
being performed with a #
15 blade on the face. The
skin is stabilized with the
non-dominant hand

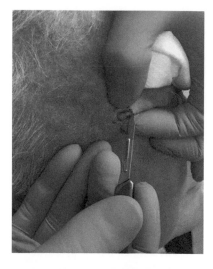

Fig. 12.4 The dermablade
is flexible and can be
grasped on both ends to
create a curved sharp for
biopsy. Shave biopsy with
a dermablade. Note again
the skin is stabilized with
the opposite hand

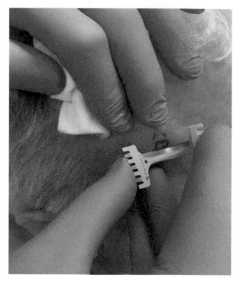

This technique of scoring allows for precision of margins, though with some neo-plasms, this may not be necessary, and this step is skipped in favor of a free-form shave. A dermablade is a device that allows for a swooping single scoop shave of a specimen, and it may be beneficial for larger lesions or for ease of use (Fig. 12.4). It is important to go as deep as the reticular dermis in order not to miss an infiltrative component of the neoplasm. Blebbing of the skin with superficial injection of anes-thetic or pinching of perilesional skin may elevate flat tissue and aid in obtaining the entire specimen including any dermal components. Forceps with upward traction may also be used but should be used with care as too much pressure on the specimen can crush it making dermatopathologic evaluation more difficult. The specimen

Fig. 12.5 A 4 mm
diameter disposable punch
instrument. Note the shape
is perfectly circular

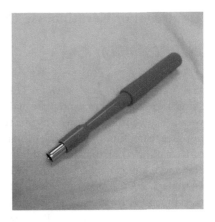

should then be placed in formalin and submitted to dermatopathology. Hemostasis may be achieved with the use of electrocautery or 20% aluminum chloride. The latter is a flammable material, so caution should be used when electrocautery is also needed, and in general their use together should be avoided, or the area should be allowed to dry prior to electrocautery. Additionally, this chemical should be avoided near the eyes. Heat cautery should be used in patients with a defibrillator or pacemaker. Alternatively, hemostasis may be obtained with direct pressure for approximately 10 min. White petrolatum and a band aid or pressure dressing should then be applied.

Punch Biopsy

A punch biopsy is generally reserved for inflammatory skin conditions. However, it may be the right technique on small lesions, under 6 mm, and those where closure with sutures may leave a better cosmetic result. The technique generally utilizes a small disposable punch instrument to take a cylindrical tissue specimen (Fig. 12.5). The same steps of marking, skin prep, and numbing as above are performed. The punch instrument is then applied perpendicularly to the skin and swiveled to the point of the hub or to desired depth. Skin forceps may be used to pick up the sample and skin scissors to cut the base and free the specimen. The specimen should then be placed in formalin and submitted to dermatopathology for processing and analysis. Most commonly a 3 or 4 mm diameter punch is used with 6 mm punch biopsies being reserved for larger lesions with two–three sutures placed for hemostasis or more if necessary. Hemostasis may be obtained with gel foam for 3 mm punches though this should not be employed in highly cosmetically sensitive areas such as the face. Generally, a suture such as 6-0 nylon or similar suture may be used on the face, with 4-0 nylon or similar suture being used on the trunk and 5-0 nylon being used on the extremities and neck. The site should then be dressed with white petrolatum and a band aid applied.

Treatment of Keratinocyte Carcinoma

Local Treatment

Electrodessication and curettage (ED & C) is a destructive technique used to treat skin cancers. The skin is prepped and numbed, as described above, and then scraped with a sharp curette followed by electrodessication. This cycle of scraping and burning is repeated up to three times on a given lesion. It is a valid option for treatment of KCs of low-risk locations and low-risk subtypes. For BCCs the subtypes superficial and nodular may be treated with this method. Overall 5-year cure rates range from 91% to 97% in patients with BCC treated by ED & C [22–24]. ED & C is not recommended for morpheaform, infiltrative, or micronodular BCC. ED & C may also be used for squamous cell carcinoma in situ (CSCCIS) and for CSCC less than 1 cm in diameter found on the trunk or extremities without high-risk features though for the CSCC treatment by surgical modality is optimal [25]. The disadvantages of this technique are two-fold. First, no tissue is submitted to pathology to confirm complete removal of the tumor. Furthermore, they heal by secondary intention which may not leave the most desirable scar. The advantage is it offers a rapid in-office minimally invasive technique.

Standard excision with postoperative margin assessment by dermatopathology is when the biopsied site and a margin of the normal skin are removed with a #15 blade and generally repaired using deep dermal sutures and superficial cutaneous sutures, depending on the area of the carcinoma and the laxity of the surround skin. The general shape of excision for best closure is elliptical [26]. This technique is appropriate for the treatment of both low-risk BCCs and CSCCs. For high-risk lesions, as defined above, delayed repair of the skin until clear margins have been confirmed should be considered in order to avoid excessive manipulation of surrounding skin with unknown margin status. In BCCs overall 5-year disease-free recurrence rate is approximately 95% [27]. In another study disease-free rates approach 98% [28] which may be the result of choosing appropriate cases for this technique. A 4 mm clinical margin for BCCs under 2 cm in diameter is recommended [29]. For CSCCs excision with a 4 mm margin is recommended or 6 mm for a high risk lesion [23]. However, Mohs micrographic surgery, discussed below, is the optimal technique when available for this subset of high risk skin cancers and for KCs in cosmetically sensitive areas such as the face. Five-year recurrence rates with standard surgical excision may be as high as 5% in primary CSCCs using the advisable margins above [30]. This number of recurrences approaches 10–18% for high risk locations such as the lip and ear and is why Mohs micrographic surgery is preferred in these lesions as discussed below [31].

Mohs micrographic surgery (MMS) is a specialized excisional technique developed by Frederic Mohs in the late 1930s, which allows for intraoperative assessment of 100% of the cancer margin [32]. The technique takes stages or serial excisions of the skin and then assesses margins with specialized processing on frozen sectioning to assess that the keratinocytic carcinoma has been removed in its entirety. The two primary advantages are that it allows for complete margin evaluation prior to closure of the skin, and MMS is a tissue-sparing technique, ideal for cosmetically sensitive areas. This type of surgery is ideal for high risk variants of both BCCs and CSCCs or for these tumors when they occur in cosmetically sensitive areas such as the face. The Appropriate Use Criteria published by the American Academy of Dermatology, American College of Mohs Surgery, American Society for Dermatologic Surgery Association, and American Society for Mohs Surgery in 2012 can aid the physician in determining which cases are appropriate for referral to this skilled excisional technique [33]. In general MMS is used for primary aggressive BCCs in immunocompetent patients except small lesions (less than or equal to 5 mm) on the trunk or extremities (excluding pretibial surfaces, hands, feet, nail units, and ankles). Nodular BCC may also be treated with MMS though lesions 1 cm or less in diameter on the trunk and extremities may be treated with standard excision. The overall 5-year cure rate of BCCs treated with MMS is over 99% [27]. For CSCCs MMS is appropriate and should be standard of care in clinically aggressive tumors, which include the aforementioned features of high risk size (equal to or over 2 cm in greatest diameter), high risk anatomic location (the scalp, ears, lip, midface, genitalia, and nail units), rapid growth, poorly defined margins, and ulceration [16]. Additionally in immunocompetent patients, MMS is the treatment of choice for all CSCCs except for those 1 cm or less in greatest diameter on the trunk or extremities (excluding the pretibial surface, hands, feet, nail units, and ankles). MMS should also be the treatment of choice for recurrent tumors. Finally tumors in immunocompromised patients, which include patients with active HIV, who had organ transplant, with hematologic malignancy, or on pharmacologic immunosuppression, are also at high risk of recurrence, and MMS may provide more definitive cure for these patients with standard excision being considered for small lesions less than or equal to 5 mm in greatest diameter on the trunk or extremities [31, 34, 35].

Radiation therapy usually delivered by a radiation oncologist may be appropriate treatment of some keratinocyte carcinomas and is most commonly delivered as electron beam radiation. Treatment considerations for radiation therapy for both BCC and CSCC include inoperable tumors and patients who are poor surgical candidates though as will be discussed later other options including systemic medications may also be used and may be preferable. Radiation as a primary treatment is reserved for these unique situations due to higher recurrence rates than surgery [36]. One disadvantage to the patient is the need for multiple successive visits to a radiation center [37]. The term inoperable is subjective, and it may be prudent to get the opinion of a skilled dermatologic or Mohs micrographic surgeon prior to initiation of radiation therapy. Five-year local control, cure, and complete response rates for both BCC and CSCC range from 92% to 96% [38–41]. Fractionated radiation may also be used as an adjuvant treatment, following surgery, generally MMS, if clear margins cannot be obtained due to invasion into the bone, parotid, or deep nerves [42–45]. Adjuvant radiation therapy may also be used if there is perineural disease which is seen more often in CSCC but may be seen rarely in BCC.

Other systemic therapies are on the horizon for inoperable or metastatic BCCs and CSCCs, which rely on the genetic profile of the tumor in concert with the hosts immune system. One such example is the immunomodulatory small molecule programmed death 1 (PD-1) ligand and receptor inhibitors, which have shown some preliminary efficacy in both advanced BCC and CSCC [46, 47]. Further investigation into the appropriate application of these modalities is underway, though the prospect of application of genomic information to treatment of skin cancer is exciting.

Superficial Therapies

Superficial therapies including topical agents, photodynamic therapy, and cryotherapy have been used in the treatment of keratinocyte carcinomas. On average, due to inferior cure rates, these modalities are generally reserved for patients for whom surgery or radiation is contraindicated [28]. Additionally, patients have the right to make informed decisions and may object to more invasive modalities of treatment.

Cryotherapy is a destructive technique utilizing liquid nitrogen at a temperature of -196 °C to bring malignant cells to the destructive temperature of -50 °C [17]. This technique may create a scar, hyper- or hypopigmentation and may obscure the ability of a dermatologist to assess for recurrence. For BCCs, cryosurgery should be reserved for the superficial subtype. In a small prospective trial, cryosurgery for BCCs has been shown to result in BCC recurrence rate of 15% [48]. For CSCCs cryosurgery of clinically less aggressive CSCCs, such as in situ lesions, has been shown to result in cure rates of 97–99% though is not a preferred treatment modality [49].

Imiquimod is a topical chemical used for treating keratinocyte carcinomas that works through activation of the immune system via TLR7. The inflammatory response created results in clearance of atypically dividing cancerous cells. Imiquimod can be used for BCCs of the superficial subtype. Studies show an 84–85% 5-year disease-free rate [50, 51]. Despite the lower cure rate, some patients may opt for this modality over excision given improved cosmetic outcomes [50]. In CSCCs treatment with imiquimod is reserved for in situ disease. In these in situ CSCCs, a 73% cure rate was demonstrated in a small double-blind, placebo-controlled randomized trial [52].

5-Fluorouracil (5-FU) is a topical cream that works as an antimetabolite through the pyrimidine nucleotide synthesis pathway to cause direct cellular destruction which happens preferentially to rapidly dividing cells causing their death. It has shown efficacy rates similar to that of imiquimod for BCCs [53]. Its use for CSCCIS is controversial, with reported clearance rates ranging from 100% to as low as 40% and recurrence rates from 9% to 42% [54]. Topical use of such agents with wraps or with Unna boots on the leg may also be considered.

Field Treatment for Actinic Damage

In patients with significant risk factors for non-melanoma skin cancer, it is common to find numerous suspicious lesions, particularly in areas of extensive sun exposure such as the face, scalp, dorsal hands, and arms. Many of these suspicious lesions, especially the small erythematous macules or papules with a gritty scale, may represent actinic keratosis (AK). The rate and probability of conversion from AK to a true CSCC are controversial. However, estimates range from 6% to 20% conversion from AK to CSCC per single lesion over a 10-year time frame [55]. In these cases of extensive actinic damage with multiple AK-type lesions, it may be prudent to initiate field therapy in an effort to prevent or decrease the risk of progression to true CSCC. Modalities for field treatment include imiquimod, 5-FU, or photodynamic therapy (PDT). The topical creams, imiquimod and 5-FU, are applied by the patient at home, according to manufacturer instructions for a period of 2–4 weeks. A newer agent ingenol mebutate may decrease application time at home to 3 days. Photodynamic therapy utilizes a chemical photosensitizer, such as methyl aminolevulinate and 5-aminolaevulinic acid, followed by irradiation with a light source, generally red or blue light. The advantage of this treatment is the entire procedure is preformed within the physician's office, increasing adherence. The disadvantage is the procedure may elicit immediate pain and requires specialized equipment. Lesion count may be reduced by 80–90% [56]. Variable rates of complete clearance from 100% down to 43% may reflect variability in individual phenotype, host reaction, and application methodology [57].

Melanoma and Melanocytic Nevi with Atypia

Malignant melanoma (MM), deriving from the melanocyte, is the type of skin cancer that accounts for most skin cancer mortality. Annually there are approximately 60,000 cases of and 9,000 deaths attributable to MM in the United States [3, 58] [4]. In 2011, the melanoma incidence rate was 19.7 per 100,000, and the death rate was 2.7 per 100,000 [3]. In recent years, the incidence of MM continues to rise at approximately 1.4% annually [59]. In some instances, this increased rate may be attributable to increased UV exposure [60].

For identification of suspicious melanocytic lesions, one may recall the ABCDE signs of melanoma: asymmetry, border irregularity, color variegation, diameter over 6 mm, and evolving [8, 9]. When identifying a suspicious pigmented lesion for biopsy, in addition to the malignant clinical features, dermoscopy can be used to obtain further insight regarding a lesion's atypia. Dermoscopy is a handheld device which combines magnification and polarized light source to visualize features of pigmented skin lesions and has been shown with proper training to improve diagnostic accuracy. This technique may also be combined with digital imaging for individual lesion short-term monitoring [61]. Short-term monitoring is only appropriate for lesions that are flat and do not have any of the published melanoma-specific criteria on dermoscopy including atypical network, negative network, streaks, crystalline structures, atypical dots and globules, irregular blotch, blue-white veil, regression structures, peripheral brown structure less areas, and atypical vessels [62]. Total body photography of patient with many melanocytic neoplasms may also aid in identification of suspicious or changing lesions which would require biopsy [63].

Patients with a personal history of melanoma should continue to follow up regularly with a dermatologist, to monitor for recurrence or development of a second primary melanoma.

Biopsy

Unlike in keratinocyte carcinomas, melanocytic lesions should be sampled in their entirety whenever possible. If clinical suspicion for melanoma is high, the initial biopsy should be a narrow excisional biopsy of the entire lesion in both width and depth [64]. An inadequate shave or punch biopsy can result in misdiagnosis and improper staging of the melanoma, which may have important prognostic implications for the patient [65]. In general, for a suspicious pigmented lesion, a 2 mm clinical margin of normal skin is biopsied with the visible lesion and sufficient dermal depth to remove all visible pigment [66, 67]. This may be accomplished in the right anatomic location and with a small enough lesion using the shave biopsy or punch biopsy technique, as described above. In some cases an excisional biopsy may be required.

For biopsies of melanocytic neoplasms, it is important to include information for the pathologist such as age and gender of patient, location of biopsy, technique of biopsy, size of lesion, and features of the lesion [69]. While controversy exists around the topic of sentinel lymph node mapping and alteration of lymphatics secondary to excision, there is currently no evidence to suggest worse outcomes when a small primary excisional biopsy is performed [70]. However, large excisional biopsies in lesions suspicious for melanoma should be discussed with the surgical oncologist prior as there is concern they may interfere with lymphatic drainage should a sentinel lymph node biopsy be indicated.

Staging of Melanocytic Neoplasms

Following biopsy and submission of tissue to a dermatopathologist, the clinician will receive the pathology report. Herein we describe some of the terminology which may arise to help decide what type of neoplasm the patient has and what are the next appropriate steps in management.

Atypia and degrees of atypia Historically described as dysplastic nevi, it is becoming increasingly common to receive a pathology report that describes a nevus as "atypical." Either way, decision management is made based on the residual clinical lesion and the pathologic grading of cytologic and architectural atypia as mild, moderate, or severe. Consensus guidelines have established the following: first mildly atypical nevi with clear margins do not need to be re-excised. Second, mildly atypical nevi biopsied with positive histologic margins without clinical residual pigmentation may be safely observed rather than re-excised. While the guidelines do not recommend re-excision of moderately atypical nevi, several concerns—including sampling error from the biopsy itself and on histopathology processing, progression of a lesion, and residual cells that may progress in atypia—support re-excision with a 2–3 mm margin of normal skin for moderately atypical nevi, and whether or not a moderately excised nevus is re-excised depends on margins taken at initial biopsy, histopathology, and clinical judgment. Severely atypical lesions should be re-excised with a margin of normal skin which is usually 5 mm [71].

Melanoma tumor thickness, also known as Breslow thickness, is the single most important factor in staging and prognosis for melanoma patients [72]. Thin melanomas, ≤ 1 mm in Breslow thickness, without ulceration and mitotic rate <1/mm^2 are considered by the 7th American Joint Committee on Cancer (AJCC) TNM Stage 1A and carry a favorable prognosis [73, 74]. However, given the rate of 10% occult metastasis in lymph nodes of patients with melanomas ≥0.76 mm with mitotic rate ≥1/mm^2 or ulceration, these exact parameters are subject to change in the upcoming 8th AJCC, such that melanomas between 0.75 and 1 mm may be considered as a higher TNM stage [75, 76]. Histologic subtype of MM may also be reported, including superficial spreading melanoma, nodular melanoma, lentigo maligna melanoma, and acral lentiginous melanoma, with superficial spreading melanoma being the most common [77].

Treatment

Surgical

Surgical treatment of localized primary MM is dependent predominately on the thickness of the tumor. Malignant melanoma in situ (MMIS) was traditionally excised with a 5 mm margin though it is now often excised with 0.5–1 cm margin. Studies using MMS for melanoma suggest that 6 mm may be insufficient, with a recent case series of 1,120 MMISs demonstrating superiority in tumor clearance with 9 mm over 6 mm [78]. Particularly, melanoma on sun-damaged skin or lentigo maligna (LM)-type MMIS may require margins closer to 1 cm for clearance, as demonstrated by Nehal et al. in a retrospective analysis of 91 biopsied "in situ" LMs, which also showed 16% of cases had unsuspected invasion [79].

For invasive melanoma, treatment depends on the stage of the tumor. Melanomas with depth ≤1.00 mm (measured from the granular layer to the deepest atypical melanocyte) should be excised with a 1 cm margin of clinically normal surrounding skin, due to decreased local recurrence demonstrated with this margin [80]. Melanomas with thickness >1.01 mm require a 1–2 cm margin depending on location and size of primary melanoma with a 1 cm margin usually being used for melanoma less than 2 mm in thickness and 2 cm being used for melanoma greater than or equal to 2mm in thickness. Even wider resections are used for melanoma greater than 4 mm in thickness [81, 82].

Sentinel lymph node biopsy (SLNB) for melanoma is a controversial topic, given that there is no survival benefit to this procedure. However, SLNB does provide significant prognostic information for disease-specific survival [83–85]. This technique is widely accepted for staging and prognosis of melanomas >1.00 mm in Breslow depth. Additionally, SLNB may be indicated for thin melanomas ≥0.75 mm with certain additional risk features such as high-mitotic index or ulceration [86]. For patients with these thin melanomas, the authors recommend referral to a surgical oncologist with expertise in SLNB for melanoma. The unpublished 8th edition of AJCC may alter current recommendations, and the reader is encouraged to refer to the most current AJCC guidelines, as research into the utility of and the indication for SLNB is ongoing (see Chap. 6 Melanoma).

Systemic Treatment Modalities

The use of systemic therapies for metastatic melanoma is a rapidly advancing field, with many promising single agent and combination regimens on the horizon. Targeted small molecule therapy against driver mutations in the RAF/MEK/ERK pathway that controls cellular response to growth stimuli is already approved for use in advanced melanoma. BRAF is mutated in approximately 66% of melanomas, and the targeted therapy BRAF inhibitor, vemurafenib, is showing excellent results in shrinking tumors [87]. However, these responses lack durability and the addition of MEK inhibitors such as trametinib is being explored to increase durability of response. An additional mechanism for targeting advanced melanoma works through modulation of the immune system. Ipilimumab, which inhibits CTLA-4, increases the T-cell immune response against the melanoma. Newer immunomodulatory agents such as nivolumab and pembrolizumab have also shown great promise and work through inhibition of PD-1 and may restore the antitumor properties of the immune system against melanoma. Further study of these agents is ongoing, and the field continues to evolve and change.

Conclusion

Skin cancer represents a large public health concern within the United States. The heterogeneity of skin cancers, from KC to MM, as well as clinical and histopathologic subtypes and certain patient characteristics will serve as guidance in the most appropriate management of a particular skin cancer. This chapter highlights the most common methods of cutaneous biopsy and treatment. Additionally, common destructive, surgical, radiotherapeutic, and chemotherapeutic options are available to the clinician and should be selected with the individual case and patient in mind.

Bibliography

1. Robinson JK. Sun exposure, sun protection, and vitamin D. JAMA. 2005;294(12):1541–3.
2. Rogers HW, Weinstock MA, Feldman SR, Coldiron BM. Incidence estimate of nonmelanoma skin cancer (keratinocyte carcinomas) in the U.S. population, 2012. JAMA Dermatol. 2015;151(10):1081–6.
3. Guy GP, Thomas CC, Thompson T, Watson M, Massetti GM, Richardson LC, et al. Vital signs: melanoma incidence and mortality trends and projections – United States, 1982–2030. MMWR Morb Mortal Wkly Rep. 2015;64(21):591–6.
4. American Cancer Society. Cancer facts and figures 2016 [Internet]. Cited 19 Nov 2016. Available from: http://www.cancer.org/acs/groups/content/@research/documents/document/acspc-047079.pdf
5. Karia PS, Han J, Schmults CD. Cutaneous squamous cell carcinoma: estimated incidence of disease, nodal metastasis, and deaths from disease in the United States, 2012. J Am Acad Dermatol. 2013;68(6):957–66.
6. Hay RJ, Johns NE, Williams HC, Bolliger IW, Dellavalle RP, Margolis DJ, et al. The global burden of skin disease in 2010: an analysis of the prevalence and impact of skin conditions. J Invest Dermatol. 2014;134(6):1527–34.
7. Guy GP, Machlin SR, Ekwueme DU, Yabroff KR. Prevalence and costs of skin cancer treatment in the U.S., 2002–2006 and 2007–2011. Am J Prev Med. 2015;48(2):183–7.
8. Stevenson ML, Glazer AM, Cohen DE, Rigel DS, Rieder EA. Frequency of total body skin examinations among US dermatologists. J Am Acad Dermatol. 2017;76(2):343–4.
9. Russak JE, Rigel DS. Risk factors for the development of primary cutaneous melanoma. Dermatol Clin. 2012;30(3):363–8.
10. Etzkorn JR, Parikh RP, Marzban SS, Law K, Davis AH, Rawal B, et al. Identifying risk factors using a skin cancer screening program. Cancer Control. 2013;20(4):248–54.
11. Karimkhani C, Boyers LN, Dellavalle RP, Weinstock MA. It's time for "keratinocyte carcinoma" to replace the term "nonmelanoma skin cancer". J Am Acad Dermatol. 2015;72(1):186–7.
12. Rogers HW, Weinstock MA, Harris AR, Hinckley MR, Feldman SR, Fleischer AB, et al. Incidence estimate of nonmelanoma skin cancer in the United States, 2006. Arch Dermatol. 2010;146(3):283–7.
13. Asgari MM, Moffet HH, Ray GT, Quesenberry CP. Trends in basal cell carcinoma incidence and identification of high-risk subgroups, 1998–2012. JAMA Dermatol. 2015;151(9):976–81.
14. Miller DL, Weinstock MA. Nonmelanoma skin cancer in the United States: incidence. J Am Acad Dermatol. 1994;30(5 Pt 1):774–8.
15. Jambusaria-Pahlajani A, Kanetsky PA, Karia PS, Hwang W-T, Gelfand JM, Whalen FM, et al. Evaluation of AJCC tumor staging for cutaneous squamous cell carcinoma and a proposed alternative tumor staging system. JAMA Dermatol. 2013;149(4):402–10.
16. Stevenson ML, Kim R, Meehan SA, Pavlick AC, Carucci JA. Metastatic cutaneous squamous cell carcinoma: the importance of T2 stratification and hematologic malignancy in prognostication. Dermatol Surg. 2016;42(8):932–5.
17. Bolognia JL, Jorizzo JL, Schaffer JV. Dermatology. 3rd ed. Philadelphia: Elsevier Saunders; 2012.
18. Alguire PC, Mathes BM. Skin biopsy techniques for the internist. J Gen Intern Med. 1998;13(1):46–54.

19. Miedema J, Zedek DC, Rayala BZ, Bain EE. 9 tips to help prevent derm biopsy mistakes. J Fam Pract. 2014;63(10):559–64.
20. Stratman EJ, Elston DM, Miller SJ. Skin biopsy: identifying and overcoming errors in the skin biopsy pathway. J Am Acad Dermatol. 2016;74(1):19–25. quiz 25
21. Steinsapir KD, Woodward JA. Chlorhexidine keratitis: safety of chlorhexidine as a facial antiseptic. Dermatol Surg. 2017;43(1):1–6.
22. Rowe DE, Carroll RJ, Day CL. Long-term recurrence rates in previously untreated (primary) basal cell carcinoma: implications for patient follow-up. J Dermatol Surg Oncol. 1989;15(3):315–28.
23. Barlow JO, Zalla MJ, Kyle A, DiCaudo DJ, Lim KK, Yiannias JA. Treatment of basal cell carcinoma with curettage alone. J Am Acad Dermatol. 2006;54(6):1039–45.
24. Goldman G. The current status of curettage and electrodesiccation. Dermatol Clin. 2002;20(3):569–78. ix
25. Kauvar ANB, Arpey CJ, Hruza G, Olbricht SM, Bennett R, Mahmoud BH. Consensus for nonmelanoma skin cancer treatment, part II: squamous cell carcinoma, including a cost analysis of treatment methods. Dermatol Surg. 2015;41(11):1214–40.
26. Zitelli JA. TIPS for a better ellipse. J Am Acad Dermatol. 1990;22(1):101–3.
27. Thissen MR, Neumann MH, Schouten LJ. A systematic review of treatment modalities for primary basal cell carcinomas. Arch Dermatol. 1999;135(10):1177–83.
28. Bichakjian CK, Olencki T, Aasi SZ, Alam M, Andersen JS, Berg D, et al. Basal cell skin cancer, version 1.2016, NCCN clinical practice guidelines in oncology. J Natl Compr Canc Netw. 2016;14(5):574–97.
29. Wolf DJ, Zitelli JA. Surgical margins for basal cell carcinoma. Arch Dermatol. 1987;123(3):340–4.
30. Brodland DG, Zitelli JA. Surgical margins for excision of primary cutaneous squamous cell carcinoma. J Am Acad Dermatol. 1992;27(2 Pt 1):241–8.
31. Rowe DE, Carroll RJ, Day CL. Prognostic factors for local recurrence, metastasis, and survival rates in squamous cell carcinoma of the skin, ear, and lip. Implications for treatment modality selection. J Am Acad Dermatol. 1992;26(6):976–90.
32. Patel TN, Patel SB, Franca K, Chacon AH, Nouri K. Mohs micrographic surgery: history, technique, and advancements. Skinmed. 2014;12(5):289–92.
33. Force AHT, Connolly SM, Baker DR, Coldiron BM, Fazio MJ, Storrs PA, et al. AAD/ACMS/ASDSA/ASMS 2012 appropriate use criteria for Mohs micrographic surgery: a report of the American Academy of Dermatology, American College of Mohs Surgery, American Society for Dermatologic Surgery Association, and the American Society for Mohs Surgery. J Am Acad Dermatol. 2012;67(4):531–50.
34. Leslie DF, Greenway HT. Mohs micrographic surgery for skin cancer. Australas J Dermatol. 1991;32(3):159–64.
35. Nguyen TH, Ho DQ-D. Nonmelanoma skin cancer. Curr Treat Options Oncol. 2002;3(3):193–203.
36. Cognetta AB, Howard BM, Heaton HP, Stoddard ER, Hong HG, Green WH. Superficial x-ray in the treatment of basal and squamous cell carcinomas: a viable option in select patients. J Am Acad Dermatol. 2012;67(6):1235–41.
37. Alam M, Ratner D. Cutaneous squamous-cell carcinoma. N Engl J Med. 2001;344(13):975–83.
38. Hernández-Machin B, Borrego L, Gil-García M, Hernández BH. Office-based radiation therapy for cutaneous carcinoma: evaluation of 710 treatments. Int J Dermatol. 2007;46(5):453–9.
39. Wilder RB, Kittelson JM, Shimm DS. Basal cell carcinoma treated with radiation therapy. Cancer. 1991;68(10):2134–7.
40. Wilder RB, Shimm DS, Kittelson JM, Rogoff EE, Cassady JR. Recurrent basal cell carcinoma treated with radiation therapy. Arch Dermatol. 1991;127(11):1668–72.
41. Childers BJ, Goldwyn RM, Ramos D, Chaffey J, Harris JR. Long-term results of irradiation for basal cell carcinoma of the skin of the nose. Plast Reconstr Surg. 1994;93(6):1169–73.

42. Han A, Ratner D. What is the role of adjuvant radiotherapy in the treatment of cutaneous squamous cell carcinoma with perineural invasion? Cancer. 2007;109(6):1053–9.
43. Mendenhall WM, Ferlito A, Takes RP, Bradford CR, Corry J, Fagan JJ, et al. Cutaneous head and neck basal and squamous cell carcinomas with perineural invasion. Oral Oncol. 2012;48(10):918–22.
44. Jambusaria-Pahlajani A, Miller CJ, Quon H, Smith N, Klein RQ, Schmults CD. Surgical monotherapy versus surgery plus adjuvant radiotherapy in high-risk cutaneous squamous cell carcinoma: a systematic review of outcomes. Dermatol Surg. 2009;35(4):574–85.
45. Geist DE, Garcia-Moliner M, Fitzek MM, Cho H, Rogers GS. Perineural invasion of cutaneous squamous cell carcinoma and basal cell carcinoma: raising awareness and optimizing management. Dermatol Surg. 2008 Dec;34(12):1642–51.
46. Falchook GS, Leidner R, Stankevich E, Piening B, Bifulco C, Lowy I, et al. Responses of metastatic basal cell and cutaneous squamous cell carcinomas to anti-PD1 monoclonal antibody REGN2810. J Immunother Cancer. 2016;4:70.
47. Chang J, Zhu GA, Cheung C, Li S, Kim J, Chang ALS. Association between programmed death ligand 1 expression in patients with basal cell carcinomas and the number of treatment modalities. JAMA Dermatol. 2017;153(4):285–90.
48. Wang I, Bendsoe N, Klinteberg CA, Enejder AM, Andersson-Engels S, Svanberg S, et al. Photodynamic therapy vs. cryosurgery of basal cell carcinomas: results of a phase III clinical trial. Br J Dermatol. 2001;144(4):832–40.
49. Sinclair RD, Dawber RP. Cryosurgery of malignant and premalignant diseases of the skin: a simple approach. Australas J Dermatol. 1995;36(3):133–42.
50. Bath-Hextall F, Ozolins M, Armstrong SJ, Colver GB, Perkins W, Miller PSJ, et al. Surgical excision versus imiquimod 5% cream for nodular and superficial basal-cell carcinoma (SINS): a multicentre, non-inferiority, randomised controlled trial. Lancet Oncol. 2014;15(1):96–105.
51. Quirk C, Gebauer K, De'Ambrosis B, Slade HB, Meng T-C. Sustained clearance of superficial basal cell carcinomas treated with imiquimod cream 5%: results of a prospective 5-year study. Cutis. 2010;85(6):318–24.
52. Patel GK, Goodwin R, Chawla M, Laidler P, Price PE, Finlay AY, et al. Imiquimod 5% cream monotherapy for cutaneous squamous cell carcinoma in situ (Bowen's disease): a randomized, double-blind, placebo-controlled trial. J Am Acad Dermatol. 2006;54(6):1025–32.
53. Arits AHMM, Mosterd K, Essers BA, Spoorenberg E, Sommer A, De Rooij MJM, et al. Photodynamic therapy versus topical imiquimod versus topical fluorouracil for treatment of superficial basal-cell carcinoma: a single blind, non-inferiority, randomised controlled trial. Lancet Oncol. 2013;14(7):647–54.
54. Shimizu I, Cruz A, Chang KH, Dufresne RG. Treatment of squamous cell carcinoma in situ: a review. Dermatol Surg. 2011;37(10):1394–411.
55. Anwar J, Wrone DA, Kimyai-Asadi A, Alam M. The development of actinic keratosis into invasive squamous cell carcinoma: evidence and evolving classification schemes. Clin Dermatol. 2004;22(3):189–96.
56. Stockfleth E, Gupta G, Peris K, Aractingi S, Dakovic R, Alomar A. Reduction in lesions from Lmax: a new concept for assessing efficacy of field-directed therapy for actinic keratosis. Results with imiquimod 3.75%. Eur J Dermatol. 2014;24(1):23–7.
57. Dodds A, Chia A, Shumack S. Actinic keratosis: rationale and management. Dermatol Ther (Heidelb). 2014;4(1):11–31.
58. U.S. Cancer Statistics Working Group. United States cancer statistics: 1999–2010 incidence and mortality web-based report. [Internet]. Atlanta: Department of Health and Human Services, Centers for Disease Control and Prevention, and National Cancer Institute. 2013. Cited 18 Nov 2016. Available from: http://www.cdc.gov/uscs.
59. National Cancer Institute. Cancer Stat Facts: melanoma of the Skin [Internet]. Surveillance, Epidemiology, and End Results Program (SEER). Cited 27 Feb 2017. Available from: https:// seer.cancer.gov/statfacts/html/melan.htmlSurv

60. Jemal A, Saraiya M, Patel P, Cherala SS, Barnholtz-Sloan J, Kim J, et al. Recent trends in cutaneous melanoma incidence and death rates in the United States, 1992–2006. J Am Acad Dermatol. 2011;65(5 Suppl 1):S17–25.e1.

61. Menzies SW, Emery J, Staples M, Davies S, McAvoy B, Fletcher J, et al. Impact of dermoscopy and short-term sequential digital dermoscopy imaging for the management of pigmented lesions in primary care: a sequential intervention trial. Br J Dermatol. 2009;161(6):1270–7.

62. Haliasos EC, Kerner M, Jaimes N, Zalaudek I, Malvehy J, Hofmann-Wellenhof R, et al. Dermoscopy for the pediatric dermatologist part III: dermoscopy of melanocytic lesions. Pediatr Dermatol. 2013;30(3):281–93.

63. Malvehy J, Puig S. Follow-up of melanocytic skin lesions with digital total-body photography and digital dermoscopy: a two-step method. Clin Dermatol. 2002;20(3):297–304.

64. Stell VH, Norton HJ, Smith KS, Salo JC, White RL. Method of biopsy and incidence of positive margins in primary melanoma. Ann Surg Oncol. 2007;14(2):893–8.

65. McCarthy SW, Scolyer RA. Pitfalls and important issues in the pathologic diagnosis of melanocytic tumors. Ochsner J. 2010;10(2):66–74.

66. Coit DG, Thompson JA, Andtbacka R, Anker CJ, Bichakjian CK, Carson WE, et al. Melanoma, version 4.2014. J Natl Compr Canc Netw. 2014;12(5):621–9.

67. Fong ZV, Tanabe KK. Comparison of melanoma guidelines in the U.S.A., Canada, Europe, Australia and New Zealand: a critical appraisal and comprehensive review. Br J Dermatol. 2014;170(1):20–30.

68. Ng JC, Swain S, Dowling JP, Wolfe R, Simpson P, Kelly JW. The impact of partial biopsy on histopathologic diagnosis of cutaneous melanoma: experience of an Australian tertiary referral service. Arch Dermatol. 2010;146(3):234–9.

69. Bichakjian CK, Halpern AC, Johnson TM, Foote Hood A, Grichnik JM, Swetter SM, et al. Guidelines of care for the management of primary cutaneous melanoma. Am Acad Dermatol J Am Acad Dermatol. 2011;65(5):1032–47.

70. Gauwerky KJ, Kunte C, Geimer T, Baumert J, Flaig MJ, Ruzicka T, et al. The outcome of patients with melanoma is not associated with the time point of lymphatic mapping with respect to excisional biopsy of the primary tumor. Dermatology (Basel). 2010;220(4):355–62.

71. Kim CC, Swetter SM, Curiel-Lewandrowski C, Grichnik JM, Grossman D, Halpern AC, et al. Addressing the knowledge gap in clinical recommendations for management and complete excision of clinically atypical nevi/dysplastic nevi: pigmented lesion subcommittee consensus statement. JAMA Dermatol. 2015;151(2):212–8.

72. Marghoob AA, Koenig K, Bittencourt FV, Kopf AW, Bart RS. Breslow thickness and clark level in melanoma: support for including level in pathology reports and in American Joint Committee on Cancer Staging. Cancer. 2000;88(3):589–95.

73. Caldarella A, Fancelli L, Manneschi G, Chiarugi A, Nardini P, Crocetti E. How staging of thin melanoma is changed after the introduction of TNM 7th edition: a population-based analysis. J Cancer Res Clin Oncol. 2016;142(1):73–6.

74. Oude Ophuis CMC, Louwman MWJ, Grünhagen DJ, Verhoef K, van Akkooi ACJ. Implementation of the 7th edition AJCC staging system: effects on staging and survival for pT1 melanoma. A Dutch population based study. Int J Cancer. 2017;140(8):1802–8.

75. Ivan D, Prieto VG. An update on reporting histopathologic prognostic factors in melanoma. Arch Pathol Lab Med. 2011;135(7):825–9.

76. Burton AL, Egger ME, Gilbert JE, Stromberg AJ, Hagendoorn L, Martin RCG, et al. Assessment of mitotic rate reporting in melanoma. Am J Surg. 2012;204(6):969–74. discussion 974

77. Feng Z, Zhang Z, Wu X-C. Lifetime risks of cutaneous melanoma by histological subtype and race/ethnicity in the United States. J La State Med Soc. 2013;165(4):201–8.

78. Kunishige JH, Brodland DG, Zitelli JA. Surgical margins for melanoma in situ. J Am Acad Dermatol. 2012;66(3):438–44.

79. Hazan C, Dusza SW, Delgado R, Busam KJ, Halpern AC, Nehal KS. Staged excision for lentigo maligna and lentigo maligna melanoma: a retrospective analysis of 117 cases. J Am Acad Dermatol. 2008;58(1):142–8.
80. MacKenzie Ross AD, Haydu LE, Quinn MJ, Saw RPM, Shannon KF, Spillane AJ, et al. The association between excision margins and local recurrence in 11,290 thin (T1) primary cutaneous melanomas: a case-control study. Ann Surg Oncol. 2016;23(4):1082–9.
81. Balch CM, Urist MM, Karakousis CP, Smith TJ, Temple WJ, Drzewiecki K, et al. Efficacy of 2-cm surgical margins for intermediate-thickness melanomas (1 to 4 mm). Results of a multi-institutional randomized surgical trial. Ann Surg. 1993;218(3):262–7. discussion 267
82. Zitelli JA, Brown CD, Hanusa BH. Surgical margins for excision of primary cutaneous melanoma. J Am Acad Dermatol. 1997;37(3 Pt 1):422–9.
83. Morton DL, Cochran AJ, Thompson JF, Elashoff R, Essner R, Glass EC, et al. Sentinel node biopsy for early-stage melanoma. Transactions of the meeting of the American Surgical Association. 2005;123(&NA):10–20.
84. Gershenwald JE, Mansfield PF, Lee JE, Ross MI. Role for lymphatic mapping and sentinel lymph node biopsy in patients with thick (> or = 4 mm) primary melanoma. Ann Surg Oncol. 2000;7(2):160–5.
85. Ferrone CR, Panageas KS, Busam K, Brady MS, Coit DG. Multivariate prognostic model for patients with thick cutaneous melanoma: importance of sentinel lymph node status. Ann Surg Oncol. 2002;9(7):637–45.
86. Wong SL, Brady MS, Busam KJ, Coit DG. Results of sentinel lymph node biopsy in patients with thin melanoma. Ann Surg Oncol. 2006;13(3):302–9.
87. Davies H, Bignell GR, Cox C, Stephens P, Edkins S, Clegg S, et al. Mutations of the BRAF gene in human cancer. Nature. 2002;417(6892):949–54.

Index